HEALTHY EATING
Changing a New Generation

Andrew St. James

ST-JUDE PUBLISHING

HEALTHY EATING:
Changing a New Generation

© Copyright 2020

First Published by St-Jude Publishing

All rights reserved
Printed in the United States of America

ISBN: 978-0-578-72667-0

Cover Image: shutterstock_1096114730 /Shutterstock.com

FOREWORD

It's been now, more than 20 years that I have been teaching undergraduate students introductory courses in nutrition. The textbooks that I have used have been big, expensive with plenty of attractive pictures, countless graphs and tables that seem to overwhelm the students with excessive minutiae, rather than help them understand and get excited to learn about the field of nutrition. The dense and detailed content became more of a distraction instead of facilitating the learning process. Consequently, I complemented my lectures with power-point presentations and movie clips, in order to summarize the most important and relevant information. My goal, as a university professor, teaching an introductory course in nutrition, was to get students engaged in the course material rather than require a mastery of the field. The textbook, I always thought, was the tool that should facilitate that process. So asking whether the course material was pertinent and usable by the students was certainly a relevant question. So at the end of each semester, I would regularly poll my students online. When asked about the textbook, used in the class, close to 40% of students would consistently admit to never opening the book, and a mere 10 to 20% of students would read most of the assigned pages. That left roughly 40-50% of the students reading the textbook occasionally. The majority of students would complain about having purchased a book they hardly ever used. In response, I began to write a textbook that was not cumbersome with details, but more focused on telling the story of nutrition in a more engaging way, capturing as it were, where nutrition fitted into the story of human health. Hence, it is preferable that this textbook not be used as an exhaustive compendium of nutritional details, for indeed, the reader will quickly find numerous details missing. Indeed, for the sake of producing a more condensed book that uses broad brush strokes to paint a colorful and understandable story, I left out details, such as the DRIs, chemical structures, and the digestion of food. Moreover, I did not include an exhaustive list of all the vitamins and minerals, but only those I thought would be of interest to the students. Forgive me of this transgression, for the purpose was not to exhaust the student with endless details, but to engage them in thinking about nutrition within broad and textured historical landscapes.

DEDICATION

If it were not for Erin, my loving wife, this project could never have been completed. She kept me laughing and smiling with silly jokes and incessant calls to walk the dogs. I also dedicate this book to Jesus Christ, Saint Joseph and Mary the mother of God.

ACCESSING THE VIDEO DOCUMENTARY:
OBESITY IN AMERICA: A NATIONAL CRISIS

ENTER the website address: https://vimeo.com/ondemand/obesityinamerica2

Register with Vimeo; it is FREE and it will give you access to the video

Click on the RENTING option and then click on the "apply promo code" option

You will find the promotional code attached to the inside of this textbook

CONTENTS

INTRODUCTION 7
CHAPTER 1 13
THE ORIGINS OF OUR CURRENT NUTRITION PRACTICES 13
CHAPTER 2 HISTORY OF NUTRITION IN HUMAN HEALTH 46
   2.1 UNDERSTANDING OF THE ROLE OF NUTRITION IN ANCIENT SOCIETIES 50
   2.2 NUTRITION AND HEALTH: HISTORICAL ROLE OF FOOD IN HUMAN HEALTH AND DISEASE 58
   2.3 NUTRITIONAL DEFICIENCIES AND FAMINES IN ANCIENT SOCIETIES 62
   2.4 THE FAMINES AND GREAT PLAGUE OF THE LATE MIDDLE-AGES 63
   2.5 EUROPE AND POST-PLAGUE RECOVERY 63
   2.6 THE BEGINNING REJUVENATION OF MEDICINE 67
   2.7 THE ENLIGHTENMENT PERIOD AND HUMAN HEALTH 72
   2.8 THE 18TH CENTURY AGRICULTURAL REVOLUTION 77
   2.9 THE ROLE OF NUTRITION IN HEALTH 80
CHAPTER 3 VITAMIN & MINERAL DEFICIENCIES 84
   3.3.1 INTRODUCTION 96
   3.3.2 THIAMIN DEFICIENCY 92
   3.3.3 NIACIN DEFICIENCY—PELLAGRA IN THE AMERICAN SOUTH OF THE EARLY 1900S 94
     3.3.4.1 *Individuals at risk of vitamin D deficiency* 100
   3.3.5 RICH SOURCES OF DIETARY VITAMIN K. 100
   3.4 MICRONUTRIENTS INVOLVED IN VARIOUS TYPES OF ANEMIAS 101
     3.4.1 Iron deficiency anemia 102
     3.4.4 Megaloblastic Anemia (B-12 & Folate) 101
     3.4.6 Copper (Cu+) Deficiency. 105
   3.7 CALCIUM, MAGNESIUM DEFICIENCIES AND PHOSPHOROUS EXCESSES 111
     3.8 Magnesium Intake 114
     3.9 Phosphorus Intake 115
   3.10 ZINC AND BETA-CAROTENE DEFICIENCIES 116
     3.10.1 Zinc Deficiency 116
     3.10.2 Beta-Carotene Deficiency 116
CHAPTER 4 EMERGENCE OF THE FOOD INDUSTRY 125
   4.1 THE BIRTH OF MANUFACTURED FOODS 125
CHAPTER 5 FAMILY AND CHILD NUTRITION 155
   5.1 THE ROLE OF NUTRITION IN PREGNANCY 155
     56.1.1 Fertility and Birth Rates in the U.S. and Worldwide 155
     6.1.3 Prenatal Nutrition 161
   5.2 THE IMPORTANCE OF INFANT NUTRITION 165
     6.2.1 Breast Milk—The Perfect Food 165
     6.2.2 Infant and Toddler Nutrition—Establishing a Quality Standard for Children 169
CHAPTER 6 FOOD SAFETY—MODERN CHALLENGE & CUMBERSOME NIGHTMARE 211
   6.1 THE FORGING OF A SAFE FOOD SUPPLY 211
   6.3 NATURAL FOODS TO SUPER FOODS: MAKING THE U.S. DIET HEALTHY 211
   6.4 FOOD POISONINGS ON THE RISE: CONSEQUENCE OF GLOBALIZATION AND EATING AWAY FROM HOME 216
   6.5 FOOD & THE CONTAMINATION OF THE ENVIRONMENT 216
   6.6 THE ORGANIC FOOD MOVEMENT 225
     6.6.1. Creating a Healthy Diet that Prevents Disease 3
   6.7 FOOD ALLERGIES & INTOLERANCES 233

CHAPTER 7 NUTRITION RESEARCH IN THE MODERN AGE: 233
    7.1 WHAT IS RESEARCH? 233
    7.2 EPIDEMIOLOGIC RESEARCH 235
        7.3.1 Lab-Based In Vitro Studies..*238*
        7.3.2 Lab-Based Animals Studies..*238*
    7.4 HYPOTHESIS EXERCISE 241

CHAPTER 8 NUTRITION AND CHRONIC DISEASE..248
    8.1 THE PREVALENCE OF CHRONIC DISEASE IN AMERICAN SOCIETY 248
    8.2 REVERSING CHRONIC DISEASE, IS ALL ABOUT NUTRITION AND EXERCISE................. 249

CHAPTER 9 THE OBESITY CRISIS..255
    9.1 THE GROWING PREVALENCE OF OBESITY WORLDWIDE & IN AMERICA........................255
        9.1.1 History of Obesity...*262*
        9.2.1 Familial Causes of Obesity: Interplay of Environment and Genetics 268
    9.3 THE MOST EFFECTIVE WEIGHT LOSS DIETS 270

CHAPTER 10 NUTRITION AND WORLD HUNGER 279
    10.1 UNDERSTANDING HUNGER 279

INTRODUCTION

America has become a sickly nation with a yearly total healthcare expenditure $3.5 Trillion dollars.[1] Most of this cost—48.6%—is driven by hospital care and physician services (Figure-1), and shockingly, roughly 75% of the US healthcare expenditure is associated with the treatment of chronic disease.[29] In fact, 71 to 86% of the national healthcare expenditure is attributed to one or more chronic disease.[8] Significant here, is that most chronic diseases—heart disease, liver, gallbladder and kidney diseases, sleep apnea and some cancers—are tagged to obesity.[25,32] A little over one quarter of the healthcare costs of the non-institutionalized population 18 years and up—roughly 28%—is dedicated to the treatment of obesity and its secondary diseases and conditions.[4] Moreover, the problem is getting worse: healthcare expenses attributed to the management and treatment of obese inpatients increased by 46% between 1998 and 2006 and by 27% for non-inpatient care of the obese; additionally, there has been an 80% jump in pharmaceutical management costs aimed at obesity.[12] This is because obesity has been steadily increasing in adults and children since the end of the 1970s.[14,15] In the US, NHANES data from 2015-2016 confirms that 71.6% of US adult men and women were considered overweight or obese, and that as many as 39.8% were obese.[14] Also, as many as 35.1 % of children aged 2 to 19 are either overweight or obese.[15] What many did not see coming was the worrisome 4-fold hike in morbid obesity in the US (Body Mass Index (BMI) ≥40) and 5-fold jump in super obesity levels (BMI ≥50) between the 1986 and 2010.[36] Additionally, pediatric obesity was barely on the radar of most pediatricians in 1960s, but quickly the prevalence of obesity rose 338% in the 6 to 11 and 348% in the 12 to 19 age groups over the following 45 years.[15]

On the international scene, overweight and obesity have more recently become pandemics with close to 1.9 billion overweight and 650 million clinically obese adults in addition to 340 million children (5-19 years of age) who are overweight or obese,[39] and there is a projected 3.28 billion adults expected to become overweight or obese by 2030.[33] What has gone wrong?

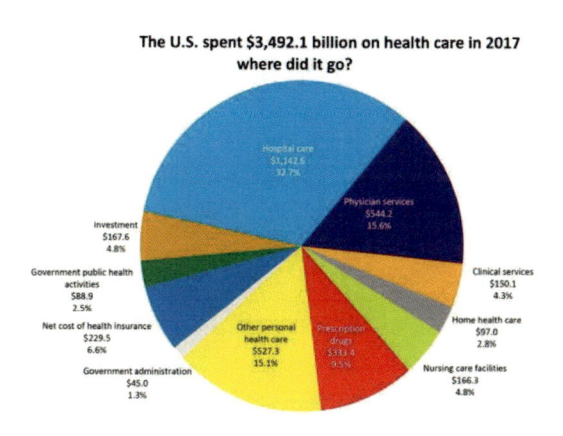

Source: American Medical Association: Trends in Healthcare Spending
https://www.ama-assn.org/about/research/trends-health-care-spending

Figure-1 US Health Expenditure 2017

Our culture is engaged in a very unhealthy relationship with food; not only do we eat large quantities of food, but individual portion sizes are significantly larger than those of the 1950s, and we are also eating more frequently; in fact roughly 20% of adult Americans eat >6 times per day.[31] This overabundance of food availability and consumption has led to the ingestion of worrisome amounts of fat, alarmingly elevated levels of sugar, and troublesome levels of sodium;[26] moreover, suboptimal fiber intakes threaten the gastrointestinal health of millions.[40]

We have supported a food industry that meticulously developed highly processed foods that have habituated the young to high taste sensations, and that have out-competed the more subtle and natural tastes of fruits and vegetables.[27] We are now looking at a generation with food habits that are so impoverished, that they are threatening its very health.[11,26]

The growing prevalence of obesity among children, in the US, is an important threat to the national wellbeing, and to our economic growth as a nation. Media coverage of diet and lifestyle has steadily increased to current fever pitch. Also U.S. society, since the 1970s, obsessed with weight loss diets, as evidenced by millions of diet book sales,[21] continues to gain weight. Studies now show that between 33 and 67% of dieters gain more weight back than they originally lost.[23] What is going on?

The main perceived causes of the obesity crisis, attributed to the overconsumption of abundant refined foods and to increased sedentarism, have distracted medical practitioners and epidemiologists from the true origins of this epidemic. Although the overconsumption of food is causative, it may only superficially address the crisis. Rather the literature posits that the breakdown of the American family makes both adults and children more vulnerable to weight gain, chronic diseases and mental illness. It is specifically the poor, representing 15% of Americans, or 46 million people, that are most vulnerable to obesity and diabetes. [22] Nutritional studies have shown that family conflict directly impoverishes the nutrition quality of foods consumed by youth, leading to less fruits and vegetables.[34] Work done by Berge and colleagues,[3] on lower functioning families, found fewer fruits and vegetables in the diet, compared to the diet of children from high function families. High functioning families, noted for being highly structured, cohesive, and having common beliefs, exhibit high resiliency and an ability to cope.[35] Gender-specific studies have identified women from low functioning families as being particularly at risk of obesity because of more junk food consumption such as chips, sodas, fast foods and processed meats,[24] whereas men from poorly cohesive homes were also subject to poor eating habits and overeating.[17] In fact, families that foster calm meal times tend to have improved eating habits[7] and more frequent family meals.[9] By contrast, when there is low family cohesion, increased conflict and household chaos, household dietary quality declines.[24] The consequence is the fragmentation of meals and the loss of family meals. Indeed, the "*snackification*" of eating habits, the preferential intake of meals limited to frozen processed dinners, quick to prepare, poor in nutritional quality and eaten in isolation, [37] have robbed the culture of the therapeutic quality of mealtime. One explanation for this would be that the family shapes the child's nutrition, [10] understood both in terms of physical and spiritual food, [20] providing calm and securing environments that favor resiliency. The impact of familial relationships is strongest in childhood with an inverse correlation between fatness and poor family relationships.[30] Mothers specifically seem to play a critical role in influencing childhood dietary intakes,[41] especially in their role as dietary gatekeepers for preschool children.[13]

Another explanation is that food, whether organic or spiritual, feeds our bodies and souls, and in both instances, the individual needs nutriture of high quality to sustain good spiritual and bodily health. Families feel the consequence of meal disruption and irregularity. This erosive process of fragmented meals characterized by eating lunch at work, alone at the desk, or dinners in the bedroom playing video games, or listening to online news, or TV,[37] are appearing more and more as significant symptoms that reveal the rather dark fate of the American family.

Everyone is rushed by so many obligations and deadlines, sacrificing as it were, the sanctity of mealtime. The consequence is that family members have become disconnected from what used to be the sacred meal hour. As a society we seem to have lost touch with our eating traditions.

Currently, the variety of vegetables, served at mealtime, has significantly declined compared to previous decades, resulting more or less in colorless plates that match the dreariness of this generation's health. The North American diet is corrupted by nutritionally inadequate processed and fast foods that predispose the consumer, over the long term, to a variety of chronic diseases.[2] Instead of preparing foods in the kitchen, our meals now are pre-packaged and reheated in the microwave for the sake of speed and efficiency in order to accommodate our fast-paced lives. [27] Are there any wonders then that the prevalence of heartburn, depression and other gastrointestinal diseases is on the rise?

As early as 1992, the National Institute of Health reported that digestive disorders were impacting Americans in significant ways. In addition, the cost to manage heart disease, obesity and type-2 diabetes has reached a level that is so preposterously elevated that it becomes questionable whether our financial system can support it. This should come as no surprised as 43 million Americans smoke, 20% of high school students smoke, more than 33% do not meet physical activity guidelines and 40% do no physical activity.[29]

Moreover, this is a time when hope is a rare commodity; depression, anxiety and mood disorders prevail and afflict a large number of people who are eager to understand what is happening to them. Is it already too late? According to the World Health Organization (Mental Health 2009 survey update), the prevalence of anxiety disorders are among the highest mental health disorders worldwide varying between 3.8% in China and 31.0% in the United

States.[19] There is also convincing evidence that depressive disorders are appearing more frequently earlier in life. Indeed, whereas the average age of onset of depression in the 1960s was 29, recent statistics indicate that more numerous cases of depressive disorders occur as early as 14.5yrs. In addition, 12.8% of US adolescents (ages 12 to 17) and 6.7% of US adults suffered from major depressive episodes in 2016 of which 64% were severely impaired.[28] This also goes hand in hand with substance abuse. As many as 14.6% of all Americans abuse some kind of substance [19] but it is specifically the 15% to 32% of teenagers (16-20 years old) and 45% of young adults (21-25 years old) who binge drank or heavily consumed alcohol regularly in 2011 that should set off alarms.[38] Additionally, illicit drug use is on the rise especially among the youth. Between the ages of 14 and 29, 9.2% to 23.8% had taken illicit drugs the month prior to taking the survey.[38] A front-page article, in the UK's Daily Mirror, dated February 10, 2014, reads: "The Generation Stress: The Scandal of Our Depressed Children." Andrew Gregory investigated the crisis. He described children under 10, tormented, anxious and worried about everything: homework, bullies, friends, appearances, sexualization and consumerism.[16] Lucie Russell, head of "Young Minds," a mental health charity, expressed her concern about these statistics. She admits: "*An increase in the number of young people under 11 in need of mental health services is a sad and very worrying accusation of the society we live in and the pressures that children face.*"
Children face pressures, but who protects them from the onslaught of demands that saturate their schedules and from the worries and fears that consume them?

It is timely to learn about nutrition, as it is the nutritional habits and overall lifestyle that we adopt, that will impact our long-term health and wellbeing the most. This is because the field of nutrition is vast, affecting so many different diseases and physical ailment, such as cardiovascular disease, renal and gastrointestinal diseases, diabetes and cancer to name but a few.

This book gives students access to a downloadable documentary that explores the impact of nutrition on the obesity and diabetes crises in the United States.[5] These are the most significant diseases afflicting our society currently, and they will likely impact student lives in some manner, either affecting them directly, or impacting family members and friends. Regardless, obesity and type II diabetes are currently driving healthcare costs and impacting American society at so many different levels. The documentary explores the prevalence, causes, assessment and the most current and effective treatments. And so the obesity documentary is valuable in forming students' critical thinking around these conditions.

This textbook is not meant to be as exhaustive, in detail and analysis, about the many facets of nutrition, as textbooks specifically framed for students in nutrition, nursing and medicine. Instead, my goal is to offer freshmen and sophomore students, who are taking general education courses, the opportunity to delve into the field of nutrition, without being overwhelmed by scientific details. This textbook attempts to introduce nutrition within an historical time-frame that follows the progress of the fields of Medicine and nutrition up to modern times. Nutrition, food and diet, from the very beginning, have been used in the treatment of disease. It is pertinent then, if we are to be successful in combating the rising prevalence of chronic diseases now afflicting the U.S., to learn about nutrition as a preventative form of medicine.

References

1. AMA (2020). Trends in Healthcare Spending. Taken from the American Medical Association website April 8, 2020: https://www.ama-assn.org/about/research/trends-health-care-spending
2. Bahadoran Z, Mirmiran P, Azizi F (2016). Fast Food Pattern and Cardiometabolic Disorders: A Review of Current Studies. *Health Promot Perspect*.;5(4):231-240. Published 2016 Jan 30. doi:10.15171/hpp.2015.028
3. Berge, J., Wall, M., Larson, N., Forsyth, A., Bauer, K., & Neumark-Sztainer, D. (2014). Youth dietary intake and weight status: Healthful neighborhood food environments enhance the protective role of supportive family home environments. *Health & Place*, 26, 69–77
4. Biener A, Cawley J, Meyerhoefer C. (2017) The High and Rising Costs of Obesity to the US Health Care System. *J Gen Intern Med*;32 (Suppl 1):6–8. doi:10.1007/s11606-016-3968-8
5. Bissonnette, D. J. Obesity in America: A National Crisis. Documentary produced by St-Jude Nutrition Medical Communications ©2010. Distributed by Films for the Humanities and Sciences. Clip segment: Interview with Dr. Barry Popkin.
6. Bissonnette, D.J. (2013). The Diabetes Epidemic: A Medical Catastrophe. Produced by St-Jude Nutrition Medical Communications © 2013. This is a 77 minute documentary that can be viewed online on demand: https://vimeo.com/ondemand/type2diabetes
7. Boutelle, K., Birnbaum, A., Lytle, L., Murray, D., & Story, M. (2003). Associations between perceived family meal environment and parent intake of fruit, vegetables, and fat. *Journal of Nutrition Education and Behavior*, 35, 24–29.
8. Chapel JM, Ritchey MD, Zhang D, Wang G. (2017). Prevalence and Medical Costs of Chronic Diseases Among Adult Medicaid Beneficiaries. *Am J Prev Med*;53(6S2):S143–S154. doi:10.1016/j.amepre.2017.07.019
9. Cooke LJ, Wardle J, Gibson EL, Sapochnik M, Sheiham A, Lawson M. (2004). Demographic, familial and trait predictors of fruit and vegetable consumption by preschool children. *Public Health Nutr; 7(2):295-302*
10. Dewan, M. (2017). Family Status: A Contributing Factor towards Childhood and Adolescent Obesity. *Bio Science Research Bulletin, 33*(1), 4.
11. Drewnowski A, Popkin BM. (1997). The Nutrition Transition: New Trends in the Global Diet. Nutr Rev;55(2):31-43.
12. Finkelstein EA, Trogdon JG, Cohen JW, Dietz W. Annual medical spending attributable to obesity: payer-and service-specific estimates. Health Aff (Millwood). 2009;28: w822–31. 10.1377/hlthaff.28.5.w822
13. Freedman, D. S., Khan, L. K., Serdula, M. K., Dietz, W. H., Srinivasan, S. R., & Berenson, G. S. (2005). The relation of childhood BMI to adult adiposity: The Bogalusa Heart Study. *Pediatrics*, 115(1), 22–27.
14. Fryar, C.D., Carroll, M. and Ogden, C.L. (2018). *Prevalence of Overweight, Obesity, and Extreme Obesity Among Adults Aged 20 and Over: United States, 1960–1962 Through 2015–2016.* URL: https://www.cdc.gov/nchs/data/hestat/obesity_adult_15_16/obesity_adult_15_16.htm
15. Fryar, C.D. Carroll, M.D. and Ogden, C.L.,. (2018b). "Prevalence of Overweight and Obesity Among Children and Adolescents Aged 2–19 Years: United States, 1963–1965 Through 2015–2016." *National Center for Health Statistics.* URL: https://www.cdc.gov/nchs/data/hestat/obesity_child_15_16/obesity_child_15_16.htm
16. Gregory, A. (2014) Generation Stress: Scandal of Our Depressed Kids as Thousands of Under 10s are Treated for Mental Health Problems. The Daily Mirror, February 10. Retrieved February 11, 2014 from: http://www.mirror.co.uk/news/uk-news/child-depression-scandal-ill-kids-3129996
17. Johnson, B., Brownell, K., St Jeor, S., Brunner, R., & Worby, M. (1997). Adult obesity and functioning in the family of origin. *International Journal of Eating Disorders*, **22**, 213–218.
18. Kessler, DA. (2009). The End of Overeating: Taking Control of the Insatiable American Appetite. Rodale Books, New York, 329pp
19. Kessler, R.C. et al., (2009b). The global burden of mental disorders: An update from the WHO World Mental Health (WMH) Surveys. Epidemiol Psichiatr Soc. 2009 Jan–Mar; 18(1): 23–33.
20. Koenig, HG (2012). Religion, Spirituality and Health: The Research and Clinical Implications. *ISRN Psychiatry*. 2012;2012:278730. Published 2012 Dec 16. doi:10.5402/2012/278730
21. La Berge, AF (2008) How the Ideology of Low Fat Conquered America, *Journal of the History of Medicine and Allied Sciences*; 63(2): 139–177 URL: https://doi.org/10.1093/jhmas/jrn001
22. Levine, J.A (2011). Poverty and Obesity in the US. Diabetes; 60(11): 2667-2668. http://dx.doi.org/10.2337/db11-1118
23. Mann, T. et al. (2007). Medicare Search for Effective Obesity Treatment: Diets are not the answer. American Psychologist; 62(3): 220-233. URL: http://janetto.bol.ucla.edu/index_files/Mannetal2007AP.pdf
24. Martin-Biggers, J. et al., (2018). Relationships of family conflict, cohesion, and chaos in the home environment on maternal and child food-related behaviours Matern Child Nutr;14(2):e12540. doi: 10.1111/mcn.12540 URL: https://onlinelibrary.wiley.com/doi/full/10.1111/mcn.12540
25. Mitchell NS, Catenacci VA, Wyatt HR, Hill JO. (2011) Obesity: overview of an epidemic. *Psychiatr Clin North Am*;34(4):717–732. doi:10.1016/j.psc.2011.08.005
26. Moss, M. (2013) Salt, sugar, Fat: How the Food Giants Hooked US. Random House, New York, 446pp
27. Nestle, M. (2002) Food Politics: How the Food Industry Influences Nutrition & Health. Berkeley, CA, University of California Press, 457pp.
28. NIMH (National Institute of Mental Health((2017). Major Depression. Retrieved from the NIH website march 29, 2018: https://www.nimh.nih.gov/health/statistics/major-depression.shtml
29. Norbeck TB. Drivers of health care costs. A Physicians Foundation white paper - second of a three-part series. *Mo Med*. 2013;110(2):113–118. URL: https://www.ncbi.nlm.nih.gov/pmc/articles/PMC6179664/
30. Padilla-Moledo, C., Castro-Pinero, J., Ortega, F. B., Mora, J., Marquez, S., Sjostrom, M., & Ruiz, J. R. (2011). Positive health, cardiorespiratory fitness and fatness in children and adolescents. *The European Journal of Public Health, 22*(1), 52-56.

31. Piernas, C and Popkin, BM. (2010) Snacking Increased among U.S. Adults between 1977 and 2006, *The Journal of Nutrition*; 140 (2): 325–332, https://doi.org/10.3945/jn.109.112763
32. Pi-Sunyer X. (2009). The medical risks of obesity. *Postgrad Med*;121(6):21–33. doi:10.3810/pgm.2009.11.2074
33. Popkin, BM, Adair, LS, and Ng, SW. (2012). "NOW AND THEN: The Global Nutrition Transition: The Pandemic of Obesity in Developing Countries." *Nutr Rev; 70(1):* 3–21. URL: https://www.ncbi.nlm.nih.gov/pmc/articles/PMC3257829/#SD3
34. Senguttuvan, U., Whiteman, S. D., & Jensen, A. C. (2014). Family Relationships and Adolescents Health Attitudes and Weight: The Understudied Role of Sibling Relationships. *Family Relations, 63*(3), 384-396.
35. Sheidow, AJ et al (2014). The Role of Stress Exposure and Family Functioning in Internalizing Outcomes of Urban Families. J Child Fam Stud ; 23(8): 1351–1365. doi:10.1007/s10826-013-9793-3. URL: https://www.ncbi.nlm.nih.gov/pmc/articles/PMC4296577/
36. Sturm R, Hattori A. (2013). Morbid obesity rates continue to rise rapidly in the United States. *Int J Obes (Lond)*;37(6):889–891. doi:10.1038/ijo.2012.159
37. The Hartman Group (2016).Table for One: Why we are Increasingly Eating Alone? Forbes, May 25th issue. Retrieved January 3, 2017 from: http://www.forbes.com/sites/thehartmangroup/2016/05/25/table-for-one-why-we-are-increasingly-eating-alone/#2f2790544112
38. USHHS (United States Department of Health & Human Services (2011). Results from the 2011 National Survey on Drug Use and Health: Summary of National Findings. Retrieved from the Center for Behavioral Health Statistics and Quality on March 29, 2018: https://www.samhsa.gov/data/sites/default/files/Revised2k11NSDUHSummNatFindings/Revised2k11NSDUHSummNatFindings/NSDUHresults2011.htm
39. WHO, (2016). "Obesity and Overweight Fact Sheet." *World Health Organization.* Accessed 05 19, 2018. http://www.who.int/news-room/fact-sheets/detail/obesity-and-overweight
40. Willett WC, Stampfer MJ, Colditz GA, Rosner BA & Speizer FE (1990): Relation of meat, fat and fiber intake to the risk of colon cancer in a prospective study among women. New Engl. J. Med. 232, 1664 –1672.
41. Yang, W. Y., Burrows, T., Macdonald-Wicks, L., Williams, L. T., Collins, C. E., & Chee, W. S. (2016). The Family Diet Study: a cross-sectional study into the associations between diet, food habits and body weight status in Malay families. *Journal of Human Nutrition and Dietetics, 29*(4), 441-448.

CHAPTER 1

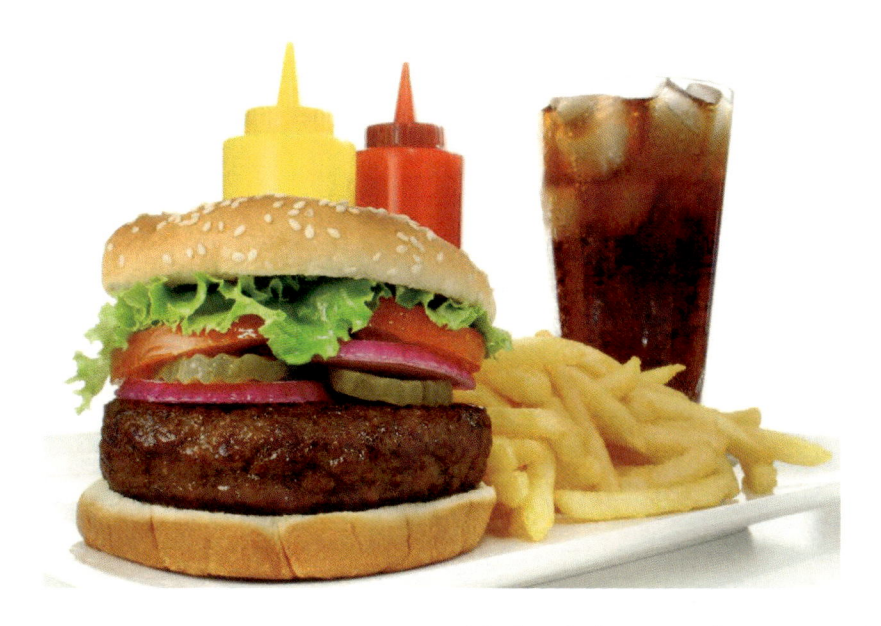

By Joao Virissimo© shutterstock_12982894/shutterstock.com

THE ORIGINS OF OUR CURRENT NUTRITION PRACTICES

Introduction
We live in a society that demands peak performance, and is intolerant of anything that is not on the fringes of excellence. Peters & Waterman introduced the notion of searching for excellence, among American companies nearly four decades ago, with their best seller—In Search of Excellence [125] —and still, it is strongly embedded in the North American psyche. It is all about finding ways to be excellent at what we do.

Consequently, we've become a culture intolerant of mediocrity when quality can be achieved; and we buy into this idea of always being at our peak level of performance, of grabbing every opportunity and seizing the day. It is a wonderful vision that leaves no room for being tired, unfocused, and moody; the solutions have been either diet and lifestyle changes, and/or an arsenal of antidepressants and antianxiety medications to deal with the rising prevalence of hopelessness and anxiety, notably in youth. [28]

1.1 Anxious and Depressed Nation—Indeed, the CDC's study of high school risk behaviors in the US between 1991 and 2013 revealed that between one quarter and one third of all students (33.33%) in grades 9 through 12 experienced significant hopelessness. Indeed, whereas the average

age of onset of depression in the 1960s was 29, recent statistics indicate that more numerous cases of depressive disorders occur as early as 14.5yrs. In addition, 12.8% of US adolescents (ages 12 to 17) and 6.7% of US adults suffered from major depressive episodes in 2016 of which 64% were severely impaired. [119] This also goes hand in hand with substance abuse. As many as 14.6% of all Americans abuse some kind of substance, [94] but it is specifically 15% to 32% of teenagers (16-20 years old) and 45% of young adults (21-25 years old) who binge drank or heavily consumed alcohol regularly in 2011. [162] Additionally, illicit drug use is on the rise especially among the youth. Between the ages of 14 and 29, 9.2% to 23.8% had taken illicit drugs the month prior to taking the survey. [162] It would seem that the practice, of chronically escaping from reality—times are indeed dark—has become significantly entrenched within our culture. We are indeed troubled and anxious, all too ready to escape reality by substance abuse and our many distractions, such as food. In fact, many are those whose intemperance of food, entertainment and work serve to mitigate on the one hand, their deep hunger to better define their purpose, and on the other hand, to alleviate their remorse of conscience emanating from the haunting echoes of their past. [13, 78] What is really concerning, however, are the 20.1 million Americans who suffer from substance use disorder. [135] The recent legalization of marijuana, in many states, is a troubling development, as it has clearly been established that continued use leads to significant declines in IQ scores. [109] Additionally, marijuana usage—24 million Americans—is linked to heightened risk of chronic obstructive pulmonary disease (COPD), [135, 152] hyperemesis syndrome, impaired coordination and performance, anxiety, suicidal ideations/tendencies, psychotic symptoms, mood disorders, withdrawal syndrome and neurocognitive impairments. [90]

Throw in the 65.3 million individuals afflicted with serious binge drinking problems, and we are looking at 93.9 million substance abusers who are in an alcoholic haze or a drug-induced brain fog for some or all of the time. There is just no way to know for sure. The reality is that if we count the legitimate psychiatric prescription drug users—21-41.1 million Americans 12 years and older of which 6.2 million misuse psychotherapeutic drugs—along with those taking illegal drugs and abusing alcohol, there is a potential 115-135 million Americans—this is 41.7% of the population—on mind-altering substances. [135, 98]

This level of drug intake is indicative of a significant malaise or unease that is pushing many towards this kind of chemical-based escapism. What are they escaping from exactly? Well nobody in the health care field is really asking that question in a meaningful way, for to do so is first, costly and second, it is very time consuming to manage the answer, and frankly, many do not want to know. The reality is that time is something the healthcare industry does not have much of, and nor is it equipped to peer deep into the individual's soul. However, if we dare to explore deeper, the guilt, disgust and shame we feel, [30, 175] as we face the sins of our past, produces stress-related behaviors, which eventually begin to feed compulsive behaviors. The obsession can be for food, drugs, or alcohol. [34] Food obsession often evolve into binge eating, and...

is associated with substantial psychiatric co-morbidities, especially those related to substance abuse and mood and anxiety disturbances." [169]

This compulsion—whether drugs or food—helps the dissonant soul to cope with the misery and troubles of life, [132] and there is plenty to go around. This misery is greatly linked to "*stressful life events*" in addition to sociocultural norms that invariably heighten anxiety when the person is unable to conform to them. [132] Hence, nobody is surprised that there are 44.7 million cases diagnosed with mental health illnesses. [135]

1.2 A Dieting Nation—America has also become a nation obsessed with dieting. This is consistent with the US obesity and overweight epidemics, [111] with as many as 71.2% of adult men and women classified as overweight or obese, and a troubling 40% who are obese. [55] The prevalence is concerning enough that the WHO now considers obesity as one of the top ten preventable cause of death, worldwide [163, 166] for which behavior and environment have been identified as primary causes. [129, 32] The epidemic status of obesity has long been established in the US, yet the 198.51% jump in obesity prevalence among adult Americans since 1960, [55] in concert with the 256% climb in children's (2-19 years) obesity prevalence since 1971, [56] paint a worrisome landscape. The 30-year linear projection for the growth of obesity in the US [49] foresees a 33% increase in obesity and a surprising 130% hike in severe obesity by 2030, with 51% of the US adult population likely to become obese. Weight loss diets have been the main behavioral therapeutic modality for weight management problems as far back as

Hippocrates, [69] and still today it is the single most utilized weight management strategy. [14, 149]

Yet studies, as far back as the late 1950s, [146] have found that caloric restrictive diets, despite causing rapid and significant weight loss, over the short term, have shown generally poor effectiveness in sustaining weight loss over long term in 2 year follow ups. [91, 124, 105] In a review of obesity treatments, Traci Mann and co-workers [105] concluded that between 33 and 67% of participants, regained lost weight and more between four to five years after dieting. Yet, millions of Americans persist in following diets for weight loss despite their many failures. In fact, of the millions in the US who are obese, roughly 50-70% are attempting to lose weight at any given time. [15]

The dieting craze really began in the 1970s with the advents of obesity and heart disease becoming more prominent in the culture. Dieting fit within the paradigm of preventative medicine, and was vigorously embraced by a public wanting to keep in check the potentially costly affair of controlling the debilitating impact of chronic disease. And so the battle was on to control hunger and slim down. [99]

Dr. Robert Atkins' *Diet Revolution* [7] and *The Super-Energy Diet* [8] revolutionized the seventies by introducing a diet formulation involving the restriction of carbohydrates. The market place of that era was invaded by other popular sages of the day like Pritikin [130] and Scarsdale, [151] who sold millions of diet books. They introduced the North American population to an obsessive preoccupation: that of pursuing optimal nutrition for weight loss and maximal health.

Hunger, has become of particular interest to the medical and scientific communities because it is the driving force behind the obesity epidemic that is now, not only sweeping America, but also the world. [165] There is something odd about this epidemic. Driven by an insatiable hunger for food, it is concerning as it knows no limitations; it can strike all ages and all nationalities. Nobody appears to be immune from its devastating grip, and all of the secondary diseases such as cardiovascular disease (CVD), coronary heart disease, stroke, type-2 diabetes, dyslipidemia, hypertension, [149, 97] depression, [140] and a variety of cancers. [38] This hunger, because of the devastation it leaves in its path, has an insatiable trait, knowing no limits, no longer regulated by temperance. These secondary diseases have become prevalent enough to set off alarms nationwide; health professionals have been warning for some time that obesity [55, 56] and type-2 diabetes [150] have reached epidemic and pandemic statuses, and will forcibly change, in a very short time, the very fabric of American society.

It is like an approaching storm, with winds blowing on the horizon, and it has gained a tremendous momentum in recent years. It is a tempest of sorts, swiftly and decisively, destroying the health of both the US adult and youth populations. Its gales are fierce, and the destruction left in its path, devastating.

This storm is troubling and destabilizing, yet, American society, warned by famed nutritionist, Adelle Davis, back in the mid-1930s, of the impoverishment of the American food supply, remained mostly silent and unruffled. Davis had written a series of diet books—*Optimum Diet, You can Stay Well, Let's Cook It Right, Let's Eat Well and Keep Fit*—that hit book stores and newspaper stands as early as 1935. It was, however, the iconic publication, "Optimum Health," that captured, what was to become, a national obsession over dieting. [36] Indeed, the pursuit of optimal health began with a natural food subculture that grew into prominence by the 1970s. Davis' nutrition publications introduced the idea that the American food supply was impoverished and, that individuals need to be diligent and smart about their food choices. She documented the excessive saturated fat, hydrogenated fats and sugar, consumed by the American public at the time. She set off alarms about the risk of vitamin deficiencies, which were already peppering the US landscape by 1934 because of the US' love affair with white bread. [18] She advised that careful food choices and proper cooking could lead to having healthy children and becoming well again. Davis was accurately capturing the clamor of the natural food movement, which was looking to achieve health through prevention. Frances Moore Lappé's "Diet for a Small Planet," published in 1971, introduced vegetarianism as a way to find that wellness. She got many to become enamored with the notion of eating healthy natural vegetarian foods to slim down and improve cardiovascular health. Her book caused many to shift away from the massive meat consumption that had defined the American diet at the time, and to embrace a more eco-friendly vegetable-based eating style. At the time, obesity was not a national epidemic, and was still under the radar of most health care professionals and epidemiologists. However, the prevalence of heart disease and overweight Americans was elevated enough for others like Nathan Pritikin, Herman Tarnower and Robert Atkins to jump into the fray with national bestsellers of their own during the 70s. In 1975, William Dufty's national bestseller, *Sugar Blues*, and many other authors, continued to capture the theme of a nutritionally suboptimal US diet right up to the present. Dufty, husband of silver screen icon, Gloria Swanson, awoke the public to the devastating impact of abundant sugar consumption on human health; it caused seismic shockwaves to run through the food industry, which had been lacing most of its products with sugar. It did not take long before the 1970's were overrun by nutrition gurus who published diet books framed to address the nutritional maladies of the time, notably, heart disease and obesity. These very popular bestsellers initiated the US population to a chronic dieting craze, focused on macronutrient manipulations for effective weight loss, that has lasted forty years, and it is still going strong. [99] The goal was to quell that hunger. Times have not really changed since the 1970s; we are still as overweight, tired and worn down, but in addition, we are now more obese, depressed and anxious. Since the new Millennium, the prevalence of obesity soared to become a national epidemic, and a pandemic. The US and the rest of the world are now grappling with an overfed population that is catapulting healthcare costs into orbit. The Zone Diet, the New Atkins diet, and the South Beach Diet, published between 1999 and 2003, embodied the zeitgeist of the dieting world. Atkins and the Zone diet continued to push the low carb diet principle. Arthur Agatston's South Beach Diet promoted healthy fat and low glycemic carbohydrate foods for good cardiovascular health and weight loss; the books offered new hope to a nation growing more obese. The public lapped up every word, as discouragement and disillusionment affected most dieters who wanted to get out from under the cloud of weight loss failures. [142,105] Most were regaining their lost weight in droves. There was, seemingly, a national resolve to fight obesity according to Dr. Richard Carmona, the Surgeon General of the United States, [136] but few were winning the battle. The problem was that there was no evidence that demonstrated that weight loss diets were effective over the long term. [105] In fact, the scientific evidence is now showing that dieting increases the likelihood of weight management problems in the future. [105]

William Dufty's description of an unhealthy food supply was spot on! It insidiously made the US population gravely ill and brought the US healthcare expenditure to the brink of insolvency. To admit that the US diet is poor is no longer shocking because of the many books that have flooded the market, starting with Harvey Levenstein's "Paradox of Plenty in 1993. [101] Then in the new millennium Aaron Bobrow Brains' "White Bread,"[18] Michael Mosse's "Salt, Sugar and Fat,"[112] Marian Nestle's "Food Politics"[118] and "Soda Politics," and Eric Schlosser's "Fast Food Nation" gave scathing depictions of the highly processed and impoverished diet consumed by the US. The situation has only gotten worse since the days of William Dufty and Adelle Davis. These books introduced the notion that food addiction and corporate complicity conspired together in sickening the US population with poor quality food for the sake of greater profits. Obesity is a real and measurable problem spawned, in part, from an overabundance of very addictive processed foods, and, paradoxically, from chronic dieting. In fact, the elevated dieting failure rate tells us something about the obesity crisis; there is more here that meets the eye. This obese culture has in fact not fully understood the depth of the problem. Some have argued that obesity presents itself more as a spiritual problem [155] of gargantuan proportion, rather than a medical enigma. The principles advanced by Michael Ozner's "The Complete Mediterranean Diet", Dean Ornishe's The Spectrum and the more recently released, "Dr. Gundry's Diet Evolution add some complexity to the solution. These authors recognize that a successful resolution of the obesity epidemic cannot take place if doctors continue to prescribe weight-loss diets that manipulate carbohydrate, protein and fat concentrations. In fact, Dean Ornishe in the "The Spectrum," proposed that there are strong emotional, sociological and psychological dimensions tied to obesity that few had been addressing. Ornishe gets it right when he describes obesity as a multifaceted problem that needs to be tackled cautiously. In the end, the poor long term success to eradicating obesity with dieting [142] may be the proof needed that the field of Medicine has been tackling this problem the wrong way.

1.3 Prevention as a Medical Strategy—Like the phoenix, prevention rises from the ashes, as the medical icon of a new era. Prevention research began as early as the 1940s, but wasn't introduced as a serious alternative medical strategy until nearly three decades later. As comprehensive knowledge was compiled, regarding the increasing risks of several prominent diseases such as lung and bowel cancers and cardiovascular disease, more strategic preventative therapies were being developed. [156, 170, 171, 172, 173]

Healthcare reforms—precipitated by rising healthcare costs in the 1980s—began to reflect a harsh order of constraint, that was called for in the eighties and nineties, [51] and that have now re-emerged again since the 2008 financial meltdown and the 2020 COVID19 pandemic. [5] These reforms, tailored to match fiscal constraint and cutback policies, dictate a new economic reality of fiscal restriction precipitated by rising costs. The Canadian solution was cost cutting, [103] whereas in the US, Managed Care— the new investor-owned- for-profit management concept—did not focus on cost control, but rather, on revenue generation. [51]

These strategies began to be seriously implemented by the late eighties, and as early as the nineties, hospital bed closures, reduced staff, overworked nurses and physicians very quickly became the norm in the health care milieu, especially in countries with socialized medicine like Canada. [103]

Though the US healthcare system stepped up to the plate, in heroic fashion, to manage the COVID-19 pandemic, the US hospitals and health systems were blindsided by what the American Hospital Association refers to as "catastrophic financial challenges" as they face estimated losses of $50.7 billion per month stemming primarily from lost revenue. [5] The reality was that, even before the pandemic outbreak, close to 50% of US hospitals were headed towards financial nose dives by 2025. [5]

In the epicentre of the shock waves, created by a tight fiscal policy and rising healthcare costs, is the strategy of preventative medicine. The goal was to manage resources in a more efficient manner, to prolong life and to curb the incidence of diseases and disabilities that were preventable. [41]

Historians almost unanimously point to Richard Mead as one of the most influential fathers of preventive medicine. [71] His reputation, driven by his recommendations, to the French government in 1720, to quarantine cities and countries as a public health measure to contain the plague, is considered today, a hallmark of strategic medical prevention. He understood the bubonic plague to be contagious, a position that contradicted the French physicians at the time, but that was grounded in the preventive measures taken to isolate towns and country during the great London plague of 1665-66 that killed 90,000-100,000 people. [114, 71] He further recommended that the French set up, in each town,

> The Health Professionals Follow-up Study recorded a 71% reduction in relative risk in subjects following a healthy diet which included none of the risks for colon cancer.

a Council of Health to manage quarantine measures and the dead. [71]

In the 19th and 20th centuries, preventive medicine strategies were rigorously implemented for the cholera epidemic (1817-1923), Spanish flue (1918), and Tuberculosis (TB) (1720-present). The first successful treatment of TB was the sanatorium, implemented in 1854, and initially described by Brehmer, a medical student who had contracted the disease. [10, 33] The cholera epidemic in London spread through the contamination of the water supply by leaking sewers, thus leading to the construction of interlocking sewer pipes to contain the spread of the cholera. [68, 106] The Spanish flue killed over 50 million worldwide [107] could only be managed by public health measures such as the tracking of cases, the surveillance of schools, boarding schools, and barracks, in addition to a second wave of measures that included closing public meeting places, cleaning of streets and sanitizing public gathering spaces. [107]

Preventive medicine continued to make significant headway since the middle of the 20th century with the use of efficacious public health strategies which contrasted with traditional Medicine's model of care that is disease-focused and thus curative rather than preventive. [52] In the new Millennium the new lingo in healthcare strategies is captured in these three terms: Lifestyle medicine, health promotion, and wellness. [43] Health promotion, a prominent strategy in smoking cessation, aimed at curbing lung disease and overall mortality, has been successful in curbing smoking through social marketing of smoking cessation, mass media campaigns and community mobilization aimed at changing social norms and practices. [62] The prevention of cardiovascular disease has also been successful. [80] Indeed, early prenatal interventions aimed at preventing obesity by ensuring good maternal nutrition and smoking cessation has lowered the incidence of childhood obesity. Moreover, breastfeeding has been linked to reduced incidence of cardiovascular disease later in life. [80] People were beginning to understand that they had the power to make concrete changes to their lifestyle, and in so doing, impact life expectancy as well as the quality of life of their children.

Nutrition has become the main focal point of preventative health care, currently being promoted in the United States, Canada, Europe and Japan. From a demographic standpoint, aging baby-boomers are especially concerned with nutritional issues, as they now begin to battle chronic diseases such as osteoporosis, cardiovascular disease and cancer; [96] these are the very diseases that threaten this age group's desire for longevity and health. King and colleagues [96] conclude:

The findings from the present study documenting poorer health status and increased rates of obesity, hypertension, diabetes, and hypercholesterolemia support an increased likelihood for continued rising health care costs and a need for increased numbers of health professionals as baby boomers age.

The association between disease and diet is so powerful, that epidemiologists have been able to establish that dietary habits, maintenance of health body weight and regularly engaging in physical activity could prevent up to 40% of all cancers. [164] Also, 14% of cancer deaths in men and 20% in women are associated with being overweight or obese. [25] Findings from the Nurse's Health Study (NHS), identified that a 45% increase of relative risk of developing colon cancer when following the typical Western diet consisting of French fries, frequent and large amounts of red and processed meats, frequent sweet desserts and abundant refined grains. [57] The Health Professionals Follow-up Study recorded a 71% reduction in relative risk in subjects following a healthy diet which included none of the risks for colon cancer. [128] American Cancer Society (ACS) indicates that 20% of all diagnosed cancers in the US are linked to fatness, physical inactivity, poor nutrition and excessive alcohol consumption. [4] The ACS affirms that the research indicates that 42% of overall cancer cases and as many as 45% of cancer deaths are preventable because most are linked to behavior and lifestyles. [3] Nutrition and physical activity is of course central to this discussion.

The World Health Organization estimates that in 2001 there were 10 million cases of cancer worldwide; they expect the number to grow to almost 20 million cases per year over the next twenty years. [172] A fear-driven population is searching for the elusive elixir that can abate the scourge that seems assured to hit. Because current statistics estimate that 38.4% of Americans will likely be stricken by some form of cancer in their lifetime—up from 25% estimated around 2010, the impetus to tackle the scourge head-on is very powerful. [117]

Diet is central to everyone's life; it is personal and so, in that sense, the consumer is now in the driver's seat, seemingly more capable than ever before of taking control of his health. This is because there is a wealth of information, easily accessed via the internet, bookstores and libraries, that is, now at the consumer's fingertips, providing the more recent advances in scientific research. However, the information is overwhelming and the interpretation difficult to confirm as there is so much disinformation.

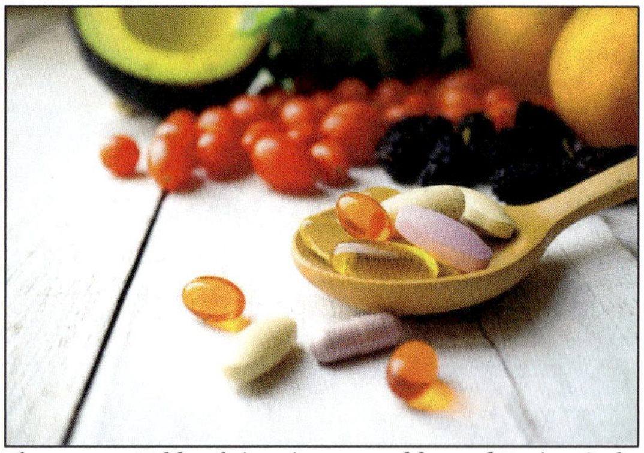

Figure 1.1: Table of vitamins, vegetables and Fruits. © shutterstock_1041373417 /shutterstock.com

There is no doubt, that popular belief supports the idea that mismanagement of diet carries repercussions that can influence the wellbeing of individuals, by permeating many facets of their active lives.

Adelle Davis popularized, back in the early 1900s, the notion of vitamins as active ingredients in food that were critical to human health (Figure 1.1). Suddenly food became, in the public's eye, a sort of medicine. She drove home an important point about food: not all food is equal. In fact, her many nutrition books helped raise the public's awareness that longevity and youthfulness could be achieved through potent food concoctions. Davis was quickly labelled as a food faddist and a promoter of nutrition quackery.

1.4 Health Reform Movement—The origins of food faddism did not, however, begin with Adelle Davis; rather it is historically linked to the 19th century *Health Reform Movement*, which consisted of alternative forms of medical practices that were made up of three systems: ***hydropathy***, ***homeopathy*** and ***Thomsonianism***.

1.4.1 Hydropathy—The notion of the healing powers of cold springs—commonly used by English peasantry—was initially investigated as a medical therapy in 1702 by the English physicians Sir John Floyer of Lichfield England and Dr. Currie of Liverpool. [44]

The idea that water could be used as a therapy was further developed into a more comprehensive system, formally named **hydropathy** by an entrepreneurial Austrian farmer named Vincenz Priessnitz (1801-51) around 1829. Hydropathy, an alternative medical treatment, used cold and hot water, either internally or externally, to treat diseases. Its popularity in Europe acted as a vector that launched it as a medical therapy here in the United States. [44]

1.4.2 Homeopathy was introduced as a formal medical therapy by Samuel Hahnemann (1755-1843), in the 18th century, based on Hippocratic notions that medicinal treatments could be made to emulate or contrast the disease. Homeopathy consisted of a novel strategy of administering medication following two concepts: **potentisation** and **provings**. [26] The former consisted of vigorously shaking and enlivening the medical properties, whereas the latter had to do with testing the medicinal concoctions on healthy people to understand the therapeutic path in unhealthy individuals. Although the method lacked scientific rigor, it nevertheless followed some kind of logical system of prescribing medicine, which appeared rooted in mystery, but nevertheless geared towards individual needs.

This organized system contrasted with spurious strategies used by contemporary doctors of that time. Thus, the patient perceived the homeopath as a thoughtful practitioner capable of titrating medicinal doses to match his or her needs. Hence, homeopathy grew in popularity with one quarter of American MDs registered as homeopaths in 1900. It was specifically the rise of pharmaceutical chemistry that brought homeopathy to a crashing end around 1935, as it could not compete with the well-standardized and powerfully effective pharmaceuticals. [24] So far, writes Cālina,

Homeopathic remedies have only been tested in little clinical trials, but no explanation was found concerning the means by which these very diluted solutions, administered orally only, can act on a molecular level, nor has it been clarified how it can interact with biologic tissue. Since there has not been a condition for which a positive or negative effect could be objectively proven, one could conclude that all the homeopathics are placebo. [24]

1.4.3 Thomsonianism (1822-1895) was founded by Samuel Thomson (1769–1843) in the 1820s, and was also known as the Thomsonian Botanical Movement. It was a popular alternative form of medicine, unique to the United States, until the Civil War (1861-65). It promoted diet, herbs and food as central components to good health, and was a movement born in opposition to the modernization of medicine and diet; [50] Flannery [50] writes:

Thomson believed that orthodox, university-trained physicians were killing their patients with toxic minerals like tartar emetic (antimony) and calomel (mercurous chloride). Convinced that he had discovered the source of health and healing in nature's apothecary, he developed a system of herbal remedies, the rights to which could be purchased.

The movement would eventually evolve to include hydropathy and homeopathy. [148] Thomsonianism, born in the Jacksonian era of populist and egalitarian beliefs, became the driving defensive force for the people's medicine. [50]

Samuel Thompson was a farmer, an amateur of medicine and a zealous critic of institutionalized medicine, who called for a return to pre-modern-day medical healing practices and food processing. Medicine, as a profession, protected by licensure, began to more formally emerge in the U.S, with English trained physicians founding, by the mid-1700s, formal medical schools. [66]

It is from these institutions that American doctors of medicine graduated, and began opening up medical practices in large northern cities like Philadelphia and New York. These kinds of doctors continued, however, to embrace the old European medical theories and practices that had been steeped for so long in stagnation and ignorance. They continued to awkwardly tackle inflammation and fevers with the practices of blood-letting and mercury-based laxatives. [66]

There was, in fact, very little evidence that these physicians were able to successfully treat disease or assist in childbirths. Yet despite their visible incompetence, it was this exclusive licensure of medical practitioners that consolidated their hold on the broad field of medicine, causing orthopedic doctors, midwives, Indian doctors, and herbalists to be forcibly reclassified as non-doctors or quacks with many of their treatments forbidden by law. [50]

This is precisely what Thomsonianism was decrying as a tragedy, as the movement believed very strongly that the plants contained true medicinal components that the standard physicians did not consider in their practice. [66] Moreover, the cholera epidemic that was raging in several large American and English cities, by the mid-19th century, [82] killed thousands of people despite the application of standard medical therapies. [37] It is not surprising then, that the field of medicine was facing quite an uphill battle to gain credibility.

Having witnessed the death of his mother, and the worsening of his wife's health, while under the care of the modern physician, Samuel Thompson began to observe the serious shortcomings of modern medicine. It was specifically the *root doctors* that healed his poor wife from post-partum (after birth) complications.[66] The botanical movement, he founded, was based on the premise that plants and herbs could restore the body's temperature balance or its *natural heat* which was lost through disease. [66]

Thus dietary practices, rooted in vegetarianism, became the central theme of his therapy; he strongly advocated for the individual to take control of his health by embracing healthy lifestyles and good food habits. [50, 148]

Thompson had seen, within the early years of the U.S Antebellum period (1812 to 1860), the impact on food habits, from the cultural mix occurring with immigration, and the more threatening dietary changes that took place with prosperity and the beginning of modernization. Thomsonianism—its hay-day lasting between 1822-1850—was a movement that was trying to guide the American diet back to a simpler and possibly healthier time period, which began with the arrival of the Puritans who sailed from England on the Mayflower. These Pilgrims arrived at Cape Cod in 1620, and introduced New England to the British Yeoman diet which consisted of wheat, barley, rye—rye was replaced by maize in the earlier years as it was a native crop—pulses (beans), beef, pork, mutton, dairy (butter & cheese), and fruits. Grains were prepared as dark breads, gruels, porridges and hasty puddings (McMahon, 1985). [104] Their main dishes were pease porridge (split pea soup), brown bread, boiled meat and vegetables, including turnips and carrots, and some fruits which they complemented with beer and fermented ciders (McMahon, 1985; Hazlit, 1902). [104, 72]

In the first great wave of immigration, in the early colonial days up to 1880, it was the populations from mostly Northern Europe, such as England, Ireland, Scotland and Scandinavia, in addition to Germany, that settled in the U.S. [85] They brought with them their rich cultural food traditions. These dietary influences began to shape the food preferences of the new settlers. Native Indian food traditions such as succotash, Indian pudding, hoecakes, popcorn, pumpkin bread and pie, cranberries and turkey were also filtering into the cultural habits (McMahon, 1985). [104]

These traditions lasted throughout most of the 17th and 18th centuries, but historians tell us that at the start of the 19th century, vegetables were more diversified and abundantly found in the diet, the consequence of maintaining side vegetable gardens—a practice that began in the early 1700s and grew in prominence by 1790. No longer were vegetables used to flavor sauces but were often served as a separate dish. Moreover, the practice of storing summer vegetables in root cellars for fall and winter consumption became prevalent by 1720—potatoes notably became popular fare in the early 18th century New England diet. [104] By 1820, large gardens of potatoes, squash and other vegetables were maintained by households. [104] From the latter half of the 19th to the beginning of 20th centuries, the second great wave of immigrants (1820-1870) arrived in the United States from mostly Ireland and Germany. The third great wave (1881-1920) and came mostly from Italy, Poland, Russia and Hungary. [1, 139] There was also a sizable influx from Japan and Mexico, [85] and because of this significant and rich change in ethnic diversity, the cultural diet of Americans dramatically changed as well.

1.5 Impact of the Industrial Revolution on US Food Consumption. The nation's population size was expanding in unprecedented ways, increasing from 9 million in 1820 to 17 million by 1840 officially naturalizing 750,949 immigrants in that period. [39] Between 72-78% of these permanent residents were from Europe, the majority coming Germany, France, Ireland and the United Kingdom. [39] The jump in the population was impressive, with 6% moving westward to Illinois and Iowa, but the most significant proportion remaining on the Eastern seaboard—roughly 94% of the increase—and a large faction gravitating towards cities. [85] They were vying for the much coveted factory jobs, and so it is in this setting that the modernization of food began. [50]

Between 1881 and 1920, the third wave of immigration occurred from South and Eastern European countries, notably, Italy, Russia and Hungry, but additionally from Mexico and Japan [39] and coincided with the height of the Industrial Revolution. [76] Prior to this period, the majority of the US population resided in agricultural households and small towns. [121] However, by 1880, even though a significant erosion of the agricultural frontier had occurred—fifty percent of US workers were still farmers—the manufacturing base, which employed less than 15% of workers consisted of small firms and workshops that relied on artisan technology for the production of tools. [2] The sawmills and grain mills—located by rivers in rural areas—depended on the flowing rivers, to run the machinery. Industrial Revolution fueled greater urbanization as more rural farm workers gravitated to the cities in order to work in the factories, [76] causing the agricultural workforce to decline from 48 to 25% and manufacturing laborers to rise from 14 to 25%. In those 40 years, the number of gainful workers rose from 18.1 to 40.5 million. [76] This coincided with technological advancements—fueled by commercial electricity—that permitted large-scale urban manufacturing. [61] Food production changed dramatically at that time to accommodate the large population base that was now conglomerating in the cities, clamoring for food. It is during that time, that food vendors began popping up everywhere along with concerns for safety and unfair selling practices.

1.5.1 Uncertainty about the Safety and Distribution of Food. The industrial production and distribution scale of milk prompted deception among some farmers and dairy producers, who would frequently dilute milk with water in order to artificially and deceptively boost volumes, thus increasing sale profits. [17] Unfortunately, the incidence of food poisonings jumped noticeably in Britain [67] and America [17, 153] by 1880 as mass food production rather than Hygiene, purity and quality of food had become the priority. Several historians claim that there was a public uneasiness surrounding the consumption of manufactured food because of the perceived deceptions wheeled by many of the food distributors. According to Gabriella Petrick, [126b] an associate professor at George Mason University, and an expert on the history of industrial foods and food technology:

… the urbanizing process made acquiring and consuming all manners of food (from meat to milk to apples, flour and canned goods) an anxiety-provoking process, especially for the women who were largely responsible for purchasing and cooking the family's meals.

The period of 1870 to 1930 favored the development of the canning industry, which gradually contributed toward making the food supply more abundant and safer. [101, 153] Indeed, by 1879 most canning of fruits and vegetables were done by hand, and involved 7% child labor, which by 1919, had fallen to 1%. Mothers often came to work in the canning industry accompanied by young children to supplement their income. [21] The canning industry, caused a revolution in the mass production and distribution of food throughout the US and the world. The mechanization of canning, at the start of the twentieth century, which rendered the capper and processing craftsmen obsolete, [22] increased canning production from 1500 to 35,000 cans per day, between 1890 and 1910. [101] The investment in canning technology by companies like Heinz, California Fruit Grower's Exchange and Campbell, in meat packing by Swift, Armour and Wilson, in flour milling by Washburn-Crosby and Pillsbury, was so extensive that big business had so transformed the food industry by 1900 that food processing represented 20% of US manufacturing. [101]

1.5.2 Impact on the Family. Nuclear families began to emerge, and the prevalence of extended families slowly faded, as urban housing was more contained and constricted; already, there were early signs of the eventual downsizing of the American dinner table that was to take place in subsequent decades as the Industrial Revolution took hold and a shift from the farm to the cities for factory jobs rapidly occurred. [133] Important changes took place in the American diet between 1900 and 1930. A downgrade in the quality of family meals ensued with several societal changes: first, the numerous white collar jobs available for women in a rapidly growing service industry; second, the servant from the middle class home was replaced by the cleaning lady, leaving food preparation to the mothers, already too busy by the clerical jobs they held outside the home. Levenstein [101] writes:

The virtual disappearance of the live-in servant from middle-class homes affected and reflected changed eating habits. While "cleaning women" may have taken over the house cleaning, laundering and even child care duties of the ex-live-in servants, food preparation was usually a casualty of the new arrangements.

The new families and homes, while benefitting from much higher standards of living and cleanliness, in addition to new economic needs and dress, both kitchens and dining rooms declined in importance. The middle class, no longer interested in cooking, sought after new interests that saturated schedules and shattered the family meal, forcing many to eat on the run, rather than dine together as a family. The fate of the American family meal was sealed when the housewives, eager to pursue their enticing new leisure activities, embraced the processed foods inventory of the new American kitchen. [101]

The American understanding of eating by the 1920s, changed with the discovery of vitamins, WW-I food rationing policies, and from the ideas propagated by health reformers and home economists. [101]

1.5.3 The New Diet & Marketplace. In the mid-nineteenth century, as technology was developing, more numerous urban centers and railroad systems began to surface—The Western Railway of Massachusetts was completed in 1843—thus fueling a **consumption revolution**. As more commodities were transported by rail between cities and counties, many cities had greater access to wheat flour, sugar, yeast, and salt. Sudden availability of white flour in the market place favored household transitions from rye, corn and whole wheat-based flat breads to fluffy white yeast-raised breads. The wheat kernel was now separated more thoroughly into the endosperm, germ and bran—this occurred because roller mills replaced stone mills—thereby creating nutritionally impoverished flour that had also lost its familiar nutty flavor. [18, 120]

Fuelled by Sylvester Graham's writings and speeches, the Health reform Movement, by the 1830s, was decrying the modernization of the food supply. Graham, having first worked in the temperance movement, evolved into more of an advocate for traditional healthy eating. He was, in fact the first American to promote vegetarianism and diet reform. [120] Graham, in his *Treatise on Bread and Bread-Making,* encouraged his readers to purchase the best unrefined flour, which, he insisted, they needed to grind up themselves in order to make homemade bread baked in their own ovens. In a time of vanishing self-sufficiency, writes Stephen Nissenbaum, [120] it was a call to return to traditional bread-making that fell pretty much on deaf ears. The American household was changing rapidly at the turn of the 19th century; it transitioned from a production unit—85% of manufactured goods were generated from the household in 1800—to a purchasing unit by 1830, with furniture, clothes and food primarily bought outside the home. The dramatic decline in household self-sufficiency within a generation, translated into a more commercial dependence on food. Between 1850 and 1900, writes Bobrow-Strain, in *Kills the Body Twelve Ways,* [19] the number of commercial bakeries increased 700 percent, causing homemade bread to drop from 80 to a mere 6 percent of all bread produced in the U.S by 1920. [19] The white sliced bread saved valuable time, was shelf-stable and safe. Bobrow-Strain [19] writes:

In an age obsessed with concerns about purity, hygiene, and sanitation, the new loaves were engineered to appear streamlined, sparkling clean, and whiter than white. After decades of enduring a reputation for filth, contamination, and foot dragging around pure-food legislation, commercial bakers had turned purity into their greatest selling point.

In the cities, the establishment of stores and shops facilitated access to readymade white wheat-raised yeast breads, pastries and cakes, stabilized with preservatives such as alum, ammonia, sulphate of zinc, and even sulphate of copper. [120]

Early in the 19th century, writes Stephen Nissenbaum,

...the marketplace was beginning to replace the household and the community as the major locus of economic activity and social relationships. [120]

The population, migrating to the US, began to spread and the emergence of new modes of transportation compounded by a new marketplace economy, fractured the family unit, but at the same created a unified interdependent network of communities that fomented commercial transactions that were mostly impersonal. [120] In this context, Sylvester Graham, decrying the lost art of homemade bread, was, in fact, romanticizing the rich traditional social environment that flourished from the community of self-sufficient families. Graham also opposed the cold and impersonal capitalist market place that dehumanized commerce. [120] Despite many of his ideas, regarding healthy eating, reemerging in populist culture, at the time, writes Nissenbaum,

Graham's eventual eclipse may have been hastened by the fact that he came to be dismissed as a charlatan by several respectable medical publications which had initially welcomed his work. [120]

The new flourishing marketplace economy could not better be exemplified but by the quickness at which meat slaughtering, packing and consumption redefined the American food inventory and diet. The railroad expansion between 1848 and 1880, with its ice-refrigerated cars and expansive rail network, transported beef, hogs and mutton carcasses from slaughter houses to meat packing facilities, which then shipped varied meat products to butcher shops for sale to the public. Between the years 1830 to 1840, Chicago was but a small meat packing hub with no railway system, overshadowed by Cincinnati's large slaughterhouse, which began in 1818 from which emerged extensive meat packing. [75] The refrigeration of the railroad cars was critical in ensuring the wide distribution of fresh meat. The American consumer, prior to ice-refrigerated rail distribution, consumed mostly meats, preserved by drying, smoking, brine or dry salt. [174] It was specifically the extensive railway network around Chicago after 1840 that made that city the largest meat packing and distribution center in the world as well as a giant commercial center. [75] In fact, by 1861 a total of 13 rail lines converged on Chicago, starting with the Galena and Chicago railways in 1848, the Michigan Southern and Northern Indiana railway in 1852, and the Chicago, Rock Island, and Pacific railway in 1854. [75] The industry, during that period, exploded into a market place that offered greater overall variety of fresh meats to the consumer. The American food industry was changing in a significant way and with it the US diet. So extensive had meat consumption become, that the dollar value of meat and meat byproducts produced in the US in 1902 was estimated at $785,500,000. [141] Also, by 1906, Packingtown—the meat packing district around Chicago—was employing 30,000 men to slaughter over 10,000 animals per day in order to keep up with the growing national and international demand for meat, representing 30 to 40 million consumers. [174b]

On the sidelines, Thomsonianism critically lashed out at the new American tradition of eating around a lavished and richly adorned dinner table with abundant meats, sauces and side dishes. Overweight Americans were already beginning to surface, and so the Health Reform Movement was attempting to awaken the public's awareness to the dangers of overindulging in rich foods and alcohol. [50, 120]

Two important events, however, caused Thomsonianism to wane. First, by the beginning of the American Civil War, American society's attention was now being diverted away from wellness issues by the internal strife and conflicts of war. [66] Second, the Thomsonian movement, consisting of many uneducated and illiterate practitioners, forcibly caused a rift with the educated medical doctors attracted to botanical healing therapies. They began dropping Thomson's name from the title of their medical societies. Hence, the Thomsonian Medical Society of the State of New York was changed, in 1849, to the New York State Physiopathic Medical Society. [66] It really wasn't until the end of the Victorian era (1901) that a preoccupation with diet resurfaced, under the umbrella of a newly formed science of nutrition, fuelled by the exciting discovery of vitamins.

1.6 The Beginning of Standard Nutrition Recommendations in the U.S

Leading the charge to help establish a scientific basis for population eating standards in order to ensure good health, was Atwater's 1894 article published in the USDA's Farmer's Bulletin. [9] Atwater was a metabolic researcher who understood the energy and macronutrient requirements of the human body. He became the first director of the Office of Experiment Stations at the USDA. He was convinced of the link between food composition and human health. He writes in 1902:

Unless care is exercised in selecting food, a diet may result which is one-sided or badly balanced that is, one in which either protein or fuel ingredients (carbohydrate and fat) are provided in excess. The evils of overeating may not be felt at once, but sooner or later they are sure to appear perhaps in an excessive amount of fatty tissue, perhaps in general debility, perhaps in actual disease. [9]

And so Atwater's work on the nutritional needs of individuals set the stage for nutritionist, Caroline Hunt's *Food for Young Children*, which was the USDA's first Food Guide published in 1916. [79] It consisted of 5 food groups: milk and meat, cereals, vegetables and fruits, fats and fatty foods, and sugars and sugary foods.

1.6.1 Food Processing & Additives.
Interest in nutrition, in the earlier part of the 20th century was quite high, as malnutrition was rampant around the U.S. Experts now believe that because Americans were consuming over 50% of their calories as white bread by the 1930s—a consequence of 1917 war rationing habits combined with the Great Depression's cheap food budgeting—that malnutrition became a prominent problem in the U.S. The white flour was so heavily processed around 1911, the consequence of the roller mills and the bleach treatments, that no nutrient in the flour could survive. [18] And, so white bread purchased in the stores could not, by today's standards, be considered a food in the strict sense. As early as the 1920s there was some suspicion, among the food reformists, that something wasn't right. Benjamin R Jacobs, a nutritional biochemist who worked for the Bureau of Chemistry (now the FDA) which came under the control of the USDA, began to document the adulteration of flour around 1906, and became a strong advocate for strict controls under the Pure Food and Drug Act. [83, 81] Then by the 1920s, he recorded the loss of nutrients with the excessive use of sodium bicarbonate—common practice at the time—in flour processing, and began experimenting on methods of enrichment. [83] As early as 1910, Harvey W Wiley, the head of the Food and Drug Administration (FDA), fought ardently against the practice of bleaching flour—a processing method that utilized nitrogen trichloride. [168] Even after he successfully got the practice of bleaching flour banned by a Supreme Court decision in and around 1911, Dr Wiley was ousted from his position in 1912; the ban on bleaching was then bypassed by an overriding Executive order. Dr Wiley later described the bleached flour in a 1914 issue of *Good Housekeeping* as *white and waxy as the face of a corpse*, according to a 1954 article by James Rorty in the National Police Gazette. [168] Nitrogen Trichloride was used in flour right up to 1948 when British Nutritionist, Lord Mellanby conducted a series of well controlled experiments on dogs, in which running fits of epilepsy-like behaviors were noted in dogs fed trichloride-bleach bread. American nutritionists, wanting to verify the findings, were able to duplicate the same worrisome outcomes in guinea pigs, rats, monkeys and rabbits. The FDA then banned the nitrogen trichloride as a bleaching agent after 40 years of use. Not long after, despite protests by U.S Army nutritionists, the FDA approved chlorine dioxide as a new bleaching agent. It is surprising that, despite the Supreme Court ban on bleach back in 1911, the practice of bleaching flour still continued and is currently permitted today. In 1926, a letter to President Coolidge from the Assistant Secretary of the USDA, R.W Dunlap, confirmed the support of Dr Wiley's findings that specific additives should not be permitted in the American food supply. He writes: *The Department and the Bureau of Chemistry share Dr Wiley's view that the use of substances such as benzoate of soda, sulphur dioxide and sulphites, saccharin, alum, chemical bleaches in flour and added caffeine in beverages, is for the most part undesirable from the broad general standpoint of human health and nutrition. The eliminations of these extraneous substances from the food supply is an object greatly to be desired.* [168]

Dr Wiley ended his career as an advocate for pure food, with the publication of his highly acclaimed and revealing:" ***History of a Crime against the Food Law***", written in 1929. [168] His efforts were for the most part in vain, as he could not overcome the strong corporate lobbyists that were pushing for the inclusion of various additives, and the continued use of sodium benzoate and bleach, despite clears signs that the practices should have been banned.

Nevertheless, mounting public concern about both the purity and safety of the food supply pushed policy makers to pass the 1938 **Food Drug and Cosmetic Act** which superseded the 1906 Pure Food Act, which could not keep up with the ever changing science of food stabilizers, moisteners and coloring agents. [81] The goal was to quell the public outcry justifiably fuelled by the frequent adulteration of food in addition to the numerous use of food additives. Under this 1938 Act, the government shouldered the responsibility to demonstrate that a product could likely injure the health of the individual and therefore restrict its use in food. [81]

It was a premarket approval system that seemed to provide the safety the public was seeking in light of the overabundance of additives flooding the market each year. [167] Food additives became historically important elements in establishing a diverse, stable and safe national food inventory. These additives facilitated the access of the population to a safe inventory. We must however question the wide assortment of additives currently used; are they really necessary?

Originally, there were only eight dyes used in food production in 1900. However, because there was no legislation regulating the quality of these dyes, it wasn't uncommon to use the same textile dyes both in clothing and in foods. The Pure Food & Drug Act of 1906, restricted such abuses, and kept the total number of dyes to seven: orange-1, erythrosine, ponceau 3R, amaranth, indigotine, naphthol-yellow, and light green. But as the number of additives grew, and the color of the products became less natural looking, public concern and awareness also grew. Many consumers suspected that there was indeed an increasing association between food and disease in the population. [81]

The truths that emerged from the work of Dr Wiley—Chief of the Food and Drug Administration (FDA)—regarding the purity and safety of the American food supply are what fuelled the counter-cultural food revolution that began to take root in the 1950s (Wiley, 1929). [168] Indeed, by the 1950s the use of chemicals in food had exploded—there were 700 chemicals used at the time in food—and as many as 39% had safety concerns. [81]

Popular radio host and self-proclaimed nutrition guru, Carleton Fredericks, stirred up public alarm about the synthetic ingredients used in white bread. The FDA was flooded with thousands of letters from an alarmed public demanding that action be taken to safeguard the wholesomeness of bread. Throughout the 1950s, writes Aaron Bobrow-Strain in his best seller: *White Bread*, [18] the U.S. Congress held hearings about the safety of many of the additives such as emulsifiers, dough conditioners and softeners that were included in industrial white bread

James Delaney chaired a select committee of the House of Representatives to investigate the safety of food additives over a two year period. [81] His 1952 report fueled the passing of two distinct amendments to the Food Drug and Cosmetic Act of 1938: first, the Miller **Pesticide Residues Amendments** of 1954 and the **Food Additives Amendments** of 1958. [81] Despite the committee advocating for laws scrutinizing the safety of pesticide residues on food and in food processing for the sake of national health, the committee report concluded:

...it is possible to utilize the poisonous properties of [pesticide] chemicals in destroying insects and controlling diseases which attack many crops, without endangering the health of the people who consume the products. [81]

Both the 1954 and 1958 bills rejected pesticide residues on food as an "*additive.*"

In the 1958 amendment, "*Congress sought to promote continued innovation in food technology by giving the FDA greater flexibility to authorize limited uses of substances in food even if shown in animal tests to be poisonous at higher levels*". [81] Interestingly, the Delaney Clause to the 1958 amendment, which prohibited the use of any additive—even in the smallest concentration—found to cause cancer in animals, showed zero tolerance for any carcinogen. [81] Bruce Wilson, writing for the National Research Council (NRC) report, concludes:

...under a standard like the Delaney Clause, or one as strict as that implied by the Delaney Committee report, few pesticides would receive approval. [116]

Equally alarming, was the commercial use of antibiotics—antibiotic growth-promoters—to accelerate the growth of domestic animals such as poultry. [23]

The question really came down to whether the public could justifiably trust corporate testing of additives.

1.6.2 Prevalence of Malnutrition. The processing of the American food supply had become so extensive between 1900 and 1940 that there were reported cases of malnutrition, even among U.S Army recruits prior to WW-I and WW-II. [134] There were suspicions, by US health authorities that malnutrition was rampant among school-aged children as early as 1920. The focus until then had been on decreasing infant mortality rates. The medical and public health effort had been promoting *"baby-saving campaigns"* aimed at educating mothers about the importance breast feeding [134] and prenatal nutrition. [147] At the start of the 20th century, as the prevalence of 19th century plagues such as cholera, yellow fever, small pox, typhoid fever and notably, diphtheria for children, significantly declined, the interest in childhood malnutrition, gained importance. It was specifically the drop in infant and childhood death rates in concert with the implementation of compulsory education laws, nationwide by 1918, and the decline in child labor (Kantor and Tyack, 1982) that opened the door to the close monitoring of, and interventions favoring, children's health in schools. In that context, lunch and milk programs were instituted, in addition to the involvement of nurses, social workers, and medical inspections (Ruis, 2013). Hastings, in 1912, writes:

With the advent of routine medical inspection, physicians and nurses working in the schools documented rampant health problems. Although many, such as poor eyesight, adenitis, and carious teeth, were relatively minor, health inspectors identified them in a shockingly high number of children; according to one report published in 1912, approximately 75 percent of schoolchildren bore at least one physical or mental defect, and most bore several. [70]

In the first decade of the 20th century, the notion of malnutrition was not clearly understood, especially by medical doctors—the science of nutrition had just begun to bloom with the discovery of vitamins—and so many definitions were floating around. Malnutrition presented itself, as it were, as a sort of "medical octopus" in that it had multiple manifestations. [147] In the early 1920s if a child had ill health, stunted growth or suffered from disability the physician would likely classify him as suffering from malnutrition. Peters, in the Report on the Committee on Medical Inspections in Schools, writes:

Based on nationwide reports, the chief medical inspector of Cincinnati thought it "fair to place the probable number of mal-nourished children in American cities at 10 per cent of the school population. [126]

But other medical presentations of malnutrition were certainly considered, notably, **athrepsia**, which is when debility in the child is rated as extreme and arising from a poor hygienic environment and insufficient food; **cachexia**, a term that refers to advanced emaciation; **dekomposition**, is a physical state of emaciation preceding death; hunger edema, describes subcutaneous and/or water accumulation in the peritoneum; **inanition**, is a manifestation of physical and mental exhaustion or unusually low zeal*;* **kwashiorkor**, is the physical manifestations of protein malnutrition, whereas **marasmus**, is the physical signs of calorie malnutrition; and finally, **poor dentition** in a child mirrored poor prenatal in-utero conditions influenced by the inadequacy of the mother's diet. [147] The absence of normative standards and quantitative techniques to identify malnutrition left health professionals with disparate estimates of the prevalence of malnutrition in schools that varied between 3 and 30%. [134] Efforts were made to simplify an approach for more uniform results. The 1912 Dunfermline Scale, developed in Scotland by Dr. Alister Mackenzie of the Carnegie Dunfermline Trust, relied on height, weight, skin complexion, mental acuity and eye sight to assess the nutritional status. The technique may have caused an overestimation of malnutrition because of some of its very subjective observations. [134, 31] Not long after, the paediatric growth charts, used by paediatricians to monitor the growth and development of children, were also found to detect feeding problems. [73] Reliance on these growth charts became more widespread after

WW-I. [134] However, leading up to WW-I, Keefer [92] writes:

Of the over three million young men who applied for military service in 1917–18, more than 30 percent were rejected on medical grounds; the fifth leading cause of rejection was underweight, and 8 percent of those rejected suffered from some physical, developmental defect.

The Surgeon General of the United States, at the time, Rupert Blue, in addition to many health authorities were clearly seeing that chronic malnutrition was at the source of the health problems and defects in these young military recruits. [16] The malnutrition statistics were seized by the then emerging Child Health Movement [102] to create a nationwide campaign to fight childhood malnutrition, making it a socio-political tool for national identity and strength. [134] During WW-I, interest in anthropometric measurements lead to the endorsement of weight to height charts, as reliable tools of nutritional health. [63] Relying on weight, public health measurements of 14 year old teenagers found that 7% were significantly underweight, whereas by 1932, the prevalence had jumped to 12.7%. [93] Despite the errors in assessment attributed to anthropometry, the National Research Council's Food and Nutrition Board's 1941 assessment of malnutrition in the US, concluded that it was vastly underreported and a problem of far greater magnitude than had been previously imagined (Jolliffe et al., 1942). By WW-II, the overall rejection rate of recruits was 45%, much higher than for WW-I. [58]

Dr W. H Sebrell, of the National Institute of Health, U.S Public Health Service, spoke about recruitment statistics before the 1941 Food and Nutrition Section of the American Public Health Association's 70th Annual Meeting in Atlantic City. [137] In his address, he cited General Hershey's report that claimed that, among 1 million men examined by the Selective Services of the U.S Army, approximately 380,000 were assessed as unfit for service. One third of those rejected, were nutritionally compromised. How could so many be affected by poor nutrition? The Chicago Tribune further investigated the claim of unfit men by breaking down the rejection rates by city wards, and found a 71% rejection rate from the poorest wards, whereas a 39.9 percent rejection rate was noted in the upper middle class sections of the city. Military recruits represented, however, only the tip of the iceberg; in 1941, a government commission was formed to investigate the prevalence of nutritional deficiencies at a much broader population level. Epidemiologists unearthed a surprisingly elevated 75% prevalence of riboflavin deficiency, among low income high school kids; 65% prevalence of scurvy or near scurvy among government administration workers; and a 54% prevalence of pre-clinical vitamin A deficiency among low income whites and blacks. In a New York City community health center that serviced low income high school students, malnutrition was identified in 37% of students by 1938, writes Bobrow-Strain in his bestseller [18] *White Bread*. Malnutrition was rampantly affecting children and adults throughout the country because of a serious failure of public health nutrition programs. It was the recognition of this failure to realign the dietary habits of Americans, throughout the 1930s, with healthy eating principles, that galvanized support for a major shift in eating practices. The goal was to alter the population's preference for white bread in favor of brown whole wheat. But the public would not budge; it held on to its beloved white bread, like a shipwrecked mariner to its buoy. It was clear that in 1941 the U.S's intention to join the war effort was driving the resolve to eradicate malnutrition nationwide one way or the other. Public health nutrition education programs and advertising could not get the masses to abandon their white impoverished bread. It became evident that the State could not impose new and healthy eating practices on the population. Such dietary shifts could only come from the inner soul of a people. That kind of change was not about to take place despite the fact that national security was at risk. Indeed, U.S soldiers were not fit enough to enter a war, let alone bring such a war to closure. The situation became so alarming, that the Food and Nutrition Board of the National Academy of Sciences sponsored the National Nutrition Conference for Defense in 1941, as a forum to study strategies that could turn the malnutrition around. The conference formulated the first Recommended Dietary Allowances (RDAs) for calories and nine essential nutrients: protein, iron, calcium, vitamin A and D, thiamin, riboflavin, niacin and vitamin C. From the conference, also arose 10 public nutrition education strategies that offered some potential for success.

In stressing the importance of a public health nutrition intervention to suppress the malnutrition, Dr. Sebrell wrote: [137]

In the field of public health, our duty is clear and well defined. We must accept the fact that malnutrition is one of the major causes of ill health and poor growth and development, and is one of the most important of the health officer's problems. We must realize that the problem of getting an adequate diet to the people is just as urgent a problem as keeping infection away from the people. That nutrition is truly the armor of robust health. With this conviction the public health workers in the United States can and will be where they should be in the very forefront of the fight to vanquish malnutrition for America-which is the greatest problem of national nutrition.

It is in this context that the USDA issued the second version of the food guide in 1921 with specific quantities from each food group recommended to be purchased on a weekly basis. By 1923 a modified version of the guide was issued to assist the non-traditional families with greater than 5 members. In the 1930s, the harsh economic realities of the 1929 crash, and the ensuing jump in food prices, invariably translated into hardship accessing good, wholesome, and affordable food. Numerous soup lines were set up to feed the many hungry unemployed men and their families (**Figure-1.2**).

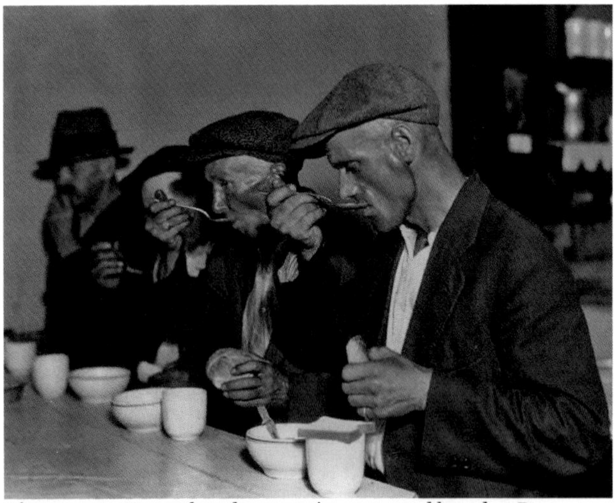

Figure 1.2: Unemployed men eating soup and bread at Bernard Macfadden's Penny Cafeteria, probably in Washington DC, USA, circa 1935. Photo by Keystone View Company/Archives Photo © iStock.com/HultonArchive

1.6.3 A New Food Guide. To address the growing prevalence of malnutrition showing up among the masses of unemployed, [143] Hazel Stiebeling, a USDA food economist, devised a new food guide in 1933, consisting of 12 food groups. [145] This third official USDA food guide, lasted until the end of the 1930s. One of the noteworthy features of this guide was that flour and cereals were encouraged to be eaten as desired. Again, the goal was to steer weekly purchases of foods in a way that would cover the nutritional requirements of families. [145]

However, this Food Guide may have misdirected the American population to liberally consume processed cereals and bleached flours that were devoid of nutrient content. Did the adoption of this Food Guide directly cause malnutrition to become rampant throughout the U.S? It is hard to say, but it most certainly did not help matters. During the depression access to protective foods such as milk, butter, tomatoes, citrus fruits, leafy, green and yellow vegetables, and eggs was rather difficult. Stiebeling, in 1939, [144] estimated at the time that the U.S diet needed to contain 20% more milk, 15% more butter, about 70% more tomatoes and citrus, a 100% increase in vegetables, and finally a 35% jump in egg intake in order to reclassify it as *nutritionally good*. Evidently, the extent to which the American diet was suboptimal in the 1930s must have been significant and worrisome enough for home economist Margaret Reid [131] to write about what she labelled as:

...a hidden hunger that threatens to lower the zest for living and to sap the productive capacity of workers and the stamina of the armed forces.

Indeed, throughout the 1930s more than 50% of calories consumed by the American public were coming from white bread. [18]

1.6.4 Revised Food Guides. From the resolutions and discussions that emerged from the National Nutrition Conference, the USDA released the 1943 National Wartime Nutrition Guide, which consisted in 7 basic food groups (**Figure-1.3**). [53, 159] This food guide had a very specific wartime focus that reflected the food rationing that was going on at that time. The government encouraged home canning, planting gardens of fruits and vegetables, buying fresh seasonal fruits, and advocated for calories consumed to equal calories expended. [84] By 1941 the first RDAs had been publically announced by the Food and Nutrition Board of the National

Academy of Science. Specific calorie recommendations accompanied 9 nutrient RDAs: protein, iron, calcium, vitamins A and D, thiamin, riboflavin, niacin, and ascorbic acid (vitamin C). [35] The government also specifically instructed farmers to direct agricultural productions towards American troops and factory workers (USDA, 1943). [160] As such, it identified the guidelines that needed to be followed in order to establish a foundational diet that maximized nutrient density and ensured complete nutrition.

This guide specified a foundation diet that would provide a major share of the RDA's for nutrients, but only a portion of caloric needs. It was assumed that people would include more foods than the guide recommended to satisfy their full calorie and nutrient needs (Davis and Saltos, 1999*)*. [35]

Notice how three of the seven groups consisted of some fruits and mostly vegetables (potatoes and other vegetables, green and yellow vegetables, and oranges, tomatoes and grapefruits).

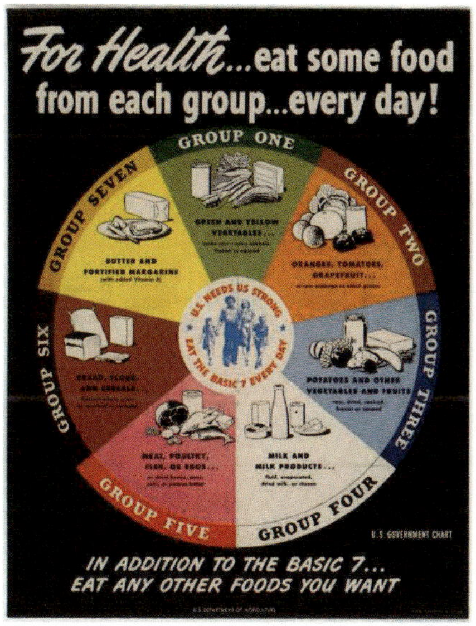

Figure-1.3 The Basic 7 Food Groups of the 1943 U.S Food Guide © National Archives, records of the Office of Government Reports

Less focus was on meeting calorie needs but rather on ensuring that the RDAs were met for the 9 essential nutrients, by encouraging the consumption of specific types of foods. [84] As such, no serving sizes were provided; the accepted assumption was that the people would naturally complete their caloric needs with *ad libitum* ingestion of affordable and available foods. Also, very little information was provided for fats and sugars, since excess caloric intakes were not yet identified as a problem at the population level. It is noteworthy to point out that one of the 7 food groups was actually butter and margarines fortified with vitamin A. [35]

As U.S soldiers were preparing to enter World War II, the only viable solution to rapidly and massively affect the nutritional status of the weakened soldiers, was the enrichment of flour and bread, with thiamine, niacin and iron; later on riboflavin was added into the enrichment mix. This policy change meant that the U.S government would only purchase enriched flour and bread—a practice that forced other milling and bakery distribution companies to follow suit with their own voluntary enrichment programs by 1942. This strategy ensured the broad distribution of white enriched bread throughout the U.S by the early 1950s. So then, as early as 1941 the U.S soldiers were already part of a public health enrichment program that could potentially improve their nutritional status by the time they were ready to enter the war in 1943. But the problem of malnutrition was widespread and affected many different strata of American life. Sebrell called on a national resolve to quell the poor nutrition of its people. He concludes: [137]

Finally, we come to problems of nutrition affecting the entire population. As health officials we must build for the future with a continuing program. Although military and defense problems are most urgent today, in time these men will again fit into the larger picture of our entire civil life, but now they must be sustained by a civil population of high morale and good health. The Secretary of Agriculture recently said." Food will win the war and write the peace." With these two goals ahead of us, the problems of better national nutrition become problems that we must solve.

After the war, the USDA generated another Food Guide in 1946, which consisted of the same 7 food groups, as during the war, except this newer version included servings. It was intended to be more practical and usable. The problem, however, was its complexity, and the fact that serving sizes were not actually defined. In the end, the population became quickly disenchanted with the guide, forcing the creation of a simpler 4 food group guide (**Figure 1.4**) 10 years later in 1956. [35, 53]

In the 1970s, a more complex and significant epidemiological problem of overeating and poor quality food consumption began to emerge. Scientists identified 4 key dietary components, which when eaten in excess, were considered deleterious to human health: saturated fat, cholesterol, fat, and sodium. It was, however, the Senate Select Committee on Nutrition and Human Needs, [161] headed by Senator George McGovern in 1977, that introduced the Dietary Goals for the United States. They represented a dramatic shift that focused on dietary excesses rather than nutrient deficiencies [35] —a reality that ravaged American society throughout the 1930s. [18]

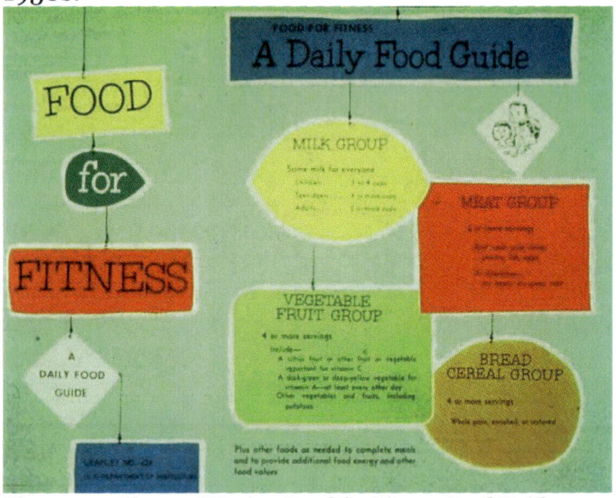

Figure 1.4 The 1956 Basic 4 Food for Fitness Food Guide. Credit to the USDAs History of the USDA food Guides.

The public was given quantitative dietary guidance [40] aimed at keeping dietary carbohydrates (including natural sugars) to 48% of calories, Protein, 12%, dietary cholesterol at <300mg /day, maintaining total fat at <30% of calories, saturated <10%, monounsaturated fat<10% and polyunsaturated fats <10% of calories, refined added sugar at <10% of calories, and finally salt at <5g/day (US Senate Select Committee on Nutrition and Human Needs Report Dietary Goals for the US, 1977). [161, 40] The main reason was that higher risks of obesity, diabetes, heart disease and stroke had been tied to high fat, sugar, saturated fat and cholesterol intakes, whereas the ingestion of high salt got tagged to hypertension. Recommendations were also made to lower salt, sugar, and meat intake specifically, in order to decrease fat and saturated fat. The committee and scientific consultants felt that the medical literature supported a diet-heart association. [122] These dietary goals met with much resistance from a food industry that did not take kindly to the recommendation to eat less. The National Dairy Council, the Salt Institute, the United Egg Producers, the American National Cattlemen's Association, and the National Livestock and Meat Board, reacted violently to the goal of eating less meat and eggs. Moreover, the American Medical Association insisted that medical issues needed to be managed by the physicians and not the government. Finally, the scientific community was not convinced that there existed sufficient data to support the cut-off goals. [122] The pressure by the food industry was powerful, and noticeably influenced the committee to sanitize the guidelines and publish an amended version in order to ensure the support of the meat and egg industries. Marion Nestle, author of Food Politics, [118] argues that the wording was significantly amended to reflect a more positive slant on meat consumption. Hence, the initial recommendation to decrease meat ingestion was changed to "*decrease consumption of animal fat, and choose meats, poultry, and fish which will reduce saturated fat intake.*" This was a positive slant that the meat industry could live with, but it poorly reflected the scientific findings that tied many cancers to populations that consume abundant meat. The meat industry insisted that the committee destroy all copies of the original report. McGovern was voted out of office not long after, and the industry made it very clear to bureaucrats never to challenge meat consumption again, writes Marian Nestle. [118] Despite the forceful hand of industry to manipulate the outcomes of the guidelines, a deleterious label did nevertheless get pinned on red meat, eggs, and whole milk—the public intuitively knew it needed to cut back on fats, and that generally meant meat. Indeed, these dietary components, were enshrined into the "foods to avoid" category of every dietitian's therapeutic pamphlet for the treatment of cardiovascular disease. Consequently, red meat and butter consumption did eventually decline over time leading to a drop in saturated fat intake, whereas poultry and fish intake increased. This shift in population eating patterns should have caused the incidence of heart disease to decline in the population, if not for the nefarious trans-fats, generated from all the margarines and shortenings that flooded the marketplace, in response to the bad press given to animal fat as early as the 1980s. The true nefarious atherogenicity of the trans-fats emerged with vengeance thirteen years later, when Willett and his colleagues [170] from Harvard, confirmed in 1993, that trans-fats did cause LDL cholesterol to increase, HDL cholesterol (good cholesterol) to drop, and markers of inflammation to increase. The Harvard group was following up on suspicions, raised by Welsh researchers in 1981 [154] that trans-fats might contribute to ischemic heart disease. Meanwhile, in 1979 two main events of significance occurred in the nutrition world. First, the USDA formulated a new food guide that was comprised of 5 food groups (**Figure 1.5**). Considered the hassle-free guide grounded on the basic four groups on the 1956 guide, it also featured an additional group (fats, sweets, and alcoholic beverages). This was an important departure from the classic role of the food guide, which was to optimize the nutrition quality of the diet. This new guide was more pragmatic in that it clearly identified, for the first time, overeating as a significant problem, and pointed the finger at a culprit food group that needed to be consumed sparingly; second, because of the controversy that emerged from the 1977 Dietary Goals for the U.S., a task force sponsored by the American Society of Clinical Nutrition [6] was established to bring scientific credence to the recommendations. It became evident from many nutrition research studies that excessive salt, fat, and sugar intakes led to chronic diseases. The findings of this task force were released by the Department of Health, Education and Welfare, now the Department of Health and Human Services (DHHS); for the first time, strong scientific evidence supported the importance of reducing excessive calories, fat, cholesterol, salt, and sugar in the diet in order to diminish the risk of diseases. The Surgeon General of the United States included the findings of this task force in his 1979 Healthy People Report, which concluded that it was indeed possible to lower disease rates by adopting healthy dietary practices.

From this report, the 1980 Dietary Guidelines for Americans was published; again it encountered considerable opposition, especially from the food industry, who opposed the extrapolations that were made in order to formulate practical ways to create a healthful diet. Consequently, a Dietary Guidelines Advisory Committee was formed to provide scientific validity to these recommendations.

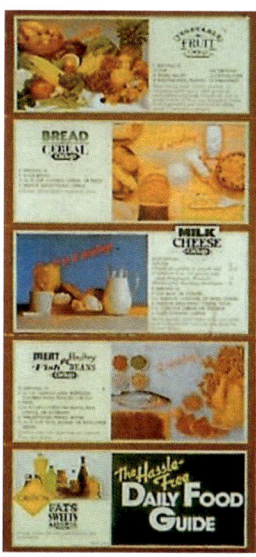

Figure 1.5 The 1979 Hassle-Free Food Guide.
© USDA. History of the USDA Food Guides

When the 1985 Dietary Guidelines for Americans were issued 5 years later, there was very little opposition from the medical community and the food industry. It just was no longer debatable that dietary intakes, at the population level, needed to be modified. Davis and Saltos [35] point out that the 1985 Guidelines resembled those of 1980, except that

Some changes were made to provide guidance about nutrition topics that became more prominent after 1980, such as following unsafe weight-loss diets, using large-dose supplements, and drinking of alcoholic beverages by pregnant women.

The Surgeon General's 1988 Report, on Nutrition and Health, emphasized the importance of embracing new dietary trends as a way of quelling the disturbing rise in chronic disease. Davis and Saltos [35] write:

Recommendations in the report promoted a dietary pattern that emphasized consumption of vegetables, fruits, and whole-grain products foods rich in complex carbohydrates and fiber and of fish, poultry without skin, lean meats, and low-fat dairy products selected to reduce consumption of total fat, saturated fat, and cholesterol.

Then, in 1989, the National Research Council's Food and Nutrition Board, [50b] reiterated the Council's Diet and Health Report that stressed the importance of decreasing total fat and saturated fat intakes to maintain a low risk of contracting chronic diseases and some cancers. The report quantified specific limits on fat, notably: <30% calories as total fat; <10% calories for saturated fat; and <300 mg for dietary cholesterol. Also, there was an emphasis to consume a minimum of 5 servings per day of fruits and vegetables, and at least 6 servings per day of breads, cereals or legumes. The USDA, in concert with the National Cancer Institute, the Produce for Better Health Foundation, CDC, and the American Cancer Society, attempted in 1991, to popularize Fruits and vegetables by instituting a nationwide EAT 5 A DAY nutrition education campaign (**Figure-1.6**). The program was an almost complete failure, as it did not manage to budge the population from its dislike of fruits and vegetables.

Meanwhile, for the very first time, the 1990 Dietary Guidelines for American, [39b] jointly produced by DHHS and the USDA, formulated a numerical goal for saturated fat: <10% of calories, and reiterated the previously established total fat cut-off of: <30% of calories.

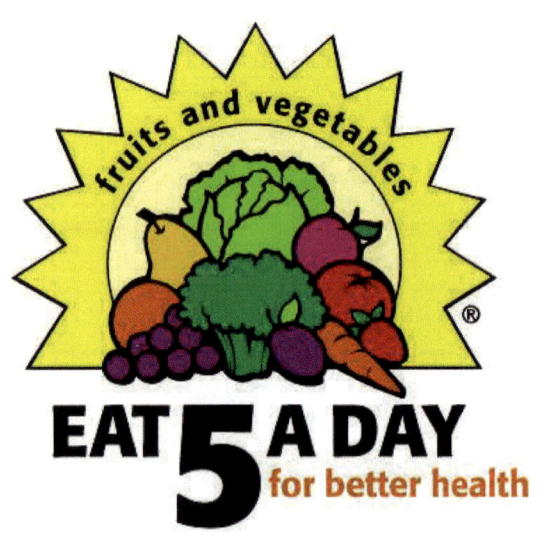

Figure 1.6 The USDA's Eat 5-A Day Nutrition campaign from 1991.

As early as 1988, the USDA began work to graphically represent the food guide, which since 1985 was known only in USDA publications as, *A Pattern for Daily Food Choices*. The decision to use the *Food Pyramid* in 1992 (**Figure-1.7**), as a visual reference to healthy eating in the U.S., was applauded as a strategic public health move that could ideally convey that breads and cereals in addition to fruits and vegetables needed to be prominent in the diet. [35, 53]

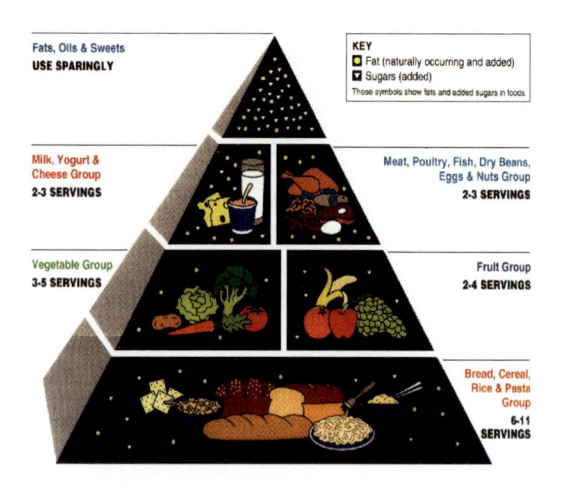

Figure-1.7 USDA 1992 Food Pyramid. © USDA History of the USDA Food Guides

The pyramid was also supportive of the EAT 5-A DAY campaign (Figure-1.6), which, when broken down, translated into a recommended minimum of 3 vegetables and 2 fruits every day. But, the pyramid situated all fats at the tip of the pyramid, thereby intimating that all fats should be minimally consumed. This was consistent with the low fat strategies, for the management of weight loss and heart disease, popular in diets. The limitation was that, even at that time, it was known that omega-3 fats were beneficial, and that omega-9 monounsaturated fats, like olive oil, appeared to provide substantive health benefits. In the end, the scientific consensus was that all fats were not equal.

In 2005, the pyramid was completely revised again (**Figure-1.8**). This time the emphasis was placed on a balance between exercise and food. A new webpage was attached to the guide, from which more detailed servings could be obtained. [35, 53]

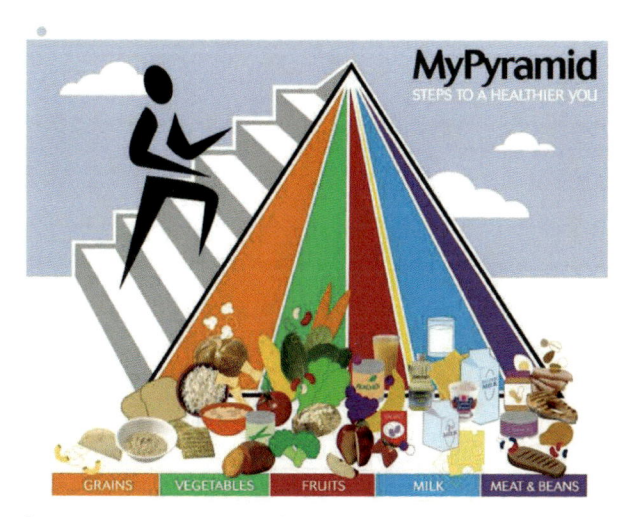

Figure-1.8 USDA 2005 Food Pyramid. ©USDA History of the USDA Food Guides

However, there were several problems that were conveyed by this rather vague, but colorful pyramid. First, it appeared to intimate that exercise allows consumers to walk right over the guide, and eat whatever they want; second, the elongated pyramid strips, did not communicate very well, that some food groups need to be consumed in greater proportion than others. Here again, the government deflected any harm away from the meat industry by creating a red strip that appeared almost equal in size to that of vegetables. The research, leading up to the 2005 publication of the pyramid, did not convincingly demonstrate that red meat was linked to colorectal cancer. At best, conclusions from the 1997 review, by the World Cancer Research Fund, could only indicate a possible association between red meat and colorectal cancer; they concluded that red meat intake should be less than 3oz-wt per day. Other reviews found moderate links. Murtaugh [113] pointed out, in a 2004 commentary, that up until that time, the data did not differentiate between the impact of regular consumption of large versus small and infrequent quantities of red meat in relations to colorectal cancer incidences. Prior to 2005 however, the research did imply that total fat and in particular, animal fat in addition to processed, salted, cured or smoked meats, subject to high temperature treatments and nitrite compounds, were tied to rectal cancer. In truth, the most convincing studies were the large scale prospective Nurses' Health and U.S. Professional Men's cohorts. The data was studied by Walter Willett and his team from Harvard in the early to mid-1990s, and showed a significant association between colon cancer and red meat specifically. [171, 60] The implications were worrisome and difficult to contest as it clearly implicated long term red meat consumption to cancer. What wasn't clearly established was whether small amounts of meat consumption were considered a risk, and whether red meat's impact was related more to a displacement of protective cruciferous vegetables out of the diet, rather than to an intrinsic problem with red meat. [113] Indeed, Trustwell [156] points out that by 2002 red meat was equivocally associated with cancer depending on exposure, quantities consumed and whether meat was lean or fatty. Not even the data linking cured and processed meats to cancer was convincing.

In 2011, the USDA came up with the MYPLATE food guide (**Figure-1.9**) in answer to the criticism that the 2005 pyramid created too much confusion. [35, 53] In this more recent version, a familiar dinner plate usurps a pyramid. Here, the consumer more easily understands that the goal is to match the MyPlate image, in which fruits and vegetables makeup 50% of the plate, grains represent 25%, and protein foods, roughly 25%.

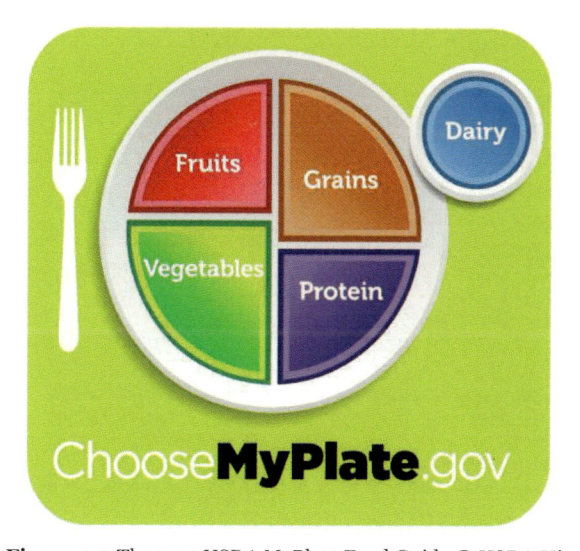

Figure-1.9 The 2011 USDA MyPlate Food Guide © USDA History of the USDA Food Guides

According to the Willett team from Harvard, there is substantial evidence now showing significant risk of diabetes, cardiovascular disease and cancers with red meat intake. [123] Analysing data from both the

Health Professionals Follow-up Study (HPFS) and the Nurses' Health Study (NHS), Willett and colleagues were able to show that both processed and unprocessed red meat intake was associated with a greater overall mortality. [123] This more recent 2006 data showed that the risk of mortality noticeably and significantly declined when fish, nuts, poultry, legumes and low fat dairy replaced red meat. Close to 38,000 men and 83,000 women were followed in the two prospective cohorts, and dietary information was compounded over time to measure the effect of long term intake. It appears that the stronger evidence, emerging since 2005, that disapprovingly waved an accusatory finger at processed and unprocessed red meats, caused the USDA to design the MyPlate image so as to emphasize protein foods rather than meat. More recently, Zheng and colleagues [177] found that a one serving increase per day of processed meat, heightened mortality by 13%, whereas a similar increased intake of unprocessed meat caused a 9% hike in mortality. [177] Using data from the Nurses' Health Study-II that followed more than 44,000 women, Farvid, et al [48] found a strong relative risk of developing pre-menopausal breast cancer among adolescents consuming larger portions of red meat. [48] The group concludes:

...greater consumption of total red meat in adolescence was significantly associated with higher premenopausal breast cancer risk (highest vs. lowest quintiles, RR, 1.43; 95%CI, 1.05-1.94), but not postmenopausal breast cancer.

The MyPlate website offers the consumer the opportunity to learn about the different food groups, and recommended serving or ounce-equivalences for each of the food groups. A **diet plan** can also be generated from the website. For instance, a 26 year old, 5 feet 10 inch adult man, weighing 179 lbs, and committed to 60 minutes of moderate physical activity per day, would require 3200 kcals per day for weight maintenance. Here are the minimal food group servings recommended for his age, weight, height, gender and physical activity.

a. **GRAINS**: 8oz equivalent/day
b. **VEGETABLES**: 3 cups equivalent/day
c. **FRUITS**: 2 cups equivalent/day
d. **DAIRY**: 3 cups equivalent/day
e. **PROTEIN FOODS**: 6.5oz equivalent/day
f. **OILS**: 7 teaspoons

This newer food guide is meant to be more interactive.

2.0 Excessive Calorie Consumption in the U.S.

The 1970s became known as the dieting era. Numerous calorie-restricted diets began popping up in bookstores and magazine stands in order to address the growing girth of Americans, who were now suffering from heart disease and diabetes in greater numbers. The foundations of, what was to be recognized as, the obesity and diabetes epidemics were being established in the mid-1970s. David Kessler in his book, *The End of Overeating*, fittingly describes the powerfully addicting unhealthy food supply created at that time. [95]

Strategies aimed at causing the growth of the U.S. food industry, in the 1980s, represented a true challenge for corporate executives. The problem was that the U.S. market was already saturated with food in the 1960s and 70s, with no visible path for growth.

The food industry, nevertheless, began to aggressively market the idea of snacking on tasty foods that were developed by the sophisticated sensory evaluation labs of food companies. Suddenly, Americans began snacking on delicious and very addictive foods in bookstores, hair salons, every corner store, school, sport facility and mall.

The idea of constant eating became such an important part of the culture that an additional 500-800 kcal per person flooded the market, going from 3300 kcal/day of available calories, in the 1970s, to 3800 kcal per day by 1994. [54, 175] The foods contributing the most to this availability of calories were singled out as added fats and oils, grains, milk and milk products, and caloric sweeteners. [158] On average, kids presently consume an additional 184-200 kcal/day, [127, 175] whereas adult caloric intake jumped from 1803 kcals/day in 1978 to 2374 kcals/day by 2003-2006, representing a 570 kcals/day increase. [42]

If we closely examine the calories right down to the most significant excess calorie contributors, salty snacks, soft drinks, burgers, French fries, and Mexican fast foods get singled out as significantly contributor in all age categories between 1977 and 1998.[115] Piernas and Popkin [127] in a subsequent investigation into the impact of large portions conclude:

Portion sizes increased across all food sources (stores, restaurants, and fast foods) for soft drinks and pizzas but only at fast-food locations for French fries.

Consider that the size of soda containers has gone from the humble 6.5fl-oz serving bottle, typically seen in the 1950s, to the 20-32fl-oz serving of the 1990s and 2000, [54] representing upwards of 400 kcal per serving. Looking at McDonald's soda servings specifically in 2000, the small was 16-fl-oz, the large 32-fl-oz and the super-size equaled 42-fl-oz. [54] The problem with consuming larger volumes of soda is that liquids also do not trigger the brain's satiety mechanisms the same way that solid foods do, thus facilitating larger calorie intakes by the end of the day. [27]

American restaurants used increased portion sizes as a successful marketing tool—as early as the 1970s—that drew customers into eating more calories by promoting a false sense of value; visibly the customer got more food at a low cost, and free refills certainly compounded the illusion. Young and Nestle [175] write:

Concern about value also drives the food service industry to offer larger products; many restaurant owners report that customers want more food for their money, and consumers increasingly choose restaurants on the basis of the sizes of food portions. Large portions often seem like a bargain: 7-Eleven's 16-oz Gulp costs just under 5 cents/oz, but a 32-oz Big Gulp is 2.7 cents/oz.

The big portion campaign was so successful that the caloric availability rose 15% between 1970 and 1994 concomitantly with the growth of portion sizes. [54]
This comes as no surprise as research clearly demonstrates that when served larger portions, the customer consumes greater calories. Obese kids appear particularly vulnerable to the negative impact of large portions, possibly because of their inability to identify normal size portions. Having been raised in the 1960s when 6-8fl-oz soda containers were the norm, a customer would be overwhelmed if presented with a 64fl-oz serving of soda. Having never seen a 6fl-oz soda bottle, American youth perceive the 64fl-oz soda as normal, and tend to consume it without too much mental anguish. [118]
Processed foods by definition had been part of our inventory for many centuries prior to the 20th century, and did not intimate impoverished food quality. Quite the contrary: processing was initially intended to make the food more digestible and shelf-stable for later use. In this way, the harsh and long Minnesota winters could be overcome by canning agricultural products harvested in August and October. Food processing artisans were very skilled as bakers, distillers and cheese makers; they processed raw products thereby making them more digestible and palatable for consumption. By contrast, our modern food supply goes through industrial food processing that manipulates white flour, sugar, and sodium in order to attain what industry experts call optimal *flavor burst*; [112] this ensures a *mouthfeel* that is pleasant to the consumer, and that arguably drives repeat consumer purchases. In the end hitting the hedonic center hard, is what the food industry is trying to achieve. It does this very well by building on 5 critical components according to David Kessler, author of: *The End of Overeating*. [95] The first is anticipation; the second is visual appeal; the third, aroma; the fourth, taste and flavor, and finally the fifth, texture and mouthfeel.

The five factors all work together in heightening the appeal of the product to the consumer. Taste and flavor are perhaps the most significant variables that help build the anticipation leading to the next purchase. Getting the public to return for a repeat purchase is what makes the product and ultimately the company successful. David Kessler [95] and Michael Moss, [112] in their best sellers, both have identified the three key ingredients the food industry manipulates in order to heighten the taste and flavor experience. Salt, sugar and fat are critical to the food industry's growing success; we consume them abundantly, despite the fact that it is these three ingredients that are making us terribly ill. The public seems incapable of resisting the fast food and snack food marketing campaigns, aimed at encouraging repeat acquisition behaviors. Public health policies, aimed at providing nutrition education to the public, appear to be powerless in causing any change in consumer eating habits. Medical science now talks about of food addictions as one of the vectors behind the obesity crisis.

Eileen Kennedy and colleagues of the Economic Research Service, in assessing government public health education interventions, concluded: [53]

Convincing people of the long run benefits of good nutrition is clearly made more difficult if immediate gratification is given higher priority.

The reality is that many people are ensnared by the very addictive taste of commercial foods, which have been enhanced by high levels of fat, sugar and salt, according to Michael Moss, author of *Salt, Sugar and Fat: How the Food Giants Hooked Us*. [112] The manipulation of these three ingredients, heighten the taste sensation to a whole new level. The consumer is also deceived by the number of calories ingested from snack or fastfoods, and even restaurant meals. This is because the foods that are consumed away from home tend to contain higher levels of saturated fat, cholesterol and total fat, compared those foods prepared at home, claims Eileen Kennedy, Deputy Undersecretary for Research, Education and Economics of the USDA's Economic Research Service. [53] Consumer knowledge about nutrition, Kennedy claims, is still pretty weak. A few years back, the USDA conducted surveys in order to measure consumer awareness about the caloric content of common foods consumed. She claims that many, including dietary experts, significantly underestimated the calorie content of several foods. Hamburger and onion rings, the majority believed, contained 863 calories and 44 grams of fat, which was far below the true content of 1,550 calories and 101 grams of fat. Tuna Salad was also incorrectly estimated. Most believed the salad was comprised of 374 calories and 18 grams of fat when in fact, it contained 720 calories and 43 grams of fat. Include next, the habits of frequent snacking and drinking copious amounts of carbonated beverages (54 gallons /person/year according to the USDA's Economic Research Service) and it becomes evident that we are consuming far more than what we actually expend in caloric output. It boils right down to the fact that, says Kennedy, Americans do not live for the future, but rather for the now. She writes: [53]

...the uncertain future benefits of better nutrition may outweigh the perceived potential benefits of healthy eating.

But in the end, the American public's attitude towards food is greatly influenced by the Madison Avenue Advertising industry that spent $7 billion in 1997 on provocative and enticing food ads that controlled and conditioned consumer behavior. This dollar amount contrasts greatly with the meager $333 million/year wielded by the USDA to promote healthy eating that same year. [59] Is anyone listening? Worldwide advertisers currently spend $2 trillion per year to influence consumer choices in a broad range of products. [77] The hay day of advertising—lasting between 1950 and 1975—saw a 490% increase in spending, reaching $28.320 billion per year by 1975 in the US. [47] Since the new Millennium inflationary forces has caused costs to skyrocket. In 2004, food corporations spend close to $900 million a year just in TV food ads for kids. [138] Ian Johnson, writing for the Baltimore Sun, convincingly argues that the Madison Avenue is successfully directing the purchases of the parents through manipulating the children to the tune of $150 billion in yearly sales. [88]

3.0 Diet Prevents Disease

From the 1950s to the present, nutrition has progressively taken on medicinal properties, as evidenced by the growth of nutraceutical industry, now estimated at $382.51 billion. [64] We are now dealing with high potency foods and supplements with the ability to treat or prevent disease.

By the 1970s traditional medicine's magic bullet treatments were beginning to be suspect, as alternative medicine advocated for a more holistic approach to treating patients, reintroducing, as it were, pre-modern medical therapies such as homeopathy, acupuncture, naturopathy, chiropractic and osteopathic medicine, [86] to address the new diseases and conditions of our age. The National Center for Complementary and Integrative Health (NCCIH) is responsible for defining through scientific inquiry alternative forms of medicine that are clearly effective. The physician's status as sole health care provider is challenged, as the individual is progressively persuaded of the viability of seeking alternative paths to manage his own health. The reason appears to be primarily tied to the medical field's mismanagement of antibiotics. [108] Indeed, evidence now emerges that methicillin-resistant *Staphylococcus aureus* (MRSA) infection and multi drug resistant (MDR) infections [100]—once limited to hospitals—are now growing in frequency at the community level. [29] Antibiotic-resistant bacteria represent a growing threat, as these bugs can quickly circumvent antibiotics and potentially override and compromise a biological system, thus leading to death. Now practitioners of alternative medicine talk more about eating well and exercising, in order to boost the immune system, and are trying to limit, rather than encourage, the use of antibiotics. [11]

In the background, while the prevalence of obesity, heart disease and diabetes is increasing, patients are now more frequently appearing in doctor's offices complaining of fatigue, back and joint pains, insomnia, sleep apnea, heart burn, migraines, depression, anxiety and difficult digestion. The pathogenicity of these conditions is less clear and not easily resolved with the magic bullet strategy. According to the National Institute of Health (NIH) 1992 statistics, digestive disorders represented 13% of all hospitalization and $87 billion U.S. in direct medical costs per year. It is the stress of the work place, of family responsibilities, the lack of sleep and exercise, and, in many instances, deplorable dietary habits that are identified as the culprits. Modern Medicine's disease model of care is limited in its ability to address the psychosocial realities that affect the patient and that ultimately influence recovery. [65] Western medicine's *scientific rationality,* stumped by these non-somatic illnesses, [74] offer little help in treating chronic fatigue, depression, anxiety, irritable bowel syndrome, lethargy, sluggishness, chronic migraines and others. The truth is that clinical medicine does not find psychological and sociocultural issues very interesting [74] nor are doctors trained or have the time to tackle them. This pure focus on physical symptomology, heavily criticized by detractors of the highly specialized nature of modern medicine like George Engel, [46] invariably leads to a neglect of the holistic view of the person. His legacy was a critique of modern medicine's materialistic, reductionistic and dualistic approaches to patient care. [46, 20] Engel's biopsychosocial model of care envisioned medical practitioners who were not cold, calculated, impersonal and purely technical in their approach to care, but rather considerate and sensitive to the human dimension and complexity of human suffering. His holistic approach struck cords with some in the medical community back in the 1980s. Borrell-Carrió et al., [20] write,

Engel provided a rationale for including the human dimension of the physician and the patient as a legitimate focus for scientific study.

He attempted to legitimize a humane and personalized approach to medical care that could still flaunt a scientific objectivity. Today, we can observe a more egalitarian approach to medical care in which the physician's face, seen as human and listening, allows patients to voice their concerns compared to times past. There is some room for negotiated therapeutic approaches between patient and physician. [20]

The MD, who generally tends to have no more than 45 hours of nutrition in a 5 year medical program, no longer carries the needed credibility to deal with the health issues, so prominent in our times. It makes sense, given that medical training has always been geared towards treating pathologies. Practically speaking, this means that if a worker accidentally cuts his finger off in a work-related accident, he's not thinking naturopath or spiritual healing, but more hospital emergency ward and critical care physician.

On issues of general health, however, some of the public has tended to no longer solely gravitate around the traditional medical practitioner, but rather to embrace alternative medicinal treatments aimed at spiritual and holistic wellbeing. These doctors of natural medicine purport to have a mastery of nutrition and the knowledge to unlock the healing powers of many of the food components of our diet. In this way, diet prescriptions are tailored to somehow maximize human health and, therefore, human performance in all facets of life.

We are experiencing a shift in health care paradigm that is guided by the very pragmatism of preventative medicine. And nutrition is indeed where the hub of activity is taking place. Is this the road less travelled that only few dare to follow because it demands a commitment to change behavior and lifestyle? Few, it appears, are willing or even able to disentangle themselves from the web of addictive foods that many have come to love. In the landscape, a golden path seemingly beckons us to follow this road to better health that demands from us, the willingness to consume foods that are unprocessed and organic.

Growing numbers are decidedly shifting their beliefs and practices, but is it already too late? In 1999, poor nutrition was already impacting Americans to the tune of $71 billion a year in lost productivity, premature deaths, and medical costs. [53] Moreover, the direct costs to manage obesity in 2010, was estimated at $315.8 billion/year. [12] The costs are so outrageously high, that it behoves us to take action and to turn this thing around.

DISCUSSION QUESTIONS

1. What have been the most significant influences to the decline of traditional medicine's legitimacy as sole healer of the sick?
2. Discuss the historical factors that have significantly influenced the changes in the dietary habits of Americans.
3. The preoccupation with diet and health resurfaced as an interest of the American population after the end of the Victorian era. Identify the 20th century influence(s) that were behind this renewed interest.
4. What were the 19th century influences that most significantly affected the American diet and caused a food consumption revolution and a modernization of food?
5. Identify the main goals of Thomsonianism.
6. Describe the historical context and circumstances leading up to the USDA's publication of the very first Food Guide.
7. Provide a critique of the second version of food pyramid that features a walker climbing steps.
8. Explain why the USDA's attempts at promoting healthy eating to the American public is more of a losing battle with no hope of succeeding.

References

1. Abramitzky R, Boustan L. (2017). Immigration in American Economic History. *J Econ Lit*;55(4): 1311-1345. doi:10.1257/jel.20151189
2. Abramovitz M., David P.A. (2000) American Macroeconomic Growth in the Era of Knowledge-Based Progress: The Long Run Perspective. In: Engerman Stanley L, Gallman Robert E., editors. The Cambridge Economic History of the United States. Vol. 3. Cambridge: Cambridge University Press; pp. 1–92.
3. ACS (2017). American Cancer Society. More than 4 in 10 Cancers and Deaths are Linked to Modifiable Risk Factors. Retrieved April 17, 2020:URL:https://www.cancer.org/latest-news/more-than-4-in-10-cancers-and-cancer-deaths-linked-to-modifiable-risk-factors.html
4. ACS (2016). American Cancer Society. Guidelines on Physical Exercise and Nutrition in the Prevention of Cancer. Retrieved April 17, 2020. URL:https://www.cancer.org/healthy/eat-healthy-get-active/acs-guidelines-nutrition-physical-activity-cancer-prevention.html
5. AHA (American Hospital Association) (2020). Hospitals and Health Systems Face Unprecedented Financial Pressures due to COVID-19. Accessed June 10, 2020: URL: https://www.aha.org/guidesreports/2020-05-05-hospitals-and-health-systems-face-unprecedented-financial-pressures-due
6. American Society of Clinical Nutrition (1979) Task Force. The evidence relating six dietary factors to the nation's health. *American Journal of Clinical Nutrition* (Supplement); 32:2621-2748.
7. Atkins, RC. (1972). Dr. Atkins' Diet Revolution. New York: D. McKay Company, 310 pp
8. Atkins, RC. (1978). Super Energy Diet Book. New York: Bantam, 331 pp
9. Atwater, W.O. (1902) *Principles of Nutrition and Nutritive Value of Food*. U.S. Department of Agriculture, Farmers. Bulletin No. 142, 48 pp.,
10. Barberis I, Bragazzi NL, Galluzzo L, Martini M. (2017). The history of tuberculosis: from the first historical records to the isolation of Koch's bacillus. *J Prev Med Hyg*;58(1):E9-E12.URL: https://www.ncbi.nlm.nih.gov/pmc/articles/PMC5432783/
11. Baars EW, Zoen EB, Breitkreuz T, et al. (2019). The Contribution of Complementary and Alternative Medicine to Reduce Antibiotic Use: A Narrative Review of Health Concepts, Prevention, and Treatment Strategies. *Evid Based Complement Alternat Med*.;2019:5365608. Published 2019 Feb 3. doi:10.1155/2019/5365608
12. Biener A, Cawley J, Meyerhoefer C. (2017). The High and Rising Costs of Obesity to the US Health Care System. *J Gen Intern Med*;32(Suppl 1):6-8. doi:10.1007/s11606-016-3968-8
13. Bissonnette, DJ. (2019). Depression: The Whole Truth. Mankato: St-Jude Nutrition Medical Communications. DVD run time: 4hr 40 min
14. Bleich, S.N. and Wolfson J.A. 2014. "Weight loss strategies: association with consumption of sugary beverages, snacks, and values about food purchases." *Patient Educ Couns; 96 (1):* 128 – 34 URL: https://www.ncbi.nlm.nih.gov/pubmed/24801411?dopt=Abst.
15. Blomain, EC., Dirhan, DA., Valentino, MA., Kim GW., and Waldman, SA. (2013). "Mechanisms of Weight Regain following Weight Loss." *ISRN Obes; 2013:* 2105-24, URL: doi: 10.1155/2013/210524
16. Blue, R. (1919). Are We Physically Fit? United States Handicapped in "Coming Period of Commercial and Industrial Competition," *Amer. J. Pub. Health* 9(9): 641–45; Taliaferro Clark, "The Need and Opportunity for Physical Education in Rural Communities," *Amer. Phys. Educ. Rev.* 24, no. 9 (1919): 436–43.
17. Blum, D. (2018). The Poison Squad: One chemist's single-minded crusade for food safety at the turn of the 20th century. New York: Penguin Press; 330 pp.
18. Bobrow-Strain, A. (2013) White Bread: A Social History of the Store-Bought Loaf. Beacon Press, Boston, pp: 272
19. Bobrow-Strain, A. (2007) Kills A Body Twelve Ways: Bread Fears and the Politics of What to Eat Gastronomica: The Journal of Food and Culture; 7(3): 45-52 retrieved August 8, 2013 from: http://comenius.susqu.edu/biol/312/killsabodytwelveways.pdf
20. Borrell-Carrió, F. et al., (2004). The Biopsychosocial Model 25 Years Later: Principles, Practice, and Scientific Inquiry. Ann Fam Med; 2(6): 576–582. URL: https://www.ncbi.nlm.nih.gov/pmc/articles/PMC1466742/
21. Brown, M., Christensen, J, and Phillips, P. (1992). The decline of child labor in the US fruit and vegetable canning Industry: Law or economics. The Business History Review; 66(4): 723-770
22. Brown, M. and Phillips, P. (1986). Craft labor and mechanization in Nineteenth century American Canning. The Journal of Economic History; 46(3): 743-756
23. Butaye P, Devriese LA, Haesebrouck F. (2003). Antimicrobial growth promoters used in animal feed: effects of less well known antibiotics on gram-positive bacteria. *Clin Microbiol Rev*;16(2):175-188. doi:10.1128/cmr.16.2.175-188.
24. Călina DC, Docea AO, Bogdan M, Bubulică MV, Chiuțu L. (2014). The pharmacists and homeopathy. *Curr Health Sci J.*;40(1):57-59. doi:10.12865/CHSJ.40.01.10
25. Calle EE, Rodriguez C, Walker-Thurmond K, Thun MJ. (2003). Overweight, obesity, and mortality from cancer in a prospectively studied cohort of U.S. adults. N Engl J Med; 348:1625–1638.
26. Cartwright, S (2006-2013) Origins and History of Homeopathy. Retrieved July 11,2012 from http://www.oxford-homeopathy.org.uk/homeopathy-origins-history.htm

27. Cassady BA, Considine RV, Mattes RD(2012). Beverage consumption, appetite, and energy intake: what did you expect? Am J Clin Nutr; 95(3):587-93.
28. (CDC). Centers for Disease Control and Prevention (2014). 1991-2013 High School Youth Risk Behavior Survey Data. Accessed on 8/4/2014. Available at http://nccd.cdc.gov/youthonline/. - See more at: http://www.childtrends.org/?indicators=adolescents-who-felt-sad-or-hopeless#sthash.kppnk4h3.dpuf
29. Chambers HF, Deleo FR. (2009). Waves of resistance: Staphylococcus aureus in the antibiotic era. Nat Rev Microbiol;7(9):629-641. doi:10.1038/nrmicro2200
30. Chao YH, Yang CC, Chiou WB (2012).Food as ego-protective remedy for people experiencing shame. Experimental evidence for a new perspective on weight-related shame. Appetite; 59(2):570-5.
31. Clark, T (1922) "Nutrition in Schoolchildren," *J. Amer. Med. Assoc.* (August 12): 519–25.
32. Cohen, DA. 2008. "Obesity and the Built Environment: Changes in Environmental Cues Cause Energy Imbalances." *Int J Obes (Lond) 32(07):* S137–S142. URL: https://www.ncbi.nlm.nih.gov/pmc/articles/PMC3741102/.
33. Daniel, TM. (2011). Hermann Brehmer and the origins of tuberculosis sanatoria. Int J Tuberc Lung Dis; 15(2):161-2,
34. Davis C. (2013). A narrative review of binge eating and addictive behaviors: shared associations with seasonality and personality factors. *Front Psychiatry*;4:183. Published 2013 Dec 27. doi:10.3389/fpsyt.2013.00183
35. Davis, C. and Saltos, E. (1999) Dietary Recommendations and How they have Changed Over Time. In: America's Eating Habits: Changes and Consequences. Frazao, E (Ed) USDA Economic Research Service, Washington, DC. USDA. Agriculture Information Bulletin No. (AIB-750): 33-50
36. Davis, A. (1935). Optimum Health. Los Angeles: California Graphic Press. 247 pp.
37. Dean ME. (2016). Selective suppression by the medical establishment of unwelcome research findings: the cholera treatment evaluation by the General Board of Health, London 1854. *J R Soc Med*;109(5):200-205. doi:10.1177/0141076816645057
38. DePergola, G. and Silvestris, F. 2013. "Obesity as a major risk for cancer." *J Obesity* 2013; doi: 10.1155/2013/291546. URL: https://www.ncbi.nlm.nih.gov/pmc/articles/PMC3773450/
39. DHS (Department of Homeland Security) Yearbook of Immigration Statistics: 2009 Data Tables (Washington, DC DHS 2010). Retrieved June 12, 2020 from: www.dhs.gov/files/statistics/publications/LPR09.shtm
39.b. Dietary Guidelines for Americans (1990). USDA and DHHS. Retrieved July 1, 2020 from: URL: https://www.dietaryguidelines.gov/sites/default/files/2019-05/1990%20Dietary%20Guidelines%20for%20Americans.pdf
40. Dietary Goals for the United States—History (1977). The U.S. Senate Select Committee on Nutrition and Human Needs, led by Senator George McGovern released guidelines. Retrieved from Dietary Guidelines for Americans website June 24, 2020. URL: https://www.dietaryguidelines.gov/about-dietary-guidelines/history-dietary-guidelines
41. Doll, R. (1985). Preventive Medicine: The Objectives. Ciba Found Symp;110:3-21. doi: 10.1002/9780470720912.ch2.
42. Duffey KJ, Popkin BM. (2011). Energy density, portion size, and eating occasions: contributions to increased energy intake in the United States, 1977-2006. *PLoS Med*; 8(6):e1001050. doi:10.1371/journal.pmed.1001050. URL: https://www.ncbi.nlm.nih.gov/pmc/articles/PMC3125292/
43. Edington DW, Schultz AB, Pitts JS, Camilleri A. (2015). The Future of Health Promotion in the 21st Century: A Focus on the Working Population. *Am J Lifestyle Med*;10(4):242-252. Published 2015 Sep 22. doi:10.1177/1559827615605789
44. Encyclopedia Britannica (1910). Hydropathy, 11th edition, vol. XIII. New York: Encyclopedia Britannica Inc. p.166.
45. Encyclopedia Britannica (1902) Hydropathy, 9th Edition (1875) and 10th Edition (1902). Retrieved July 11, 2012 from: http://www.1902encyclopedia.com/H/HYD/hydropathy.html
46. Engel, GL. (1980). The clinical application of the biopsychosocial model. Am J Psychiatry; 137(5):535-44.
47. Farmer, M. (2019). Madison Avenue Manslaughter: An inside view of fee-cutting clients, profit-hungry owners, and declining ad agencies. Third edition. New York: LID Publishing
48. Farvid MS, Cho E, Chen WY, Eliassen AH, Willett WC (2015). Adolescent meat intake and breast cancer risk. *Int J Cancer*; 136(8):1909-1920. doi:10.1002/ijc.29218
49. Finkelstein, E. A., Khavjou, O. A., Thompson, H., Trogdon, J. G., Pan, L., Sherry, B., & Dietz, W. (2012). "Obesity and severe obesity forecasts through 2030." *American Journal of Preventive Medicine, 42(6),* 563-570, URL: 10.1016/j.amepre.2011.10.026.
50. Flannery, MA. (2002) The early Botanical Medical Movement as a Reflection of Life, Liberty, and Literacy in Jacksonian America. J Med Libr Assoc. October; 90(4): 442–454. Retrieved on September 10, 2013 from: http://www.ncbi.nlm.nih.gov/pmc/articles/PMC128961/
50b. FNB (1991) Food and Nutrition Board. Institute of Medicine. Washington: National Academy Press. URL: https://books.google.com/books?id=-EMrAAAAYAAJ&printsec=frontcover#v=onepage&q&f=false
51. Frakt, A. (2018). Reagan's deregulation and America's exceptional rise in healthcare costs. New York Times. The Upshot, June 4. URL: https://www.nytimes.com/2018/06/04/upshot/reagan-deregulation-and-americas-exceptional-rise-in-health-care-costs.html
52. Frank, AL (1996). Prevention into the 21st century. *Mt Sinai J Med*; 63(3-4):236-240. URL: https://pubmed.ncbi.nlm.nih.gov/8692170/
53. Frazao, E. (1999) America's Eating Habits: Changes and Consequences. USDA Economic Research Service. USDA. Agriculture Information Bulletin No. (AIB-750) 494 pp, May Retrieved Sept 10, 2013 from: http://www.ers.usda.gov/publications/aib-agricultural-information-bulletin/aib750.aspx
54. French, SM., Story, M. Jeffery, WM. (2001). Environmental influences on eating and physical activity. Annual Reviews of Public Health; 22: 309-335. URL: https://www.annualreviews.org/doi/full/10.1146/annurev.publhealth.22.1.309
55. Fryar, C.D., Carroll, M. and Ogden, C.L. (2018). *Prevalence of Overweight, Obesity, and Extreme Obesity Among Adults Aged 20 and Over: United States, 1960–1962 Through 2015–2016.*URL:

56. Fryar, C.D. Carroll, M.D. and Ogden, C.L.,.(2018b). "Prevalence of Overweight and Obesity Among Children and Adolescents Aged 2–19 Years: United States, 1963–1965 Through 2015–2016." *National Center for Health Statistics.* URL: https://www.cdc.gov/nchs/data/hestat/obesity_child_15_16/obesity_child_15_16.pdf
   https://www.cdc.gov/nchs/data/hestat/obesity_adult_15_16/obesity_adult_15_16.pdf
57. Fung T, Hu FB, Fuchs C, Giovannucci E, Hunter DJ, Stampfer MJ, Colditz GA, Willett WC. (2003). Major dietary patterns and the risk of colorectal cancer in women. Arch Intern Med;163:309–314.
58. Ciocco, A. Klein, H and Palmer, CE. (1941)"Child Health and the Selective Service Physical Standards," *Pub. Health Rep.* 56, no. 50 (1941): 2365–75; *Our Country's Call to Service* (Washington, D.C.: U.S. Office of Education, Federal Security Agency, 1942).
59. Gallo, AE. (2000). Food advertising in the United States (Chapter-9). In: AIB-750. USDA/ERS: 173-180. URL: https://www.ers.usda.gov/webdocs/publications/42215/5838_aib750i_1_.pdf?v=41055
60. Giovannucci E, Rimm EB, Stampfer MJ, Colditz GA, Ascherio A & Willett WC (1994): Intake of fat, meat and fiber in relation to risk of colon cancer in men. Cancer Res. 54, 2390 – 2397.
61. Goldin C., and Katz L.F. (1998). The Origins of Technology-Skill Complementarity. The Quarterly Journal of Economics;113:693–732.
62. Golechha M. (2016). Health Promotion Methods for Smoking Prevention and Cessation: A Comprehensive Review of Effectiveness and the Way Forward. *Int J Prev Med*; 7:7. Published 2016 Jan 11. doi:10.4103/2008-7802.173797
63. Gordon. MB and Elias H. Bartley,EH (1919) "Malnutrition in Children: A Study of the Examination of Nine Hundred Children under Eight Years of Age," *Arch. Pediatr.* 36: 257–67, quotation on 266.
64. Grand View Research (2020). Nutraceutical Market size share & trends analysis report by product (dietary supplements, functional foods, and functional beverages) by region and segment forecast, 2020-2027. URL: https://www.grandviewresearch.com/industry-analysis/nutraceuticals-market
65. Green, AR, et al. (2002). Why the disease-based model of medicine fails our patients. Western Journal of Medicine; 176(2): 141–143. URL: https://www.ncbi.nlm.nih.gov/pmc/articles/PMC1071693/
66. Haller, JS.Jr. (1994). Medical Protestants: The Eclectics in American Medicine (1825-1939). Carbondale (IL): Southern Illinois University Press, 340 pp.
67. Hardy A. (1999). Food, hygiene, and the laboratory. A short history of food poisoning in Britain, circa 1850-1950. *Soc Hist Med*;12(2):293-311. doi:10.1093/shm/12.2.293
68. Harris JB, LaRocque RC, Qadri F, Ryan ET, Calderwood SB. (2012).Cholera. *Lancet*; 379(9835):2466-2476. doi:10.1016/S0140-6736(12)60436-X
69. Haslam D. (2016). Weight management in obesity - past and present. *Int J Clin Pract*; 70(3):206-217. doi:10.1111/ijcp.12771 URL: https://www.ncbi.nlm.nih.gov/pmc/articles/PMC4832440/
70. Hastings, RW. (1912). "Medical Inspection of Schools," *Amer. J. Pub. Health* 2(2): 971–76, data on 973.
71. Hattie, WH. (1928). A Father of Preventive Medicine. Can. Med Assoc.J. 19(1): 101-105. URL: https://www.ncbi.nlm.nih.gov/pmc/articles/PMC1709743/?page=3
72. Hazlit, WC. 1902). Diet of the Yeoman and Poor in England *in "Old Cookery Books and Ancient Cuisine", edited by Henry B. Wheatley, London, 1902. E-text prepared by David Starner, Alicia Williams, and the Project Gutenberg Online Distributed Proofreading Team. Adapted and illustrated to be posted by Leopoldo Costa.*
73. Heffron, JL.(1900) "The Diet of School Children," *J. Pedagogy* 12 (1900): 285–94,
74. Helman, CG. (1994). Culture, Health & Illness. 3rd edition. Boston: Butterworth-Heinemann, 446 pp
75. Hill, HC (1923) "The Development of Chicago as a Center of the Meat Packing Industry," Mississippi Valley Historical Review 10 (3): 253.
76. Hirschman C, Mogford E. (2009) Immigration and the American industrial revolution from 1880 to 1920. *Soc Sci Res*;38(4):897-920. doi:10.1016/j.ssresearch.2009.04.001
77. Hough, J. (2018). Madison Avenue's comeback campaign. Barrons Feb 24. Retrieved June 25, 2020 from: URL: https://www.barrons.com/articles/madison-avenues-comeback-campaign-1519437814
78. Horvat-II, J. (2013). Return to Order: From a Frenzied Economy to an Organic Christian Society. York, PA: York Press, 381 pp.
79. Hunt, C.L. (1916) *Food for Young Children.* U.S. Department of Agriculture, Farmers. Bulletin No. 717, 21 pp
80. I.O.M (Institute of Medicine) (2010) (US) Committee on Preventing the Global Epidemic of Cardiovascular Disease: Meeting the Challenges in Developing Countries; Fuster V, Kelly BB, editors. Promoting Cardiovascular Health in the Developing World: A Critical Challenge to Achieve Global Health. Washington (DC): National Academies Press (US); 2010. 6, Cardiovascular Health Promotion Early in Life. Available from: https://www.ncbi.nlm.nih.gov/books/NBK45695/
81. I.O.M (Institute of Medicine) 1999 (US) Food Forum. Enhancing the Regulatory Decision-Making Approval Process for Direct Food Ingredient Technologies: Workshop Summary. Washington (DC): National Academies Press (US); 1999. APPENDIX A, Legal Aspects of the Food Additive Approval Process. Available from: https://www.ncbi.nlm.nih.gov/books/NBK224037/
82. I.O.M (Institute of Medicine). (1988) (US) Committee for the Study of the Future of Public Health. The Future of Public Health. Washington (DC): National Academies Press (US); 3, A History of the Public Health System. Available from: https://www.ncbi.nlm.nih.gov/books/NBK218224/
83. Jacobs, BR. (1922). Self-Rising Flour: What is it? Am. Food Journal; 17: 9-11.
84. Jahns L, Davis-Shaw W, Lichtenstein AH, Murphy SP, Conrad Z, Nielsen F (2018). The History and Future of Dietary Guidance in America. *Adv Nutr*;9(2):136-147. doi:10.1093/advances/nmx025
85. Jiménez, TR. (2011) Immigrants to the United States: How Well Are They Integrating Into Society? Washington DC: Migration Policy Institute, 25pp.
86. Johns Hopkins University. (2020). Types of complementary and alternative medicine. Health> Wellness and Prevention. Retrieved on June 25, 2020 from Johns Hopkins Medicine webpage: https://www.hopkinsmedicine.org/health/wellness-and-prevention/types-of-complementary-and-alternative-medicine
87. Jolliffe, N., McLester, JS., and Sherman, HC. (1942) "The Prevalence of Malnutrition," *J. Amer. Med. Assoc.* (March

21, 1942): 944–50, quotation on 950. See also "Recognition of Early Nutritional Failure in Infants, Children, Adolescents and Adults," *J. Amer. Med. Assoc.* (February 21, 1942): 615–16; John F. Kendrick, "A Cooperative Nutrition Program in North Carolina," *Pub. Health Rep.* (May 21, 1943): 797–803; H. D. Kruse, Otto A. Bessey, Norman Jolliffe, James S. McLester, Frederick F. Tisdall, and Russell M. Wilder, *Inadequate Diets and Nutritional Deficiencies in the United States: Their Prevalence and Significance* (Washington, D.C.: National Research Council, 1943).

88. Johnson, I. (1993). Kids influence $150 billion in spending, so Madison Ave aims at them "Mom can we buy a…" Baltimore Sun Nov 7. URL: https://www.baltimoresun.com/news/bs-xpm-1993-11-07-1993311080-story.html
89. Kantor, HA. and Tyack, DB. (1982) "Introduction," in *Work, Youth, and Schooling: Historical Perspectives on Vocationalism in American Education*, ed. Harvey A. Kantor and David B. Tyack (Stanford: Stanford University Press, 1982), 1–13, data on 7–8.
90. Karila, L. et al. (2014). Acute and long term effects of cannabis use: A review. Curr Pharm Des; 20(25):4112-8.
91. Kassirer J, Angell M. (1998). "Losing weight—an ill-fated New Year's resolution." *N Engl J Med;338:* 52–4.
92. Keefer, FR. (1920) "Causes of Army Rejections: What Health Officers Can Do to Remedy Conditions," *Amer. J. Pub. Health* 10 (3): 236–39, data on 237. See also *Defects Found in Drafted Men* (Washington, D.C.: Government Printing Office, 1919); Frederick L. Hoffman, *Army Anthropometry and Medical Rejection Statistics* (Newark: Prudential Press, 1918).
93. Kerr, AM. (1933) "Effect of the Economic Crisis on the Nutrition of School Children," *Pennsylvania Med. J.* 37 (1933): 232–34.
94. Kessler, R.C. et al., (2009). The global burden of mental disorders: An update from the WHO World Mental Health (WMH) Surveys. Epidemiol Psichiatr Soc. 2009 Jan–Mar; 18(1): 23–33. URL: https://www.ncbi.nlm.nih.gov/pmc/articles/PMC3039289/
95. Kessler, DA. (2009b) The End of Overeating: Taking Control of the Insatiable American Appetite. Rodale Books, New York, 329pp
96. King DE, Matheson E, Chirina S, Shankar A, Broman-Fulks J. (2013) The Status of Baby Boomers' Health in the United .: The Healthiest Generation? *JAMA Intern Med.*;173(5):385–386. doi:10.1001/jamainternmed.2013.2006
97. Klein S, Burke LE, Bray GA, Blair S, Allison DB, Pi-Sunyer X, Hong Y, Eckel RH. and American Heart Association Council on Nutrition, Physical Activity, and Metabolism. (2004). "Clinical implications of obesity with specific focus on cardiovascular disease: a statement for professionals from the American Heart Association Council on Nutrition, Physical Activity, and Metabolism: endorsed by the American." *Circulation. 110(18):* 2952-67 URL: https://www.ncbi.nlm.nih.gov/pubmed/15509809/
98. Kupelian, D. (2014) 70 million Americans taking mind altering drugs. WND Weekly. Feb 9, 2014. Retrieved Feb 11, 2014 from: http://www.wnd.com/2014/02/70-million-americans-taking-mind-altering-drugs/
99. La Berge, AF (2008) How the Ideology of Low Fat Conquered America, *Journal of the History of Medicine and Allied Sciences*; 63(2): 139–177 URL: https://doi.org/10.1093/jhmas/jrn001
100. Labruère R, Sona AJ, Turos E. (2019) Anti-Methicillin-Resistant *Staphylococcus aureus* Nanoantibiotics. *Front Pharmacol*;10:1121. Published 2019 Oct 4. doi:10.3389/fphar.2019.01121
101. Levenstein, H. (1988). Revolution at the table: The Transformation of the American Diet. New York: Oxford University Press. 275 pp.
102. Lindenmeyer, K. (1997). *"A Right to Childhood": The U.S. Children's Bureau and Child Welfare* On the child health movement, see, *1912–46* (Urbana: University of Illinois Press, 1997).
103. Macdonald, C. and McIntyre, M. (2018). Realities of Canadian Nursing. 5th Edition. Toronto: Wolters Kluwer Publishing.
104. McMahon, SF. (1985). A comfortable subsistence: The changing composition of diet in rural New England 1620-1840. The William and Mary Quarterly; 42(1):26-65
105. Mann T, Tomiyama AJ, Westling E, Lew AM, Samuels B, Chatman J. (2007). "Medicare's search for effective obesity treatments: diets are not the answer." *Am Psychol. ;62(3):* 220-33 URL: https://www.ncbi.nlm.nih.gov/pubmed/17469900
106. Margotta, R. (1996). The Hamlyn History of Medicine. Paul Lewis (ed) London: Institute of Neurology, 192 pp
107. Martini M, Gazzaniga V, Bragazzi NL, Barberis I. (2019). The Spanish Influenza Pandemic: a lesson from history-Published 2019 Mar 29. doi:10.15167/2421-4248/jpmh2019.60.1.1205
108. Mayo Clinic. Staff Antibiotics: Misuse Puts you and Others at Risk Retrieved July 13, 2012from: http://www.mayoclinic.com/health/antibiotics/FL00075
109. Meier, MH. et al. (2012) Persistent Cannabis users show neurophysiological decline from childhood to midlife. Proceedings of the National Academy of Science. Retrieved Feb 12, 2014 from: http://www.pnas.org/content/early/2012/08/22/1206820109.abstract
110. Milner, J. A. (2000) Functional Foods: the US perspective. The American Journal of Clinical Nutrition 71(6):1654s-1659s.
111. Mitchell, N., Catenacci, V., Wyatt, HR., and Hill, JO. (2011). Obesity: Overview of an Epidemic. Psychiatr Clin North Amer; 34(4): 717-732. URL:https://www.ncbi.nlm.nih.gov/pmc/articles/PMC3228640/
112. Moss, M. (2013) Salt, sugar, Fat: How the Food Giants Hooked US. Random House, New York, 446pp
113. Murtaugh, MA (2004) Meat Consumption and the Risk of Colon and Rectal Cancer. Current Medical Literature: Clinical Nutrition; Vol. 13 Issue 4, p61
114. National Archives (UK). Great Plague of 1665-1666: How did London Respond to it? Accessed June 10, 2020 from: https://www.nationalarchives.gov.uk/education/resources/great-plague/
115. Nielsen SJ, Popkin BM(2003). Patterns and trends in food portion sizes, 1977-1998. JAMA.22-29; 289(4):450-3.
116. NRC (1987). National Research Council (US) Committee on Scientific and Regulatory Issues Underlying Pesticide Use Patterns and Agricultural Innovation. Regulating Pesticides in Food: The Delaney Paradox. Washington (DC): National Academies Press (US). A Legislative History of

116. the Pesticide Residues Amendment of 1954 and the Delaney Clause of the Food Additives Amendment of 1958. Available from: https://www.ncbi.nlm.nih.gov/books/NBK218051/
117. NCI (2018). National Cancer Institute. Cancer Statistics. Retrieved April 17, 2020. URL: https://www.cancer.gov/about-cancer/understanding/statistics
118. Nestle, M. (2002) Food Politics: How the Food Industry Influences Nutrition & Health. Berkeley, CA, University of California Press, 457pp.
119. NIMH (National Institute of Mental Health (2017). Major Depression. Retrieved from the NIH website march 29, 2018: https://www.nimh.nih.gov/health/statistics/major-depression.shtml
120. Nissenbaum, S. (1980) Sex, Diet, and Debility in Jacksonian America. Chicago: The Dorsey press. American Society and Culture: The Dorsey Collection, 198pp.
121. Olmstead A. L., and Rhode P.W. (2000). The Transformation of Northern Agriculture. In: Engerman Stanley L, Gallman Robert E., editors. The Cambridge Economic History of the United States. Vol. 3. Cambridge: Cambridge University Press. pp. 693–742.
122. Oppenheimer GM, Benrubi ID. (2014). McGovern's Senate Select Committee on Nutrition and Human Needs versus the meat industry on the diet-heart question (1976-1977). *Am J Public Health*;104(1):59-69. URL: https://www.ncbi.nlm.nih.gov/pmc/articles/PMC3910043/ doi:10.2105/AJPH.2013.301464
123. Pan A, Sun Q, Bernstein AM, Schulze MB, Manson JE, Stampfer MJ, Willett WC, Hu FB: (2012) Red meat consumption and mortality: results from 2 prospective cohort studies. *Arch Intern Med* 172:555-563
124. Perri, M.G. 1998. "The maintenance of treatment effects in the long-term management of obesity." *Clin Psychol: Sci Pract* ;5: 526–43.
125. Peters, T. and Waterman, RH Jr. (1983). In Search of Excellence: Lessons from America's Best Run Companies. New York: Harper-Collins Publishing. pp. 400.
126. Peters, WH. (1916). Report of the Committee on Medical Inspection of Schools. Am J. Pub. Health; 6(6): 589-9.
126b. Petrick, G. (2011) Purity as life: H.J Heinz Religious sentiment and the beginning of the Industrial Revolution. History & Technology.; 27(1): 37-64
127. Piernas C, Popkin BM.(2011). Food portion patterns and trends among U.S. children and the relationship to total eating occasion size, 1977-2006. *J Nutr*;141(6):1159-1164. doi:10.3945/jn.111.138727
128. Platz EA, Willett WC, Colditz GA, Rimm EB, Spiegelman D, Giovannucci E. (2000). Proportion of colon cancer risk that might be preventable in a cohort of middle-aged US men. Cancer Causes Control;11:579–588.
129. Popkin, BM, Adair, LS, and Ng, SW. 2012. "NOW AND THEN: The Global Nutrition Transition: The Pandemic of Obesity in Developing Countries." *Nutr Rev; 70(1):* 3–21. URL: https://www.ncbi.nlm.nih.gov/pmc/articles/PMC3257829/#SD3
130. Pritikin, N. and McGrady, P (1984). Prikin Program for Diet and Exercise. New York: Random House Publishing, 464 pp
131. Reid, MG. (1943) Food for the People. New York, John Wiley & Sons, 653pp.
132. Rosenbaum DL, White KS. (2013). The Role of Anxiety in Binge Eating Behavior: A Critical Examination of Theory and Empirical Literature. *Health Psychol Res*;1(2): e19. Published 2013 Jun 18. doi:10.4081/hpr.2013.e19
133. Ruggles S.(2009). Reconsidering the Northwest European Family System: Living Arrangements of the Aged in Comparative Historical Perspective. *Popul Dev Rev*;35(2):249–273. doi:10.1111/j.1728-4457.2009.00275.x
134. Ruis, AR. (2013). Children with half-starved bodies and the assessment of Malnutrition in the United States 1890-1950. Bulletin of the History of Medicine; 87(3), Fall 2013
135. SAMSHA (Substance Abuse and Mental Health Services Administration. (2017). Key substance use and mental health indicators in the United States: Results from the 2016 National Survey on Drug Use and Health (HHS Publication No. SMA 17-5044, NSDUH Series H-52). Rockville, MD: Center for Behavioral Health Statistics and Quality, Substance Abuse and Mental Health Services Administration. Retrieved from https://www.samhsa.gov/data/sites/default/files/NSDUH-FFR1-2016/NSDUH-FFR1-2016.htm
136. Sansom, W. (2005). The US Surgeon General Carmona calls obesity the terror within. UT Health. Accessed June 20, 2020 from: https://news.uthscsa.edu/u-s-surgeon-general-carmona-calls-obesity-the-terror-within/
137. Sebrell, WH. (1942) Urgent Problems in Nutrition for National Betterment. American J. Publ. Health 32:15-20
138. Shields, M. (2004). Madison Avenue offers junk food for thought: Study illustrates Industry restraint. Media Daily News, June 3. Retrieved June 25, 2020 from: https://www.mediapost.com/publications/article/4396/madison-avenue-offers-junk-food-for-thought-study.html
139. Shirey, W. (2015). Immigration Waves. Retrieved June 22, 2020 from: URL: https://immigrationtounitedstates.org/603-immigration-waves.html
140. Simon, G.E., Ludman, E.J., Linde, J.A., Operskalski, B.H., Ichikawa, L., Rohde, P., Finch, E.A., and Jeffery, R.W. 2008. "Association between obesity and depression in middle-aged women." *Gen Hosp Psychiatry* 30(1): 32–39 URL: https://www.ncbi.nlm.nih.gov/pmc/articles/PMC2675189/
141. Smith, D.I. (Spring 2019) "19th Century Development of Refrigeration in the American Meat Packing Industry," Tenor of Our Times: 8 (1): article 14. Available at: https://scholarworks.harding.edu/tenor/vol8/iss1/14
142. Soeliman FA, Azadbakht L. (2014). Weight loss maintenance: A review on dietary related strategies. *J Res Med Sci*;19(3):268-275. URL: https://www.ncbi.nlm.nih.gov/pmc/articles/PMC4061651/
143. Stiebeling, HK. And Leverton, RM (1941). Nutrition. Annu. Rev. Biochem. 10:423-448. Downloaded from www.annualreviews.org Access provided by 64.254.187.112 on 06/11/20.
144. Stiebeling, HK. (1939) Better Nutrition as a National Goal: The Problem, Year Book of Agriculture p 380
145. Stiebeling, H.K. and M. Ward.(1933) *Diets at Four Levels of Nutrition Content and Cost*. U.S. Department of Agriculture, Circ. No. 296, 59 pp.,
146. Stunkard, A.J. and McLaren-Hume. 1959. "The results of treatment for obesity." *Archiv Intern Medicine* 133: 75-85 URL: https://jamanetwork.com/journals/jamainternalmedicine/article-abstract/562795?redirect=true
147. Sutherland, JP. (1937). The Medical Octopus. Boston: Meador Publishing, 333 pp.
148. Suzuki, N. (2010) Popular Health Movement and Diet Reform in 19th Century America The Japanese Journal of American Studies 21: 111-137

149. Swift, D.L. (2014). "The Role of Exercise and Physical Activity in Weight Loss and Maintenance." *Prog Cardiovasc Dis.* 56(4): 441–447 URL: https://www.ncbi.nlm.nih.gov/pmc/articles/PMC3925973/
150. Tabish SA. (2007). Is Diabetes Becoming the Biggest Epidemic of the Twenty-first Century?. *Int J Health Sci (Qassim)*;1(2):V-VIII.
151. Tarnower, H. and Sinclair-Baker, S. (1980). The Complete Scarsdale Medical Diet. New York: Random House Publishing, 240 pp
152. Taskin, D.P (2009). Does Marijuana increase the risk of chronic obstructive pulmonary disease? CMAJ; 180(8): 797–798. doi: 10.1503/cmaj.090142 Retrieved August 26, 2017 https://www.ncbi.nlm.nih.gov/pmc/articles/PMC2665954/
153. Tauxes, RV., and Esteban, EJ. (2007). Advances in Food Safety to prevent foodborne disease in the United States. In: Silent Victories: The History and practice of public health in the 20th century (Ward, JW. And Warren, C eds). New York: Oxford University Press, p: 18-43
154. Thomas LH, Jones PR, Winter JA, Smith H. (1981) Hydrogenated oils and fats: the presence of chemically-modified fatty acids in human adipose tissue. *American Journal of Clinical Nutrition*; 35:877-86.
155. Tilney, J. (2017). Is your weight problem actually a spiritual problem? Charisma/Health. URL: http://www.charismamag.com/life/health/33006-is-your-weight-problem-actually-a-spiritual-problem
156. Trustwell, AS. (2002) Meat Consumption and Cancer of the Large Bowel. European Journal of Clinical Nutrition 56, Suppl 1, S19–S24
157. USDA. History of the USDA Food Guides. Retrieved from USDA/Choosemyplate.gov website on June 24, 2020 from: https://www.choosemyplate.gov/eathealthy/brief-history-usda-food-guides
158. USDA (2010). : U.S. Department of Agriculture and U.S. Department of Health and Human Services. Dietary Guidelines for Americans, 2010. 7th Edition, Washington, DC: U.S. Government Printing Office, December 2010. URL: https://health.gov/sites/default/files/2020-01/DietaryGuidelines2010.pdf
159. USDA (2005). Nutrition and your Health: Dietary Guidelines for Americans. Appendix G-5 History of the Dietary Guidelines for Americans. United States Department of Agriculture (USDA). Retrieved on September 16, 2013 from: http://www.health.gov/dietaryguidelines/dga2005/report/HTML/G5_History.htm
160. USDA (1943). Food for Freedom Informational Handbook 1943. Historical Dietary Guidance Digital Collection [Internet] [cited 2017 Dec 2]. Available from: https://nutritionhistory.nal.usda.gov/download/1789419/PDF.
161. U.S. Senate Select Committee on Nutrition and Human Needs (1977). Dietary Goals for the United States, 2nd ed. Washington, DC, U.S. Government Printing Office. URL: https://thescienceofnutrition.files.wordpress.com/2014/03/dietary-goals-for-the-united-states.pdf
162. USHHS (United States Department of Health & Human Services (2011). Results from the 2011 National Survey on Drug Use and Health: Summary of National Findings. Retrieved from the Center for Behavioral Health Statistics and Quality on March 29, 2018: https://www.samhsa.gov/data/sites/default/files/Revised2k11NSDUHSummNatFindings/Revised2k11NSDUHSummNatFindings/NSDUHresults2011.htm
163. Wakefield, J. (2004). "Fighting Obesity Through the Built Environment." *Environ Health Perspect; 112(11):* A616–A618. URL: https://www.ncbi.nlm.nih.gov/pmc/articles/PMC1247493/
164. WCRF/AICR (1997). Food, nutrition and the prevention of cancer: a global perspective: World Cancer Research Fund / American Institute for Cancer Research. 1997.
165. WHO, (2016). "Obesity and Overweight Fact Sheet." *World Health Organization.* Accessed 05 19, 2018. http://www.who.int/news-room/fact-sheets/detail/obesity-and-overweight
166. WHO, (2003). "The Global Strategy on Diet, Physical Activity and Health." *World Health Organization.* Accessed 05 22, 2018. http://www.who.int/dietphysicalactivity/media/en/gsfs_general.pdf
167. WHO/ FAO (1956) Report of the Joint Expert Committee on Food Additives, General Principles Governing the Use of Food Additives.
168. Wiley, HW. (1929). The History of a Crime Against the Food Law. Milwaukee, WI, Lee Foundation for Nutritional Research, 413pp.
169. Wilfley DE, Friedman MA, Dounchis JZ, Stein RI, Welch RR, Ball SA. (2000). Comorbid psychopathology in binge eating disorder: relation to eating disorder severity at baseline and following treatment. J Consult Clin Psychol. 2000; 68(4):641-9.
170. Willett WC, Stampfer MJ, Manson JE, et al. (1993) Intake of trans fatty acids and risk of coronary heart disease among women. *Lancet*; 351:581-5.
171. Willett WC, Stampfer MJ, Colditz GA, Rosner BA & Speizer FE (1990): Relation of meat, fat and fiber intake to the risk of colon cancer in a prospective study among women. New Engl. J. Med. 232, 1664 –1672.
172. World Health Organization (2001) Cancer Strategy [Online] Available: retrieved August 2012 http://www.who.int/ncd/cancer/strategy.htm
173. Wynder EL, Gori GB. (1977) Contributions of the environment to cancer incidence: an epidemiologic exercise. J Natl Cancer Inst. 58: 825-32.
174. Yeager Kujovich, M. (1970). The Refrigerator Car and the Growth of the American Dressed Beef Industry. The Business History Review 44 (4): 465.
174b. Young Lee, P. (2008) Meat Modernity, and the Rise of the Slaughterhouse, (New Hampshire, Durham: University of New Hampshire Press) 34 pp.
175. Young LR, Nestle M. (2002). The contribution of expanding portion sizes to the US obesity epidemic. *Am J Public Health*;92(2):246-249. doi:10.2105/ajph.92.2.246
176. Zeeck A, Stelzer N, Linster HW, Joos A, Hartmann A Emotion and eating in binge eating disorder and obesity. Eur Eat Disord Rev. 2011 Sep-Oct; 19(5):426-37.
177. Zheng Y., Li Y., Satija A., Pan, A., and Sotosrieto, M., Rimm E. et al.(2019). Association of changes in red meat consumption with total and cause specific mortality among US women and men: two prospective cohort studies. *BMJ*; 365 :l2110

Comments

The main philosophy of constraint advocated by government had two main objectives: first, to reduce the duplication of efforts or in other words to consolidate services; and second, to adapt to a new mandate of government policies.

The new mandate that was developed in the early part of the this millennium in Canada, was framed by the "*Commission on the Future of Health Care*" and driven by the public's concern over a progressively apparent disabled health care system. It is a little bewildering, to say the least, to witness these changes especially in countries like Canada with government-supported health care systems that have, in the past, been able to deal with the public's health in a timely manner and with quality of care. Now, financial constraints make accessibility more difficult as evidenced by the long waiting lines in many of Canada's emergency rooms. The impetus now is to embrace the concept of "Integrated Care for Integrated Health." This notion of integration translates into an insidious systemic infiltration of management devices geared to control health care cost through an orchestrated and disciplined use of resources.

CHAPTER 2

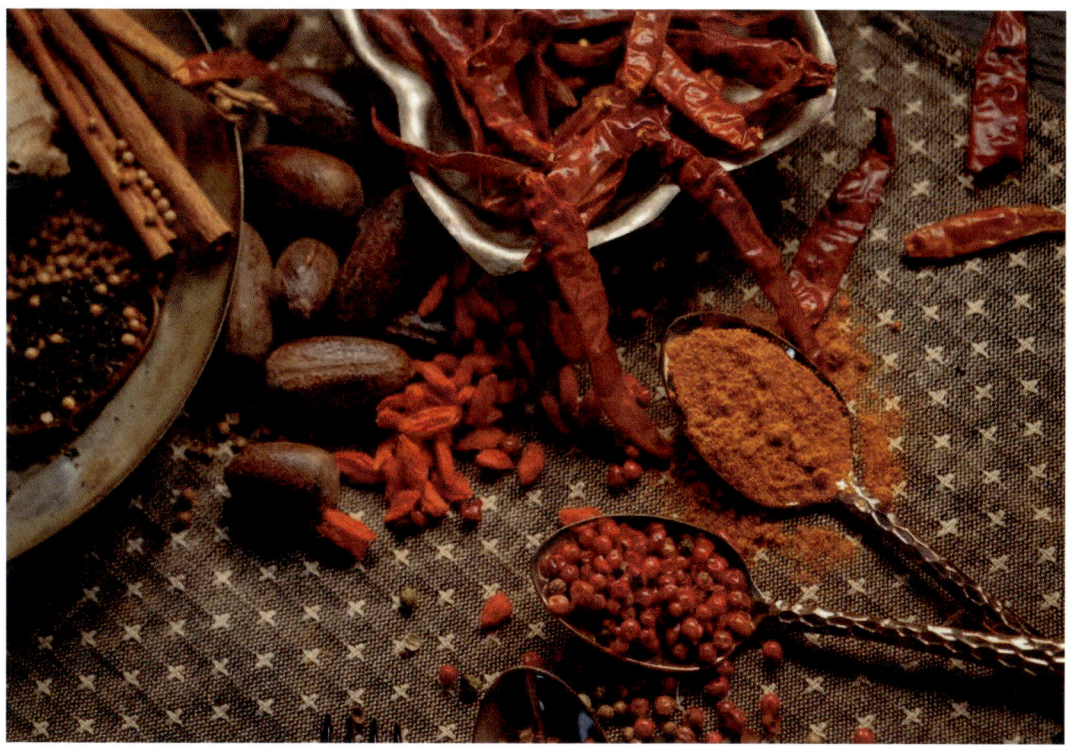

HISTORY OF NUTRITION IN HUMAN HEALTH

Born in Amburg Bavaria in 1831, Carl Von Voit, (1831-1908) would go on to become a doctor of Medicine, a professor of anatomy and physiology in addition to being a notable chemist who advanced new and compelling theories about human metabolism and nutrition.[41] Intrigued by the output of the four elements, oxygen, hydrogen, carbon and nitrogen, and their relations to food intake, Dr Von Voit, pioneered the first nitrogen balance studies, and the first experiments involving oxygen and carbon dioxide exchange during exercise. He also created the first respiration chamber that permitted key observations that were helpful in understanding the biochemistry of human metabolism. He noted, for instance, that CO_2 was abundantly produced when carbohydrates and fats were consumed. [41] His discoveries along with other notable scientists of the time—Liebig, Jean-Baptiste Boussingault, Friedrich Bidder and Carl Schmidt, and Bischoff—enveloped the field of nutrition and medicine in an aura of mystery and scientific paradoxes. These discoveries took place concomitantly with Louis Pasteur's and Joseph Lister's work on fermentation and putrefaction that gave rise to a new etiology of disease: bacteria. [72]

By the early 20th century, nutrition emerges, with the discovery of vitamins, as field vitally important for population and individual health.
The quest to maximize the human diet for optimal health—a preoccupation that has taken the last three decades of the twentieth century by storm—is about as old as man's quest to acquire food.

Archeobotanists have argued that sparse populations during the Palaeolithic period—roughly 3 million people—may well have been caused by the nomadic lifestyle, which occasioned malnutrition. [12] The hunter-gatherer of this period, consisted of men and boys hunting for prey; the elders instructed the young, made medicinal concoxions and tools, which left women to gather foodstuffs such as snails, small turtles, plants, roots, acorns, nuts and berries. [79] The Neolithic period, characterized by farming and the domestication of animals, coincided with major climatic changes involving the retreat of glaciers and subsequent exposing of fertile lands. This favored the beginning of agricultural practices and a population explosion, over a 7000 year period, totalling 100 million.[12] Tannahill[79] refers to this period of 10,000 to 3000 BC as:

the gestation period of modern civilization.

Farming assured the availability of food in sufficient quantities and quality, creating as it were, surpluses of food used likely to feed the agricultural workers and builders of towns and communities. [79]

It was clear that satisfying the worker's hunger impacted physical performance. The rationale was that hunger, a physiologically driven mechanism for survival, becomes at the same time a powerful impetus to work and to eventually initiate progress. This idea that privation is a strong impetus for change is very much a primary idea that was carried forward from ancient Greek thinkers and philosophers. [48] Aristotle argues that for substantive change to unfold, *form, matter and privation* make up the essential tripod needed to foster this change. [78]

William Hazlitt, a 19th century English journalist and writer also understood the importance of pri-

> We should nevertheless question whether newer and improved diet strategies can be implemented in our lives that will shield us from the diseases of our time.

vation and avoiding overindulgence in food. He writes:

Prosperity is a great teacher; adversity is a greater. Possession pampers the mind; privation trains and strengthens it.

The Ancient Greek thinkers also advocated for the need in restraint and selectivity of food as a means of acquiring and maintaining good health. We have presently lost touch with this deeper understanding of our human vulnerability to excessive intake of food. The U.S. has possibly become obese because of unchecked desires for unhealthy foods, consumed in overabundance.

The purpose of exploring eating habits of Ancient societies is primarily driven by our thirst for knowledge of our own origins, and understanding the evolutionary steps of man. In this age of exponential growth and accelerated lifestyles, the pace of societal change has taken place at such a heightened rate, that one wonders whether we have adopted lifestyles, and specifically eating habits, that are at all compatible with our capacity as a species to survive.

There is a popular and well accepted view that nutrition is central to our wellbeing. At the most elemental level, we have come to understand that eating from the five food groups will provide us with the essential nutrients needed for growth and good health. The consumer should nevertheless question whether newer and improved diet strategies can be implemented that will shield him from the diseases of our time. This is a valid question indeed, as the public wonders about the pesticide residues in fruits and vegetables, the purity and nutrient content of milk; they are concerned about the antibiotics and hormones used on dairy herds for accelerated milk production and growth, to control mastitis and other infections. They are troubled by the health repercussions arising from genetically modified foods creeping into grocery stores. At one end of the spectrum, we are suspicious about the safety of the food supply. Some are choosing to purge meat and milk from their diet, relying strictly on organically grown fruits, vegetables, legumes and nuts for complete and safe nutrition. At the other end of the spectrum, food scientists are isolating the chemical and bioactive constituents of foods, encapsulating the protective phytochemicals, vitamins and minerals, and marketing supplements that offer promises of improved and unfailing health.

We are all too often convinced by the latest media soundbite that we should be altering our food purchasing practices in order to safeguard our families. Have we become too reactionary? Is there not a more fundamental and immovable set of nutrition principles that can ensure individual and population health?

How do we know if our decisions are wise? Our Ancestral heritage provides us with dietary traditions, key understandings of the foods we ought to be consuming and of those we should be avoiding. In a civilization that manages to survive wars, famines, plagues and austerities of the land, diet becomes part of a sort of collective unconscious, a truth deeply rooted in tradition, and thus requiring no further discussions or debates. Dietary practices follow a rhythm that is intuitively reassuring. We know simply that it is right, but how?

The answer may well be that we have come to trust the legacy of our forefathers. Has that legacy been somehow broken? The cultural practices of our families were grounded in a knowledge that was dutifully passed on through generations of reliable and stable family structures, rooted in experiences that tested the knowledge, and found it to be true over time. Have divorces and separations interfered with the passing on of that knowledge? Have we lost the enduring wisdom that sustained the societies of old because of the growing numbers of shattered families?

2.1 Understanding of the Role of Nutrition in Ancient Societies

In Ancient civilizations, foods were perceived as a source of nourishment with no real therapeutic value per se, but certainly they had a preventative feature. Prominent in the diet of man from the very beginnings of the Neolithic Age, were carbohydrate-rich cereals **(Figure-2.1)**. Archaeobotanical findings in mainland Greece and in Macedonia reveal a preponderance of carbohydrate-rich cereals in the diet of the common person, consisting primarily of barley and wheat. [79]

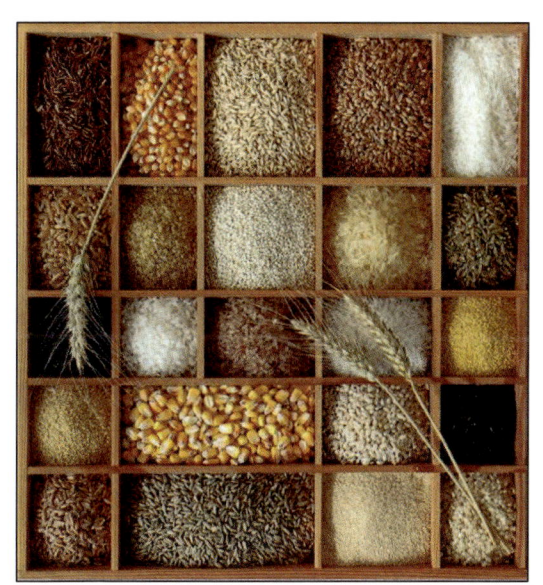

Figure 2.1: Cereals in Wooden Box. © Elena Schweitzer © Shutterstock.com

Emmer wheat, known also as two grained spelt or starch wheat, was first cultivated in Palestine, Syria and Asia Minor, with evidence of its use in Neolithic

European cultures as well. Club wheat, characterized by the whiteness of its endosperm, was popular in Mesopotamia in 3000 BC and progressively surpassed Emmer wheat in most of Europe by AD 1000 and onwards. [12]

Egyptian and Roman societies relied on bread as a staple of their diet, and were producing varieties of cakes and pastries. Historians estimate that the first leavened bread probably originated in Egypt; in fact millers and bakers had reached professional status by 2000 BC. [12]

In addition to wheat and barley, Ancient cultures, found in Italy and in China around the 100s BC, appeared to cultivate millet. Evidence of rye was found in the more northern wintery locations such central Europe, Hungary and Britain as well as in Afghanistan. Many varieties of oats were cultivated in western and eastern Europe, and were indigenous to areas of North Africa. Rice, however, was a dominant crop in Asia as early as 2800 BC. Some have argued that its origins stemmed more likely from India and moved into China during the Bronze Age.[51]

The oldest form of cultivated Indian maize is attributed to southern Mexico around 4500 BC. The Maya and Incas were greatly dependent on maize, as a primary foodstuff, but it was the Peruvians that became the most skilled cultivators of maize by the time Hernando Cortes lead the Spanish conquest of the Aztecs in 1521. [12]

In pre-Hellenic Greece, the Mycenaean civilization, known also as the Aegean civilization, lived in proximity to the Aegean Sea at around 3000 BC.

The Aegean people had a rich diet of vegetables, fruits and legumes, which included celery, chicory, cucumber, garlic, leeks, pumpkins, water parsnips, pears, chick peas, Anis seeds, coriander, lentils, peas, vetch, olives and olive oil, in addition to varieties of fruits such as figs, pears, plums, pomegranates, and apples. The entire base of their agricultural system was founded on what some historians have referred to as the "***eternal trinity***" which consisted in olives, cereals and wines. The only beverages consumed were water, milk, wine and fruit juices; historians seem to agree that wines were moderately consumed, and only during feasts or festivals.[82]

In recent times much attention has been given to the idea that, rather than consuming a diet based on the USDA's MyPlate food guide, we should be rethinking our dietary habits along the lines of the Palaeolithic diet. The Palaeo-diet is rooted in the belief that our prehistoric ancestors were primarily meat consumers and very healthy. The suggestion that we should become dependent primarily on meat sources for protein is controversial, as red meat has, over the last two decades, received so much bad press. The American Cancer Society has taken a strong position against red meat, in light of the abundance of epidemiological research that associates higher risks of some cancers with frequent and abundant meat consumption. These are findings that put into question the importance that meat should hold in the human diet for optimal health. A recent review by Lippi et al., [50] concludes:

Convincing association was found between larger intake of red meat and cancer, especially with colorectal, lung, esophageal and gastric malignancies. Increased consumption of processed meat was also found to be associated with colorectal, esophageal, gastric and bladder cancers. Enhanced intake of white meat or poultry was found to be negatively associated with some types of cancers.

From an evolutionary stand point, archaeologists have advanced four lines of evidence that support meat-based diets as part of the survival and evolution of the *Hominid* species that was present in Africa 4 million years ago (Australopithecines and Kenyanthropicenes). The first is the progressive decrease in mandible size as the diet changed from vegetarian to mostly carnivorous foods. The large massive mandibles were supposedly needed to crush and grind the plant food. The eating habits of modern primates, like the gorilla or chimpanzee, are studied to understand the possible significance of the massive mandible and crania of the early hominids such as the Australopithecines. Indeed, gorillas have large mandibles and crania to accommodate the extensive chewing associated with vegetarian eating, inferring that likewise the early Hominid's diet would have been made up of mostly plant food. [71]

The second line of reasoning is the cranial size of the hominid, which gradually increased to house a large brain and higher intelligence. In fact, subsequent slender and slight species (Australopithicus africanis and Homo habilis (2.5-1.8 million years ago), characteristically had finer cranial features (including a slighter mandible and smaller teeth), and a larger brain. Richards [71] argues that many assume, perhaps incorrectly, that the anatomical adaptation reflected a greater meat-based diet that no longer required extensive chewing. Later on, the *Homo erectus* emerged out of Africa about 1.8 million years ago, and was singled out by archaeologists as the only generally accepted hominid specie from which would have emerged the archaic Homo sapiens, roughly 400,000 to 200,000 years ago—the likely descendent of the modern human (Homo sapiens sapiens) of the Holocene. Archaeologists estimate that the archaic Homo sapiens appeared in Africa about 200,000 to 100,000 years ago, and eventually spread through Europe some 60,000-40,000 years ago. Survival of the archaic line of Homo sapiens, such as the Neanderthals, would have depended on their ability to adapt to colder climates through the use of fire and sophisticated tools that would have been instrumental in cutting, chopping and cooking plant food, in addition to butchering and slicing meat. The broader and more diverse diet, embraced by this hominid line, is evidence of a greater intelligence, but according to Richards,[71] does not necessarily mean less vegetables and more meat, but rather more manipulation of the foods, through cooking and improved processing techniques. In fact, Milton [54] supports the idea that the mandible would have decreased in size concomitantly with more calorically dense plant foods such as fruits. This is pretty much consistent with the long-held belief that humans are more adapted to be vegetarians, according to Marion Nestle, [57] based on the known fact that most living primates are vegetarians. From a health perspective, Dr David Jenkins, a professor and nutrition researcher at the University of Toronto, promotes the importance of a vegetarian diet in order to maintain a healthy gut microbiota. His research team [86] clearly shows significant declines in blood cholesterol with increased consumption of plant foods, soluble fibers and fermentable substrates, considered essential in maintaining this healthy symbiosis with gut bacteria. The highly processed foods and meat-based Westernized diet is actually responsible for a high prevalence of chronic diseases such as diabetes, obesity and cardiovascular disease. [19] Moreover, this diet is changing the makeup of gut microbiota with potentially disastrous health consequences. Shi, [77] in a review of the impact of the Western diet on the gut microbiota and the incidence of chronic disease writes:

Our diet provides not only the nutrients we need but also the material and medium for sustenance and growth of gut bacteria. The composition of the diet will inevitably affect selective growth of types of bacteria in the gut. High consumption of ultra-processed food can change the gut microbiota and lead to inflammation. The effects can even be transferred to later generations via epigenetic change.

The third argument for a carnivorous diet is based on the "**expensive tissue hypothesis**" proposed by Leslie Aeillo and Peter Wheeler [5]. It suggested that the increasing brain size of the hominids, through time, required more calories and nutrients. They argue that this larger brain could only be supported by calorically-dense animal tissue rather than low calorie plant foods. Cordain [22] and his research colleagues, further complete this line of thinking, by inferring that the increased brain size of the Hominid would have necessitated the consumption of two specific fatty acids. The first, docosahexaenoic (DHA), and the second, arachidonic acids, both abundantly found in bone marrow and ruminant brains. Broadhurst [11] points out that it is common for all mammals to have a central nervous system that is dependent on a 1:1 ratio of DHA to arachidonic acid to the almost total exclusion of other long chain fatty acids. As a counter argument, these fatty acids can also be easily derived from vegetable oils not just animal fats. Furthermore, Chamberlain [15] stresses the importance that omega-3 fatty acids would have had on the expanding brain and its neurological network. This is a fatty acid abundantly found in plant oils such as flaxseed and soybean oil, in addition to being highly concentrated in fish oils. [87]

The abundant African fauna was likely a very rich supply of meat for the earlier *Homo sapiens* (Pleistocene Hominids) of the Palaeolithic (Old Stone Age) communities. The success of the hunt was dependent on the level of skill and on opportunity. In the beginning, the desire for meat likely originated from easily killed tortoises, lizards, porcupines and small mammals such as squirrels. Eventually, as hunting skills were perfected, larger mammals were pursued and killed.[72]

Here Aeillo and Wheeler (1995)[5] propose the fourth argument in support of the hypothesis that these early Hominids were mostly meat consumers. They advance that the gut size of these Hominid ancestors would have gradually decreased in size to accommodate the transition from plant foods to meats. Aeillo and Wheeler[5] advance that the gut would not have needed to work as hard on a meat diet compared to a mostly plant food diet, which contains a lot of indigestible fibrous components. However, the conclusion that daily subsistence of the early Homo sapiens was meat based, around the middle Palaeolithic period, has been regarded, by experts in the field, as biased and weak. Although sophisticated butchering tools and fauna skeletons, from that period are evident, the more rudimentary tools for processing plants may not be recognizable to the modern archaeologist. Moreover, the absence of organic plant matter, that has long ago decomposed, can lead archaeologist to overzealously conclude that meat was predominant in the diet.[51] Richards[71] writes in his 2002 article, published in the European Journal of Clinical Nutrition:

To summarize, the archaeological record, consisting of stone tools and animal bones, is most likely biased and unrepresentative of the daily subsistence practices of hominids. Our inferences, from what we do have, is of a strongly meat-based subsistence, starting with the appearance of our line, Homo, in Africa, as evidenced by the remains of butchered animals and increasingly sophisticated stone tools.

The problem is that organic plant materials decompose so readily, leaving no artefacts for archaeobotanists to collect from the Palaeolithic period, and thus creating a significant gap in archaeological records. This is in stark contrast to the significant skeletal remains, and cave drawings (**Figure 2.2**) which the zooarchaeologists have access to from that era. It is therefore unreasonable to assume that prehistoric man did strictly rely on land mammals for protein; in fact, it is well known that late Stone Age communities, right up to coastal settlements in Europe and North America, relied on seal meat.[12] The Dorset site of Phillip's Garden in Newfoundland provides evidence that harp seal hunting was a popular activity near the end of the ice Age.[40] As the end of the Pleistocene era drew near, and the Mesolithic period commenced (10,000-6,000 BC), the Ice Age and the dominance of the Mammoth fauna gradually faded, forcing populations, of the periglacial zone of Europe, to not only adapt to faster and smaller mammals, but also to improve fishing skills and bird hunting.[40] Reliance on freshwater fish would have been especially true in South Eastern Europe near the Danube gorge, and also near the Baltics. Indeed, archaeological finds in northern Latvia—The Zvejnieki Stone Age complex—convincingly points to the dependence on freshwater fish as the primary source of protein.[31] Eriksson[31] and colleagues write:

It is clear from the stable isotope analyses that the Zvejnieki people were heavily reliant on freshwater fish until the end of the Early Neolithic, when the consumption of fish declined somewhat, although it still made an important contribution to the diet.

Although the Neolithic period is recognized as the transition to agriculture and animal domestication, it has been argued that earlier domestication would have occurred among the Upper Paleolithic hunter-gatherers. Scant evidence implies that the reindeer, during the upper Palaeolithic period, would have been the first case of domestication.[56] Evidence for the domestication of the dog, between 18,000 and 10,000 BC is very convincing,[56] and would have taken place for companionship[56,42] and to assist man in the hunt[66]. Peri[66] writes:

...these "Paleolithic dogs" were used to haul mammoth meat and recently Shipman hypothesized that they helped humans actively hunt mammoth, leading to their outcompeting Neanderthals

Interestingly, cave drawings of the Neolithic period (~7000 BC) from the at Catal Hüyük site in the Near Orient, support the notion that dogs would have only assisted in the hunt during the Neolithic.[42] By contrast, others have seen no evidence of domestication at any time during the Palaeolithic period.[70]

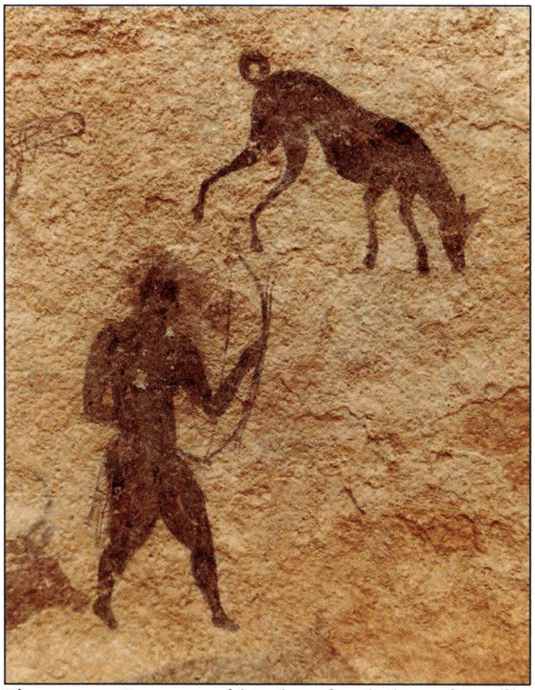

Figure 2.2: Famous prehistoric rock paintings of Tassili N'Ajjer, Algeria. © Pichugin Dmitry/shutterstock.com

Meat and Fish

The archaeological evidence does appear to indicate that small, as opposed to the large, animals, such as tortoises, lizards, porcupines and squirrels, occupied a more prominent position in early man's menu.[12] The love for meat would have begun in this context of easy prey, and would have evolved to larger mammals as hunting techniques were perfected.[79] Even as prehistoric man transitioned to more of a Neolithic period, hunting still persisted. For instance, wealthy Aegean people would have depended on the hunting of wild game like antelope, deer, rabbit, boar and wild goats for protein.[75] Scholars[51] who have analysed the writings of Homer conclude that, while meats and breads would have made up the menu of choice of the Hellenic heroes, but rarely fruits or vegetables, the common folk, by contrast, would have had a sparse diet made up of mostly vegetables and breads—meat in the Aegean era would not have been in abundant supply. Archaeological findings do, in fact, support the understanding that Aegean peasant society would have consumed more vegetables and grains than animal remains; there is but scant evidence in support of chickens in the prehistoric Aegean diet, however wild duck may have enjoyed some popularity. Craik[24] contends that fowl would have likely been cooked privately in homes for individual consumption, but that oxen, lamb, swine and fat goats would have been menu items of choice for public feasts and festivals.

The Neolithic Revolution in Europe, around 10,000-3000 BC,[39] was characterized by the domestication of livestock and the cultivation of specific plants in order to ensure the provision of foodstuffs for a growing population. This was a turning point as the modern man began building fundamental dwellings, and developing a hunting-fishing economy in addition to lithic technology (tools made of stone). Within this growing community context, the modern Hominid began to refine the techniques of grinding, sawing, boring and polishing. Richards[71] argues that the move, from hunter-gatherer to an agricultural-based society, was prompted by severe climate fluctuations that made the once sufficient food supply, suddenly scarce, and not so dependable. The Hominids of the early Palaeolithic period, according to Molleson,[55] would have greatly depended on hunting gazelle in addition to gathering plant foods, in the early Holocene (10,000 BC). At that time, when climate changes and overhunting, began to threaten the availability of these important food sources, these early ancestors to man, by necessity, would have been obliged to domesticate sheep and goats. It would have also been necessary to more heavily process plants in order to produce breads and porridges. In Old Europe, nomadic groups transitioned to sedentism, at which point populations grew in size. This necessitated the planting of crops and the domesticating of animals as food sources. Food became more available, and so the population increased, affecting an inevitable move towards urbanization and crowding conditions. It is at this point, that archaeologists[71] claim that population health began to decline, as evidenced by the prevalence of dental caries in addition to more numerous artefacts of pitted dentition, resulting from poorly ground-up flour. Hence, some scholars propose that once the modern human began to consume porridge and breads in Europe, rice in Asia, and maize in the New World, human health and stature began to deteriorate.

Although domestication of animals, by the Aegean people, such sheep, swine, goats and cattle would have likely been practiced, it would appear that the meats were consumed only on special feasts.[51, 79] Also, the proximity of Aegean people to the sea, should have reasonably translated into abundant supplies of fish contributing to the common diet of the people. Similarly, Cycladic people of the Late Bronze Age in the Aegean Basin (1600-1100 BC), consisting of Mycenean and Minoan people, [6, 63] should have been great vertebrate fish consumers because of their costal proximity, however, write Petroutsa and Manolis: [63]

Isotopic data to date suggests a rather homogeneous diet mainly based on C₃ plant and animal protein. There are no individuals with δ¹³C and δ¹⁵N values that could represent important marine protein intake, despite proximity to the Aegean Sea.

In Neolithic times, there is lasting vestiges of shells that support a dependency on the sea. Nevertheless, considerable evidence supports wheat, barley and beans as having been the staples of the Greek daily menu. This means that for a Greek family, around 3000 BC, right up to around 500 BC, typical daily rations of food would have been the same for both rich and peasant. Their diets would have revolved around, barley paste, barley gruel, or barley flatbread, complemented by some olives, figs and goat's milk cheese with periodic use of salted fish to enhance the savoring experience. Goat, mutton or pork would have been consumed more frequently by the rich, in addition to drinking more wine than water compared to the poor. [79] At around 4000 BC chick peas and lentils were grown in Assyria, and evident in the Greek diet at that time. [12] They would have complemented their diet by bread, mixed with olive oil and goat cheese and served with wine.[49]

There is the possibility that Homeric Greeks may have only considered fish and shellfish as delicacies [24, 51] and thus, were rarely included as part of the regular menu. Vickery [82] proposes that there was likely a prejudice against fish in some regions; there is, for instance, the possibility that near Smyrna, fish would have been seen as not fit to eat. Vickery [82] advances, however, that the long-held belief that Homeric Greeks rarely ate fish may, in fact, be erroneous. Indeed, by the 4th century BC the famous Greek chef, Archestratus, referenced the Athenians' love of dried or salted tuna caught from the Black Sea; he preferentially identifies fresh Byzantium fish as ideal for his dishes. [79] While the Greeks preferred dried and salted tunny, the Romans, greatly involved in fish breeding, preferred wrasse, and engaged in significant fish trade aimed at stocking waters. [12]

For the Greeks and the Romans, it has been argued that fish were mostly looked upon as inedible by the

> While the Greeks preferred dried and salted tunny, the Romans, greatly involved in fish breeding, preferred wrasse, and engaged in significant fish trade aimed at stocking waters

inland populations; the coastal people of the Mediterranean, by contrast, did eat an abundance of fish, although the price of fish would have made it somewhat prohibitive. There is nevertheless a paradox that puts into question the importance of fish in the early Greek diet, and it is this: of the animals that could be eaten by man in the Mediterranean, fish could also eat man; some experts have argued that eating fish therefore, could have been considered a morally ambiguous and reprehensible practice. [69]

Purcell[32] argues that this moral conundrum surrounding the consumption of fish is supported by cultural symbolism associated with fish in antiquity; one of these symbols is "*death,*" argues Berg.[10] Pre-historic Greeks appear to have both a positive and negative impression of fish. Berg writes:

On the one hand, the sea and the animals residing in it are strongly associated with death. On the other hand, the sea's positive dimensions, such as fertility and rebirth, are expressed in conspicuous marine consumption events.

Vickery [82] contends, however, that the spread of Christianity would have brought clarity to this moral ambiguity, and greatly contributed to an increased consumption of fish.

Richards and colleagues [71] also write about the Atlantic coastal regions of Europe, during the late Mesolithic period, greatly relying on marine fish as their main source of protein.

Dairy Products

In Neolithic communities, the domestication of animals, such as goats, cows and pigs, led to the consumption of goat and cow's milk, and milk products, dating back to the Ur (2900 BC). More recently, Charlton [16] uncovered evidence of milk consumption as early as 4000-2400 BC among farmers in Britain, using lactoglobulin proteins embedded in the teeth plaque. Given the abundance of goats, archaeologists are of the opinion that Ancient Greek society likely consumed mostly goat milk.[82] The Scythians, by contrast, who were a group of nomadic tribes that roamed the grassy steppes of Eurasia, between 700 and 300 BC, drank reindeer and elk milk.[12]

Butter probably occurred by accident with the transportation of milk over long distances. It is not clear if butter was used in Egypt, although a fatty-like substance, resembling butter, was found in mummified remains. Archaeologists are however certain that butter played an important role in the Mesopotamian Civilization, which began around 3500 BC. It is quite certain that Northern European tribes extensively used butter, which was easily produced because of the colder Northern climate.[12]

In 1500 BC, biblical writings, of the time of Abraham, also confirm the familiarity of the Israelites with butter, whereas Classical Greece and Rome did not appear to use butter because of the preponderance of olive oil in those regions.

The consumption of sour milk, curds and cheese was likely widespread, covering Mesopotamia, Egypt, Palestine as well as Greece and the Roman Empire. The first cheese-making in Greece and Crete likely took place during the end of the Neolithic and start of the Bronze Age as evidenced by pottery cheese strainers.[12]

Honey and Cane Sugar
Early Stone Age paintings in caves provide evidence of an early interest in honey. Archaeo-botanists contend that most hominin species would have had seasonal access to honey as the preferred concentrated sugar.[19] The earliest record of honey is from Mesopotamia (3000 BC), although it would seem that date syrup held a more prevalent place in the diet.[12] The Maasai, an East African people, would have relied on a pastoral diet consisting of meat, milk and blood, strictly restricting vegetables from the diet, but giving significant importance to honey in the diet.[7] Maasai warriors of East Africa use to strictly rely on honey as their sole source of food during their long journeys.[7] Its popularity grew, to such an extent, that it became the main source of sugar for the Egyptians, Greeks and Romans. The earliest practice of beekeepers can be traced back to Egypt sometime between 2560-2420 BC.[12] Many times in the Bible, notably in the Book of Kings ~550BC: (2Kings: 18-32), honey is referred to as a part of the common diet:

Until I come and take you away to a land like your own land, a land of grain and wine, a land of bread and vineyards, a land of olive trees and honey, that you may live, and not die.

Again in around 750BC Isaiah 7:15: *He shall eat curds and honey when he knows how to refuse the evil and choose the good.* To a lesser degree, sweetness in food preparations was also provided from dates, figs, grapes, sweet oils from the palm, and sugary sap from trees.[12]

Greece, Crete, Cyprus and Palestine would have inherited the practice of beekeeping. Greek mythology makes a reference to honey and milk being fed to Zeus. By the time Aristotle (384-322 BC) refers to the honey as a medicinal agent, beekeeping in Greece has already been established since the 8th century BC. It is clear that honey remained the main sweetener of foods for the Greeks, Romans and Egyptians, despite grapes, figs and dates occupying, it would seem, but occasional substitutes.[12]

The plant species of sugarcane originated in New Guinea and began to spread worldwide with the beginning of massive human migration at around 8000 BC.[9] Sugar juice extraction from the cane possibly originated in India early on in prehistory (500 BC),[12] and was used as a drink. There is some evidence that India began to synthesize sugar crystals, between 400 and 600 AD, likely only to flavor spices for some kind of a milk curd recipe popular in India and Persia.[9] Between 200-300BC historical records confirm that sugarcane was just getting introduced to the Western world. The observations of Pliny the elder (21-77 AD) reveal that sugar cane in his time was primarily used as a medicine. While honey was initially the sweetener of choice, it was used along with sugar up until AD 300—by this time sugar and honey were equally popular as a sweetener for 700 years—after which time the role of honey was reserved only for rituals and etiquette in gatherings of social or political importance.[12]

The actual cultivation of the sugarcane in Mediterranean Europe did not take place until after the arrival of the Moors in Spain around the 8th century, but even then it the cane was often chewed and the juice extracted from the cane was not added to food, but strictly used as a medicine.[12] The Moors became the primary vector for disseminating sugarcane throughout the West beginning in Morocco, Sicily and Spain between 800 and 1000 AD, having already establish centers in Egypt and Palestine as early as 750 AD. Spain eventually became the pivotal export center of the sugarcane plant back to North Africa and to the New World. The Mediterranean region, right up to the 13th century, became heavily focused in perfecting sugarcane agriculture with experimentation. [33] The winters in the northern Mediterranean regions shortened the growing season resulting in a lower quality sugarcane that eventually could not compete with the tropical areas of the New World. [33]

Europeans began refining cane sugar around the 15th century in Venice, [12] thanks to the invention of the Trappetum by Pietro Speciale, [9] described as a three-roller sugarcane mill, a technical advancement contested by some scholars [24b, 9] who advance that Brazilian inventors were the true originators of the device. Nevertheless, this new milling technology was responsible for reviving the sugar industry in Venice up until the sugar cane production in the Americas outperformed the poorer quality Mediterranean plant. [33] The use of white sugar as a sweetener did not occur until the popularization of coffee and tea in England by the 17th century. [12]

Coffee and Tea
Coffee and Tea were two significant products that greatly influenced many cultures. Coffee is of particular interest in light of the extent of its worldwide consumption. There are, however, various conflicting historical accounts about the origins of the coffee bean and the drink itself, thus making, even the most popularly accepted claims, unreliable. The first appearance of the coffee plant was reported in Kaffa, a specific region of Ethiopia, around the 6th century AD [65] and perhaps as late as the 9th century.[85] The most popularly reported account revolves around Ethiopian shepherds noticing that when their goats ate the berries, from this strange bush, they would not sleep at night. Legend has it that the Ethiopians likely had, not long after in the region of Kaffa, begun to chew the berries, and then brew both the leaves and the berries in hot water, so as to experience their stimulating effect. A somewhat popular treat, for the Galla tribe, was to make the berries into a paste by mixing it with animal fat, and then eating it.[65] Later on, perhaps by the 8th century, the coffee plant was intentionally grown, and the bean adopted, into the main stream culture in one form or another.[65]

The Ethiopian coffee plant was then likely brought to Yemen, Saudi Arabia, by Arab traders around AD 900, thus the origin of the *Arabica* genus. This transition seems historically accurate, as Rhazes, an Arabian physician, makes some mention of coffee in official 10th century writings.[65]

The practice of roasting, grinding and brewing the grounds in water to make the coffee beverage, likely began in the Yemini city of Mocha around the 14th or early 15th century.[76, 85] A popular story recounts how, nearby *Sufi* monks, began to boil the berries and leaves in hot water, immediately discovering that the beverage was beneficial in sustaining them in night prayer vigils.[76, 85] One monk, disturbed by the excitability of the drink, threw the branches of the coffee plant into the fire, claiming the berries to be evil. It is at that point that he noticed an attractive smell emanating from the burnt berries in the fire. Several monks, who had gathered to appreciate the aroma, took the roasted berries (**Figure 2.3**) and began to ground them in order to make an improved beverage.[76]

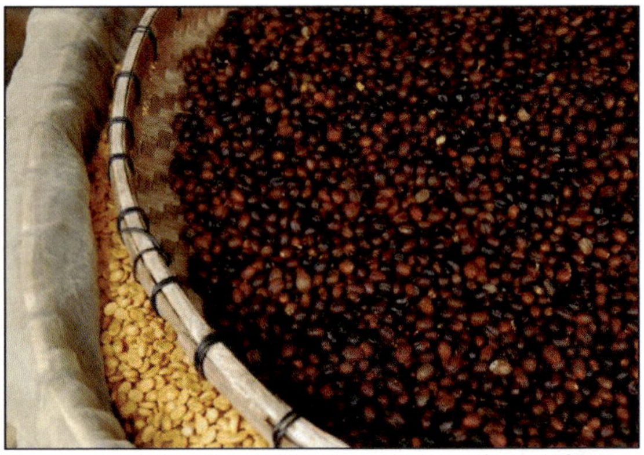

Figure 2.3: Ethiopian Coffee Beans © JoanChang/ Shutterstock.com

It eventually became a much appreciated beverage, by the Arab world, as well as a heavily guarded secret. In 1536, the Turkish Ottoman Empire, occupied Yemen, and so coffee beans were exported, from the Yemini port of Mocha, to numerous Turkish territories such as North Africa, Egypt, Turkey and Persia, around the end of the 15th Century. [65] Not long after, the first coffee houses began to spring up in Constantinople. Recognizing how lucrative coffee exports could become by 1600, the Ottoman empire, wanting to maintain the exclusive monopoly of its distribution, decided to only ship infertile coffee beans—the Turks boiled the beans to prevent germination—to warehouses in Alexandria, Egypt, and from there, Venetian traders brought the beans back to Italy in 1600. Shortly after, in 1616, coffee houses had already become popular in Venice; similarly, they spread to France by 1644, then to England and Vienna by 1650.[85] North America had its first taste of coffee in 1668, as a cargo of coffee beans travelled, with Captain John Smith, to Jamestown. Around the early 17th century, Yemen lost the exclusivity of the coffee plant, as pilgrims to Mecca, began to bring back intact beans to places like India and Indonesia, in order to develop their own sustainable coffee plantations.[85] Also, during the 17th century, the Dutch controlled shipping trade, throughout the world, and were very dominant in the East Indies. Their navy was larger than France's, England's and Italy's, combined.[49] It was inevitable, that Dutch ships would also get hold of coffee trees, which they shipped back to Amsterdam in 1616, and then transplanted to Java, Sumatra, Timor and Bali, where coffee plantations have flourished ever since.[65]

Tom Standage, an historian and author of *The History of the World in Six Glasses,* [76] argues that it was the use of coffee in the 17th Century that inspired the Enlightenment period. He writes:

The impact of the introduction of coffee into Europe during the seventeenth century was particularly noticeable since the most common beverages of the time, even at breakfast, were weak 'small beer' and wine. ... Those who drank coffee instead of alcohol began the day alert and stimulated, rather than relaxed and mildly inebriated, and the quality and quantity of their work improved. ... Western Europe began to emerge from an alcoholic haze that had lasted for centuries.

Tea, Camellia Thea, is indigenous to China; the origin of tea drinking varies depending on whether you listen to Chinese, Indian or Japanese legends. Nevertheless, history accurately describes tea as the favorite drink of China, by the 5th and 6th Centuries AD. At that time, the leaves were made into cakes and boiled using rice, ginger, salt, orange peel, pine kernels, milk, walnuts and onions.

The practice of steeping the leaves into hot water did not begin until the 15th Century Ming Dynasty. Europeans finally began the tradition via the Dutch traders in 1610.[76]

2.2 Nutrition and Health: Historical Role of Food in Human Health and Disease

The oldest document in existence that represent a reliable historical record of disease is the Ebers Papyrus dating back to 1552 BC. It clearly describes conditions such as depression, dementia, and heart disease, and is concerned about the diagnosis of pregnancy, skin conditions, intestinal diseases and parasites to name a few. However the remedies for this conditions are almost entirely wrapped up in magical formulas and incantations. [74] For this reason, historians, interested in the history of Medicine, write primarily about the Classical Greek period beginning roughly around 500 BC. Hippocrates (460-375 BC), Plato (427-347 BC), Socrates (470-399 BC), and Aristotle (384-322 BC) were very significant figures in shaping Western traditional thought, but it was Hippocrates and Aristotle who set the foundation for Western Medicine. [74] It is important to note that philosophy, at that time, was an essential discipline in the physician's formation, allowing conclusions to be drawn on the basis of logic and common sense, rather than superstitions. Sallam [74] writes:

In the field of medicine, physicians were always described as philosophers-physicians and medical knowledge thrived under these circumstances.

Hippocrates, considered the father of Medicine, provided the foundation to the discipline of Medicine, a knowledge base and an ethic of practice, compiled in the *Hippocratic Corpus*, which were to last right until modern times. He taught that the doctor's place was at the bedside of the patient, and that the lifestyle of a patient, which included diet, be closely documented. He writes: [46]

In the same way, he (doctor) must observe how men live, what they like, what they eat and what they drink, whether or not they take physical exercise or are idle and gross. All this a doctor must know; in order to understand local complaints and be in a position where he can prescribe suitable treatments."

Diet, in the Classical Greek period, was promoted by the doctor as a sensible approach to disease prevention and correction. Plato in his document, The Timaeus, argues that balance is integral to achieving a state of "wellbeing". He writes:[67]

The only way, in fact, in which good health can be maintained, is for replacement and waste to be uniform, similar, and of the same scale; any trespass beyond these limits in the process will give rise to all kinds of change, and to endless disease and deteriorations.

Specific foods were therefore prescribed with the intention of realigning the imbalances. Hippocratic authors further define disease as arising from the biological imbalances of the four humors (**Figure 2.4**): blood, phlegm, black bile and yellow bile. [74] This was a formidable departure from conventional thinking which ascribed to the notion that all diseases were from God. This mystical influence of the deities on disease can, in fact, be traced back to Egypt. [74, 67]

Hippocrates introduced the importance of making objective medical observations, and of finding natural causes and treatments; he discouraged the practice of attributing illnesses to supernatural origins.[51]

Aristotelian medical theory advanced that disease originated from 3 basic causes which impacted the humors: First, excesses or deficiencies whether they be in diet, drink or exercise; second, from violent causes such as wounds, trauma, or extreme fatigue; and third, atmospheric conditions which, it was believed, could predispose the individual to disease. The notion that disease could be explained by 4 humors (Figure 2.4) stemmed from the pre-Socratic philosopher, Empedocles of Agrigentum (500-430BC) who advanced that the entire universe could be explained by the 4 elements of water, fire, earth and air. There was a big picture of universal organization and symmetry that was drawn from this Empedoclean model, which was seen as the root of all things.[51] And so, nature and man appeared to be intertwined, connected to the four seasons, and the four characteristics of these seasons: cold, hot, moist, and dry (Figure 2.4).

These natural systems were based on the principles of balance, and thus offered a rational structure that accommodated the idea that there were inherent dangers associated with excesses or clear deficiencies. He derived maxims that were grounded in common sense, enduring and eventually shaped modern Medicine. For instance, he stated that all excesses therapeutically require measures to deplete or diminish the excess. Hippocrates writes: [67]

Diseases that are generated by repletion are cured by depletion, and all which arise from deplete on are cured by repletion; all which arises from exertion are cured by inactivity and all which arises from inactivity is cured by exertion

Socrates also refers to the essentiality of food in replacing water and heat losses, a concept of balance greatly advocated by the Greek Masters. Consistent with this idea of equilibrium, Plato, in the Timaeus, [67] describes the origins of disease from four perspectives: first, as an imbalance between 4 elements: fire, water, earth and air. It was understood that any excesses or deficiencies in these elements would result in changes in the cold, hot, moist, and dry properties of the body, thus affecting the humors, and leading invariably to disease (Figure 2.4).

Plato then describes diseases of the "secondary formations" when there is insufficient food or drink to replenish the blood; the consequence is disease resulting from disturbances in marrow, bone, flesh, sinew and blood, consequently leading to *anemia, diabetes, and heart disease* (Figure 2.4).

> Hippocrates introduced the importance of making objective medical observations, and of finding natural causes and treatments; he discouraged the practice of attributing illnesses to supernatural origins

Conceptually, Plato writes of a decomposition or catabolic breakdown of flesh, and of blood changing to a black discharge in deficient diets, typically representative of constipation and stomach ulcers (Figure 2.4). It is interesting that one method of recognizing stomach ulcers in contemporary Medicine is black tarry stools called *melena*. In a similar way, yellow bile can be a symptom of jaundice or gallstones (Figure 2.4).

A third origin of disease is considered from breath, phlegm, and bile. Here Plato recognizes the importance of lung diseases resulting in coughs, colds and asthma (figure 2.4) and of the transformation of body fluids during the disease processes as visible signs of the loss of body balance. Fourth, he accepts the notion that diseases can be caused by the soul and mind, and stresses the importance of balance between mind and body for achieving health.

UNDERSTANDING THE HUMORS & RELATIONSHIPS TO DISEASE		
BLOOD	HEART DISEASE, ANGINA, NOSE-BLEEDS, ANEMIA, DIABETES	HOT / WET
YELLOW BILE	GALLSTONES, JAUNDICE, MIGRAINES	HOT / DRY
BLACK BILE	CONSTIPATION, STOMACH ULCERS	COLD / DRY
PHLEGM	ASTHMA, COUGHS, COLDS, BRONCHITIS, DISEASES OF THE LUNGS	COLD / WET

Figure 2.4 The Graphic Representation of the 4 humors. Permission granted from St-Jude Nutrition Medical Communications. Figure adapted from writings published in Irwin, 1947.

It is surprising that the Ancient Greek Masters conceived such principles as "biological balance" and "co-dependency of mind and bodily disease", for they devised their paradigms from rational thought and observations rather than from experimentation; the dissection of animal and human remains was strictly forbidden by Greek society.

Although their beliefs were somewhat rooted in some element of truth in so far as there were homeostatic (equilibrium) mechanisms in the body, it is clear that the Masters' understanding of the pathophysiology of diseases was fundamentally flawed.

The belief that nutrition was an integral part of an individual's health, or for that matter, of the collective health, was certainly understood and practised in the Classical Period, and seemed to be advocated within a paradigm of balance and temperance.

Elizabeth Craik, a reputed British Classics scholar, who teaches at the University of Saint Andrews, writes about Hippocratic balance, describing it in terms of a balance for the individual's physical condition, and elements in diet and in food.[23] The physicians understood that balance for the individual was dependent on routines for eating frequencies and on types of foods that varied with seasons, customs and geography.

The idea that what we are, conditions what we should eat, was central to the belief that our biology basically commands what we should be eating; not providing what it needed was seen as problematic. This physical balance referred to a needed equilibrium in body function, which was achievable so long as excesses in food intake were balanced with abstinence, and increases in weight gains were tempered by weight loss.

The Greek writings speak of "Diaita" or of a regimen, as a way of living with a specific focus on diet, exercise, baths and emetics.[24] It had a strong therapeutic meaning, quite unlike the notion of nourishment or "trophe" which was more akin to food. Diet and food were thus seen as distinct. However, for the Hippocratic physician, the idea of diet was not at all tied to enjoyment, nor to anything attractive or good-tasting, but more to a regimented austerity. Foods and concoctions were prescribed without any practical preparation or cooking guidelines; these food and plant mixtures were purely medicinal in nature. Diet and medicines were, in fact, considered of equal importance by Greek and Roman physicians in battling the diseases of the time.[24] In Oribasios' *Medical Complications*,[35] a recipe for insomnia, written by Dieuches—a 3rd Century BC physician—illustrates that the poppy seed was well known in Ancient Greece to have soporific properties:

It is sufficient to put into a pint and a half of the finest and ripest barley four and a half pints of milk and water, in the proportion of two-thirds of milk to one-third of water, and the head of a poppy that has been toasted; and after mixing in by the fire one tenth of an ounce of pounded figs, boil the ingredients together, and serve after cooking to the consistency of soup; it provides some respite and also sleep for those who are convalescent.[35]

Similarly, a mixture of cheese, barley and poppy seeds was prescribed by Hippocrates in order to displace the womb. A plant called *asafetida*, was also commonly used to control flatulence and indigestion.

The critical step in understanding the transfer of Greek medical knowledge to Europe, is the invasion of Egypt by Alexander the Great around 331 BC and the subsequent construction of Alexandria. Indeed as the city Alexandria grew in size, so it did also in importance—becoming second only to Rome. It was after the construction of the great Library and museum of Alexandria by Ptolemy-I that the works of Aristotle, brought over to Alexandria by both Alexander and Ptolemy-I—both were students of Aristotle—were included in the Library. [74] After the University of Alexandria was built—the first university of knowledge in the world—Greek philosophers began to converge on Alexandria, teaching the principles of Aristotelean medical theory. The school of medicine remained active until the fall of Alexandria around 300 AD and the subsequent burning of the Alexandria Library in 391 AD. [74]

Early on, before the end of Alexandria, Claudius Galen (AD 129-199), born in Pergamum, Greece had studied medicine at the University of Alexandria, learning the Aristotelean principles which were to make him a great medical physician. He then travelled to Rome where he became a surgeon to the gladiators and eventually the physician of Emperor Marcus Aurelius. His fame grew as he expanded his study of animal dissections—a practice that was not permitted in Ancient Greece.[52] Considered a Giant in the history of Western Medicine, he ventured forward with scientific queries, moving beyond the confining limits of dialectics, but remained nevertheless loyal to the teachings of Hippocrates and other ancient Greek thinkers, thus promulgating through his writings, fundamentally inaccurate precepts that went unchallenged all through the Dark Ages (5th to the 8th century), and into the early period of the Renaissance around the 14th century. He wrote about four hundred treatises during the apex of the Roman Empire and was acclaimed as a gifted diagnostician. [51]

Galen embraced Hippocratic medicine and the doctrine of the four humours (blood, phlegm, yellow bile and black bile), deciding to formulate treatments based on the principle of opposites. For instance, a patient with fever was thought to result from excessive yellow bile and to be in the element of fire, thus necessitating the consumption of cool liquids and foods.

Galen was, however, not permitted, by the Christian Church, to dissect human corpses for the sake of a precise study of anatomy and of the pathophysiology of the disease; the Church considered such a practice disrespectful towards God and the dead. He consequently wrote 16 books on human anatomy, which were based on inferences made from animal anatomy (mostly monkeys) that were erroneous in many cases. The main problem was that none of Galen's anatomical findings could be verified, nor could there be independent and innovative breakthroughs in physiology and pathology (the study of disease). The absence of challenges to Galen's medical treatise precipitated medical science into a slow and long decline.

The Dark Ages, which historically began in 415AD with the murder by marauding crowds of the great Alexandrian philosopher and mathematician, *Hypatia*, was characterized by an almost total absence of scientific progress. No significant findings or changes in practices were added to the Classical Greek doctrines of Medicine. This period of medical and not to mention, intellectual stagnation, lasted for about one thousand years. Carl Voit refers to this period as:

...intellectually barren, during which only a blind imitation of the old and senseless scholasticism prevailed....there were not enough new facts to create new ideas. Satisfaction was sought in acute dialectics.

Although there were no advancements in knowledge, this became the period of Monastic Preservation of scientific information (AD 400-1100) as well as a period of Monastic Scholasticism (AD 1100-1300) supported mostly by the Catholic Church. Sallam writes: [74]

Meanwhile in Europe, some of this work was preserved and/or translated from Greek or Arabic to Latin by various Christian monks and physicians, most notably St Isidore of Seville (560-636), St Benedict of Nursia (480-547), Cassiodorus (490-573), Bertharius of Monte Cassino (810-883), Walafrid Strabo of Reichenau (808-849), St Hildegarde (1099-1179) and Marbodus of Angers, Bishop of Rennes (1035-1123).

2.3 Nutritional Deficiencies and Famines in Ancient Societies

Since the Neolithic Revolution, some 8000 years ago, the human diet has been founded on simple food habits, consisting of a wide diversity of cereals, fish, domesticated animals, fruits and vegetables. Despite the availability of a broad but simple diet, nutritional deficiencies were still fairly common in some populations. Vitamin A deficiency causing night blindness was documented in an Egyptian medical treatise named the *Ebers Papyrus* that dates back to 1600 BC, in which the recommended treatment was ox liver. [12]

A similar treatment was also found in Hippocrates' writings, in Roman texts, and in Galenic prescriptions, as well as in Chinese literature dated AD 610. (Brotwell and Brothwell, 1998). Thanks to pioneering work by Wald in the 1930s, we now understand that night vision requires the presence of vitamin A in the eye pigment, rhodopsin, and that liver is a rich source of vitamin A. [28] What is clear is that ancient civilizations comprehended that diet could play a therapeutic function in curing diseases.

Other nutritional diseases like Beriberi, which resulted from thiamine deficiency, was also documented in China during a nine month siege of the city of Tsai Chseng around AD 529; there is evidence that the deficiency may well have been known in China as far back as 1000 BC, [12] although the evidence is less convincing. It wasn't until the 19th Century that it became clear that meat and whole grains could cure the symptoms of Beriberi. [8]

Rickets, a disease resulting in the bowing of the long bones—the consequence of vitamin D deficiency—caused insufficient calcification of the bone matrix. The earliest signs of rickets in skeletal remains were unearthed in Denmark, during the Neolithic Age. [12] Rickets seems, however, to have occurred quite infrequently among the early populations of China, Scandinavia, and Egypt, as evidenced by archaeological findings of the last century, which uncovered a small number of slightly bowed long and pelvic bones. This was not an unexpected finding, given the abundant fish oils and fish consumed by these populations. [12]

The frequency of bowed legs seems, however, to have increased in first and second Century Rome because of poor child-rearing practices, which involved keeping the children indoors and away from the sun more than they should have. Considering the abundance of fruits and vegetables, available to most hunting and collecting communities, it would have been quite unusual to find cases of vitamin C deficiency until after the Neolithic revolution. Hippocrates does document a condition involving the bleeding and ulceration of the gums, typical of scurvy.[12]

More threatening than some of the nutritional deficiencies, were the famines, which wiped out large segments of the populations. There were numerous famines documented in Egypt many of which were caused, according to early Egyptian texts, by detrimental climactic changes, frequent flooding of the Nile, and the destruction of food. Significant as well was the influence of political strife on poor farming practices, the impact of overpopulation, the devastation of disease, and the collapse of food distribution systems—usual in war-torn countries. [12]

A famous 7 year famine, depicted at the causeway of Unas at Saqquara Egypt, showed a scene of severely malnourished people, which would have taken place during the Third Dynasty. [12]

Between the years 100 BC and AD 1910, China would have experienced more than 1800 famines, and the British Isles, a total of 200 famines between the years AD 10 and 1850. In Mesoamerica, between 1451 and 1456, storms, frosts would have caused crop shortages and subsequent malnutrition. [12] In 1505, just prior to the small pox epidemic hitting the Aztecs in 1521, famine caused widespread devastation, arguably making the population more vulnerable [61] to the diseases brought to the continent by Hernando Cortés and his Spanish troops. Cortés' men decimated 75% of the Aztec population. [58] Together with the military assaults, most of the population was effectively wiped out, leading to important food shortages which led to malnutrition among the Aztecs. [12, 61] Historians have clearly recognized the impact of the epidemics in the success of Cortés' military campaign against the Aztecs. They write:

The other two epidemics, of smallpox (1545–1548) and typhus (1576–1581) killed up to 75 percent of the population of Mesoamerica. The population before the time of the conquest is estimated at 15 million; by 1550, the estimated population was 4 million and less than 2 million by 1581. Whole towns disappeared, lands were deserted, roads were closed, and armies were destroyed. The "New Spain" of the sixteenth century was an unpopulated country and most Mesoamerican cultures were wiped out. [58]

Cortés' defeat of the Aztecs was so extensive that their labor intensive agricultural system—artificial floating islands called *chinampas* [58]—could not survive such an extensive slaughter of their workforce.

Plant diseases, in human history, were also responsible for major crop failures, such as rust disease in cereals; Aristotle (384-322 BC) recorded yearly variations of rust disease, which he attributed to warmth and moisture. [12]

The Roman Empire began to decline between the second and fifth centuries AD because of barbarian attacks on an immense Roman territory, widespread poverty and oppression of minorities, private and public corruption, and a series of ravaging plagues and epidemics. These slowly ate away at the fiber of a powerful Empire. The plagues were often carried by invaders and by Roman armies, returning from war, causing alarming death rates in the general population.[49]

The term "plague" described a multitude of conditions and diseases with high death rates such as smallpox, scarlet fever, cholera, typhus and diphtheria, for which there were no cures. Within this terrible context of human suffering and devastation, arose a new meaning to life, which was grounded in the mystical beliefs of Christianity.[61] Indeed, the idea of redemptive suffering, espoused by the early Christians, resurfaced in this time of human despair, and gave hope to a downtrodden populace. The Church taught that the individual could unite his suffering with that of Jesus on the cross, becoming, as it were, complicit with Christ, in the salvation of humankind, through which he could share in the redemption of mankind by his suffering in the Church. (Cf. Colossians 1:24).

Individuals began to put more trust in mystical cures, achieved by anointing the sick with holy oil, prayer and the laying of hands. Christianity also promulgated the moral obligation of helping the sick; it argued that caring for the sick was a duty, and was thus responsible for the building of hostels, which eventually became hospitals. The first great Christian hospital was established by St Basil, at Caesarea in AD 370.[49]

Among the many plagues that pillaged the Roman Empire, none were more effective and decisive, in provoking the rapid Roman demise, than the pandemic plague of 542-543 A.D during the reign of the emperor Justinian. [84] Medicine was essentially powerless in stopping the human devastation.

The rational and deductive reasoning, typically assigned to science, was no match to the pestilence that was killing so many people. Witchcraft, magic and Christian mysticism became alternatives for a population that began to mistrust medical science, which was still stagnating in the Greek doctrines of the humors, and limited to the examination of body fluids such as blood, urine and sputum. [61]

The death rates were exceedingly high during this apocalyptic era of plagues and epidemics, and Medicine crumbled under the weight of its inadequacy. The Christian Church, in contrast, increased in popularity—for a time—because it regarded caring for the sick a moral obligation of its people, thus discouraging the emergence of doctors as paid professionals. [61] Historical records confirm that the rise of Christianity in the early centuries played a significant role in introducing a moral standard to caring for the sick. Buklijas writes: [13]

While institutions providing some form of medical treatment existed in ancient Greece and Rome, neither of these cultures organized community care for the sick, poor, and needy. A radical change occurred in the late Antiquity, with the rise of Christianity, which embraced charity as one of its basic doctrines. The first hospitals were founded when Christianity became the state religion of the Roman Empire.

By the Middle Ages (476 to late 15th century), Europe had been struck by successive wars, epidemics and famines, which carried a terrible price of human suffering. The Benedictine order had instituted, by the 8th-9th centuries, many monastic infirmaries and hospitals which were thriving during the Crusades (1095-1492 AD) [13] and which used medicines, prepared by the monks from the plants and herbs grown in their gardens, to treat the sick.[49]

Throughout the middle Ages, hundreds of hospitals, founded by the Benedictines on the principle of Christian charity, emerged all over Europe in an attempt to care for the victims of leprosy and various other epidemics. Historical documents confirmed the existence of about two hundred hospitals throughout England and Scotland, and over two thousand all around France. Those monks devoted to Medicine eventually emerged from the confinement of their monasteries to make home visits; they became recognised as healers, and their popularity grew.[49]

The Church, meanwhile, began to frown at the practice of Medicine by its religious brothers, because they were breaking the rule of the monastic order, by exposing themselves to the temptations of the world. Pope Honorius III (1215-1222) eventually forbade the clergy from practising Medicine, leaving a very dormant lay medical profession to rise from somnolence to treat the sick.[52]

The laity tried to claim ownership over the domain of Medicine, founding in 1220 the first faculty of Medicine in Montpellier, France. It was Europe's first medical school, but this early version of medical education offered very little in terms of new science; its knowledge base was still shaped by the many inaccuracies of Claudius Galen's translation of the classical Greek masters. Indeed, once the many translations of Aristotle's writings were translated from Greek the teachings of Aristotelean medical principles became the foundations of the first secular medical schools. Sallam writes:[74]

The most famous of these were the medical school of Salerno (Scuola Medica Salernitana founded in the 9th century), the University of Bologna (founded in 1088), Oxford University (founded c. 1096), the University of Paris (founded c. 1165), Cambridge University (founded in 1209), the University of Montpellier (founded in 1220), the University of Padua (founded in 1222) and the University of Naples (founded in 1224).

It was the Salerno School of Medicine, founded in the 10th century, which was the oldest of the modern world and recognized at the forerunner to the model of modern universities. It subsequently became a government-sponsored academy under the rule of Frederick II in 1224 AD,[26] requiring that all those who desire to practice Medicine be trained by the great masters at Salerno. Certainly, Salerno's influence grew substantially, between the 11th and 13th centuries, under the influence of Benedictine monasticism. Indeed, translations of the Greek classics in the 12th century by the monk, *Constantinus Africanus*, significantly broadened the school's knowledge base.[64] Hence, from this school a more credible physician began to emerge. Consequently, lay Medicine resurfaced in the social fabric, and doctors organized themselves into professional bodies, which were protected by law.[52]

This reorganization allowed the status of the medical physician to grow, but Medicine was still held hostage by the old teachings of the school of Salerno, and so advances in Medicine were still greatly hindered. Situated at the bottom of the medical hierarchy was the barber-surgeon, whose activities were mostly focussed around blood-letting, tooth extractions, treating and cauterizing wounds, lancing abscesses and applying ointments.[52]

It was however, during the Renaissance (13th-17th centuries) that universities became more grounded in Aristotelean principles and universities distinguished themselves as, *religious* or *free*.[74] Why this fascination with old Greek medical theory? The scholars left Greece as the Turks conquered Constantinople in 1453; they fled to Italy, bringing with them the writings of Plato and Hippocrates. In its romantic fascination with the classics, European culture ensnared Medicine in old age thinking and beliefs that were still rooted in the middle Ages. Many hospitals, originally founded by religious orders like the Sisters of Mercy opened the door not only to the sick but also the poor, abandoned children, and travellers.[13] In this period, writes Buklijaz,

Hospitals preserved both the symbolic and material link to the Church and religion, based on the idea that the body and the soul were closely connected and mutually influenced.

Hospitals eventually moved to the cities, having fallen under the auspices of public authorities,[13] who oversaw the wealthy civic coffers. Buklijas writes:

Italian merchant urban communes, such as Florence, Padua, and Venice, spearheaded urbanization and partial secularization of hospitals, which were being increasingly established by local governments, confraternities, and rich individuals.

They loosened up the purse strings for the building, expansion and renovation of urban hospitals. This new kind of hospital-directed patronage resulted in the creation of the famous Hôtel-Dieu in Paris, the Santo Spirito in Rome and St. Bartholomew's and St. Thomas' in London.[49] However, it is of historical significance to point out that the original Hôtel-Dieu hospital in Paris was founded in the 7th century by St. Landry, the bishop of Paris, making it the first religious-based hospital in the West, and the oldest hospital in the Western world. It was subsequently demolished for renovations in 1184. [59]

However, despite the revival of learning and the foundation of such great universities as Cambridge (1229) and Oxford (1249), the science of Medicine was not moving ahead rapidly; progress was not taking place, and the significance of this stagnation soon impacted on a society devastated by great famines, and the second pandemic in the Christian era: the bubonic plague. [61]

2.4 The Famines and Great Plague of the Late Middle-Ages

The medical doctrines and medicinal practices had very little to offer a population faced with the devastating famines that ploughed through Europe from 1308 to 1332. Food was so scarce that people were forced to rely on dogs and cats to fill their cooking pots. When food became even more difficult to obtain, they ate dove excrement and even children.[49]

The years 1250 to 1270 represented a period abundant births and booming economic growth that drove up the quality of life all over the Europe. It was a period that also foster urbanization. In fact, between 1086 and 1300s the population in England doubled and the urbanites grew from 10 percent to 15-20 percent of the population. The cities became the hub of agricultural markets. [73] Deforested lands gave way to numerous farms, which painted a new European landscape and drove a strong agricultural economy. However, by 1300, over farmed lands became underproductive and a downturn in the economy was further precipitated by a mini Ice Age. [45] The winters were particularly cold, and the summers, wet and cool, conditions unfavourable for a rich harvest—the harvest of 1315 was the poorest in memory. [45] Food became scarce and hyperinflation made prices beyond the reach of the peasants. Malnutrition became a widespread problem, as people lived in misery. [45] Mass hysteria drove crowds of hungry people to attack condemned prisoners in the gallows and hack away at their flesh. The numerous deaths that arose from these famines were often seen as provoked by the wrath of God or Satan. Hence, priests and witches were, in fact, perceived as the most effective healers because they claimed to know how to appease such a wrath by urging confessions and prayers. They also claimed to possess an empirical knowledge of sacred plants, which they used in medications.[61]

The witches were close to the earth, and with their potions, were seemingly capable of appeasing the perceived devastating evil spells. The popularity of witchcraft continued up until the seventeenth century despite the emergence of 17 medical schools by the fourteenth century. Faith in magic and miracles became even more strongly embedded in human belief, as Europe witnessed Medicine's inability to control, ever so slightly, the scourge of pneumonic and bubonic plagues that visited the continent first, between 1358-1351, wiping out roughly 24 million people, and second, in 1362 and again in 1369, killing primarily children.[61]

The plague continued its infectious roaming, but with less virulence, for the following 100 years up to approximately 1469, killing about 13% of every new generation. The historical medieval documents that describe these times, speak of intolerable levels of human suffering and fear. The plague made several visits before its final retreat from Europe in 1720, hitting Venice in 1575 and in 1630—killing one third of its population. It then visited Marseille in 1720, decimating 80,000 people (**Figure-2.4**). The only truly effective and honest advice that could be given at the time to diminish a person's chances of contracting the plague is described in Nikiforuk's *The Fourth Horseman*: [61]

Flee quickly, go far, come back slowly

Despite the overwhelming evidence that no effective remedy existed that could change the deadly path of the plague, physicians, still limited by restrictive and archaic knowledge as well as by practices and remedies that held little therapeutic value, persisted in dispensing medical treatments and advice. The most popular antidotes included: (a) consuming figs with two filberts; (b) the avoidance of lettuce; (c) chewing food slowly and leaving the table hungry. Light wine mixed with spring water was encouraged as a way to keep the body cool and able to fight disease. None of these antidotes worked, of course, which discredited the physicians. In fact, the doctors' plague remedies, if anything, were more likely to bring death on more rapidly.[61]

So drastic was Medicine's approaches at trying to curb the relentless scourge of the plague, that physicians would recommend drinking liquid gold depending on the phase of the moon. It is certainly arguable that medical science, at this point in its history, was but in its infancy. The body of knowledge surrounding human physiology was insufficient to expect physicians to prescribe effective treatments; too much of science was based on alchemy, which was to impede any significant advancement in chemistry for about 300 years (1400-1650).[61]

Yet like quacks and charlatans, they tried all sorts of remedies. This left the door wide open for uneducated charlatans to spin their own webs, and brew potions that were as ineffective as those concocted by the physicians. Hence, there was insufficient evidence to sway an individual towards a physician rather than towards a healer.

The healers and charlatans were mostly found in the rural areas, as most physicians practised Medicine in urban settings, which was conducive to maintaining their social standing. This trend was so popular, that by the beginning of the French Revolution, in 1789, 80% of physicians lived in cities.

The healers came under different titles, and their gifts for healing, touching, and setting bones were considered innate and tied with heredity. They were generally simple farmers or tradesmen, but very effective in healing. These healers were surrounded by a mystical aura that gave them unexplainable powers. The mysterious nature of their ability suggested divine or spiritual intervention. They were essentially the physicians of the peasants, and because no social status was involved, as it would be if higher education was associated with their abilities, the healers remained close to the people and were trusted.[49]

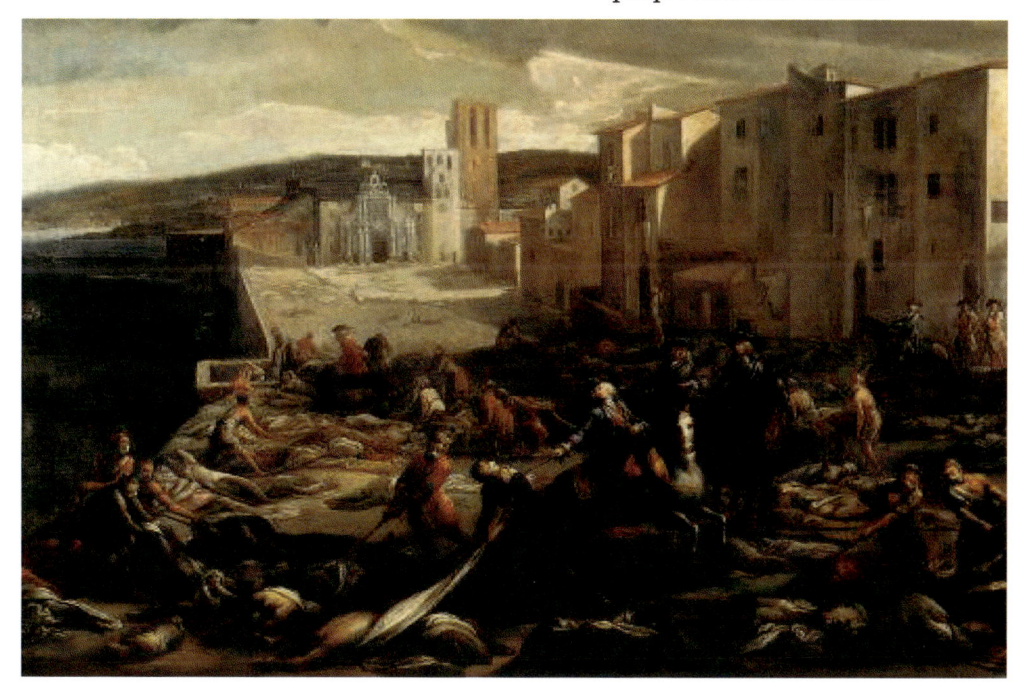

Figure 2.4: Michel Serre (1658-1733) - The plague in Marlles in 1721. De Agostini Picture Library images Collection ©Getty

2.5 Europe and Post-Plague Recovery

In the fifteenth century, following the most devastating period of the plague, European society began a slow recovery phase; its resilience was aided by the Renaissance, which was a period during which numerous wars were gradually ending, and humanity was celebrating and exalting itself. Renaissance actually means: rebirth. And so humanity was being reborn into a new understanding of self. The survivors of the plague found it easier to get jobs because of a much smaller population base; the economy overall remained stagnant, as there was no real population growth until the mid-16th century. In fact, a noted further population decline occurred after 1377. [73] There were two main reason for this decline: first, between the years 1350 to 1450, epidemics and plagues decimated the population every six years. [49] The periodic waves of unpredictable epidemics created psychological fear from which arose an ardent interest in meeting immediate rather than future needs. Luxury items were purchased by the rich and poor who espoused the 20th century's dictum of living for today. Agricultural production began to diversify, yielding specialty crops like sugar, saffron, fruits and wines; in addition, imported exotic goods from the Far East spilled over into the market place.[49] Second, the greater availability of jobs in the post-plague period, incentivises women to join the job market, causing a significant drop in birth rates. [73] Rigby writes:

Most historians would accept that, under the impact of repeated outbreaks of epidemic disease (and, more controversially, because of lower fertility rates as women postponed marriage to take advantage of their increased employment opportunities in an age of labour shortage), England's population declined after 1377.

Once the population began to grow, early in the 16th century, so did the economy in response to increased demand. [73] Life expectancy was improving and the population was healthier because of an improved diet that included greater varieties of foods. The agricultural surplus of grains, in the late 15th century, in addition to better transportation and communication systems improved the individual's access to food. Medicine's archaic practices, however, still lingered and so did the people's mistrust of doctors. The most potent enemy of the people was considered nature, as the public avidly remembered the lethality of the unpredictable plagues.[49]

Cities grew as cohesive social and political centres, with the market place being at the epicentre of human activity. The cities were however, made of dark and narrow streets that stunk of raw sewage, rotting foodstuff, and an overbearing stench emanating from animal slaughterhouses. The largest cities were mostly found in Italy, with approximately 5 cities populated with 50,000 to 100,000 souls, and one large city, Naples, estimated at over 125,000 souls.

Over the course of the 15th century, the market place became diversified in an unprecedented way: meat and dairy products were abundantly and frequently part of the diet. Consumption of such quantities of pork and lamb would not be seen again until the 19th century. Vegetables, however, were not found much in the diet of the lower classes, whereas sweet wines and citrus fruits were eaten by the rich to compensate for the lack of vegetables.

Both an improved economy and diet contributed most significantly to population health, whereas Medicine remained profoundly challenged and inefficacious because of its un-founded treatments.[49]

2.6 The Beginning Rejuvenation of Medicine

It wouldn't be until the 16th century that Galenism would begin to slowly come to an end, and that anatomy would get rejuvenated with the brilliant work of Leonardo da Vinci (1452-1519 AD) (**Figure 2.5**)—known as the artist-anatomist who created the science of anatomy[44]—and Andrea Vesalius (1514-63 AD). They did extensive dissections of human corpses and pictorially represented their detailed study of the human anatomy with an amazing genius and skill[52] (**Figure 2.6**). These works brought to light the many anatomical errors that had been reported one thousand years earlier by Galen. Historically, this was an important time of change, as monasticism's almost exclusive hold on knowledge was gradually loosened—monks throughout the dark ages securely held ancient writings in their libraries, thus preserving them from the marauding Goths and Visigoths. This facilitated a greater access to previously hidden documents; also Gutenberg's printing press in 1440, opened the doors to a much greater distribution of knowledge. [80] Prior to that time, Catholic monks copied and translated books by hand. Afterwards, discoveries and dialectic arguments could be more widely available for erudite discussions. In the era of academic conservatism that loomed over universities, there was great resistance to da Vinci and Vesalius' new findings; surgeons, least of all, benefited from the redefined scientific know-ledge as they were unable to implement the new anatomical findings into their practice of surgery. The problem was that they did not have any kind of scientific education. More stunning still was the fact the both da Vinci and Vesalius undertook the dissection of human corpses despite the Church's condemnation of such practices—a position maintained right up until the 19th century.[52]

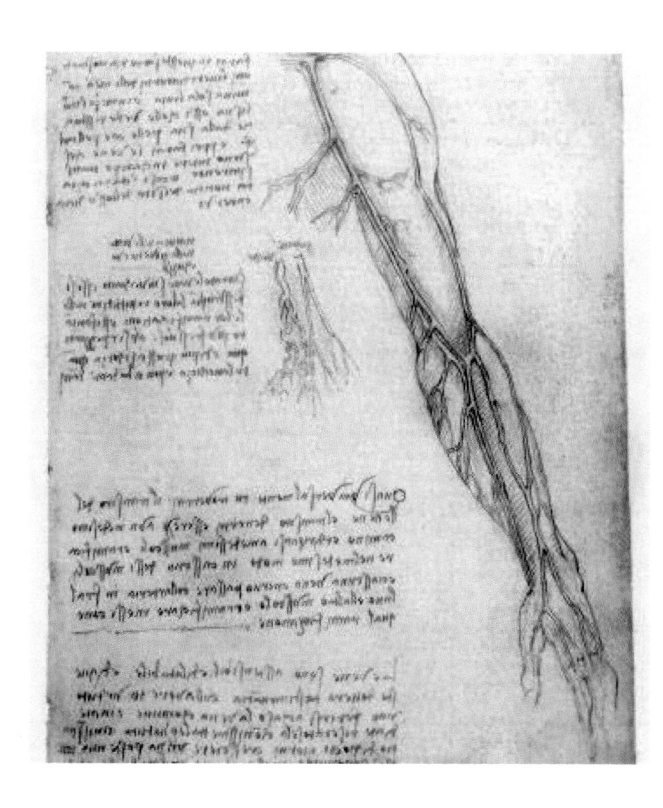

Figure 2.6: Da Vinci Superficial Vessels of the Arm Vessels. Credit: Science Source. © Getty Images

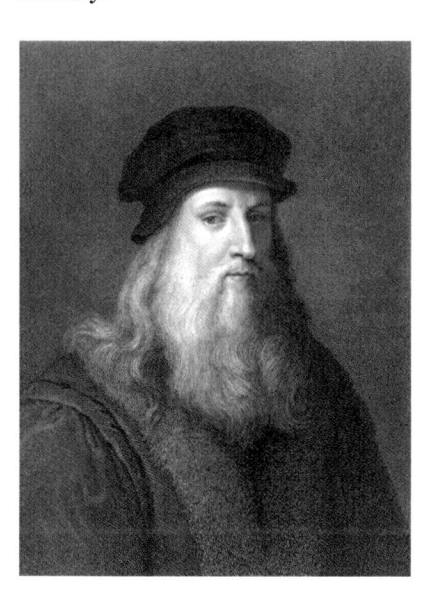

Figure 2.5: Leonardo da Vinci. Credit: shutterstock_81841951

Their work was done under a shroud of darkness, and the origin of their findings could therefore not be fully disclosed. Mesquita et al., write:[53]

By identifying "the anatomical errors" present in Galen's book and speech, he challenged the dogmas of the Catholic Church, the academic world and the doctors of his time. However, the accuracy of his findings and his innovative way to disseminate them among his students and colleagues was essential so that his contributions are considered by many the landmark of modern medicine.

It is noteworthy that no dogma of the Catholic Church ever pertained to concepts of anatomy. It was rather the practice of digging up the dead that infuriated the Church.

Contributing further to Medicine's stagnation, was the fact that the Renaissance, that golden age lasting between 1350 and 1550 AD, was characterized by renewed fascination for the great Greek classics, and an experimental mind-set in poetry, painting, sculpture, architecture and music. And so the lack of medical progress persisted right into the 17th century, and this despite the emerging know-ledge of the golden age of science.

2.7 The Scientific Revolution of the 17th Century

This was a period when experimental research and the natural sciences began to develop broadly. The scientific revolution of the 17th century introduced the "Scientific Method," which proposed using inductive and empirical experimentation that were reliable and repeatable. In this way it was possible to unravel the great mysteries that had, until then, prevailed under a shroud of mysticism.[49]

Scientific societies were established such as "The French Académie des Sciences (1666) and the English Royal Society (1662) of which Sir Isaac Newton was a member. They fostered many discoveries to practical problems, and these findings fuelled tremendous progress in technology and in the natural sciences. The new scientific revolution, headed by René Descartes (1596-1650), Galileo (1564-1642), Sanctorius (1561-1636) and Gian Alfonso Borelli (1608-1679) offered the hope of a new system of thought that would permit man to finally gain control over the environment and nature's deadly forces. The scientific revolution began with the intent of breaking down false perceptions based on objective, observable and repeatable research. Galileo essentially proved Copernicus' theory, that the sun rather than the earth was the center of the universe, by directly observing the planetary system with his telescope.

It was inevitable, that from the infancy stages of Medicine and Chemistry would emerge a number of hucksters, charlatans and quacks, trying to push remedies and elixirs with no proven track records and low success rates. Such a quack hit the scene in 1653, and attained world recognition as an expert in scurvy.

Dr Everard Maynwaringe was a brilliant graduate from Cambridge University's School of Medicine. He promoted a "Scorbute" pill as well as a "Catholick (universal) elixir" none of which worked very effectively. He published in 1665 *A Treatise of the Scurvy*, work that, in later years, did not hold much credibility as a research document. The publication of his Treatise also coincided with the plague in London. True to form, Maynwaringe peddled his elixir as an effective cure for the plague. He claimed that out of 86 plague victims that were treated, 56 survived, representing a 65% success rate. Later in his career, in order to better market himself and confuse the public, he changed his title to: "Doctor of Hermetic Philosophy and Physick". By the time he died in 1699, he was poor and the public opinion had turned against him.

Medicine, its most potent therapies stemming from the strategic use of herbs, was not much better than Maynwaringe's cures. Herbalists strongly believed in the magical properties of the various elixirs; the leading physicians of the day prescribed mixtures and concoctions that contained ingredients like worms, foxes' lungs, lozenges of dried vipers, oil of wolves, moss from the skull of a victim of violent death and crab's eyes. Despite Medicine's stagnation, the new science eventually had repercussion in the field of Medicine, which until then, had been based on classical 2nd century Greek Galenism.

The new science was materialistic, in the sense that it believed the universe to be composed of matter in motion; it was also mathematical, in that calculations, rather than common sense, were being advocated as the basis for understanding the universe.[49]

It was a European-wide phenomenon that moved beyond the academic spheres to the public domain, because of the creation of the printing press; suddenly access to information was no longer, strictly limited to the centers of higher learning. Physicians, however, did not seem to immediately benefit from this revolution; doctors remained stuck in prescribing old age remedies such as purging, bloodletting, enemas and various elixirs.

Galenic theories of Medicine were essentially based on Aristotle's 4 elements (earth, fire, water and air). They explained disease by the imbalance of the "4 humors": the red of blood, the yellow of bile, the black of black bile, and the white of phlegm. Paracelsus (1493-1541), a trained alchemist, was convinced that disease did not stem from an imbalance of the humors, but rather that each disease had its own cause.[52]

Paracelsus, strongly opposed Aristotelean and Galenic principles of the humoral imbalances and maintained specific poisons in the body could be cured by similar poisons. Grandjean writes: [34]

> **The 17th century ignited the belief that the threatening forces of nature could be finally mastered.**

It is an important tenet of Paracelsian medicine that the cure must conform to the body: the principle of 'like cures like'.

He created various preparations from the distillate of many types of metals, and ended up giving patients oral doses of purified mercury, arsenic and antimony at times that coincided with notable astrological events. [34, 60] Although his ideas and remedies were strange—a sort of incoherent mix of astrology, philosophy and alchemy—he did successfully manage to change some very inflexible notions in both Chemistry and Medicine. The tendency of doctors to treat diseases with bloodletting and sweating had begun to shift towards a strategy of prescribing the ingestion of chemicals to address the accumulation of poisons in the body, the consequence of failing organs. [60] The Paracelsians argued the body/organic matter consisted of salt, sulfur and mercury, [68] and that the more violent diseases of the time—notably syphilis—required stronger chemical treatment compounds. [60]

Oddly enough, miraculous cures had been ascribed to Paracelsus's secret concoctions, but so had many deaths. Nevertheless, the Paracelsian system did influence the scholastic formation of an Englishman by the name of Robert Boyle (1627-1691), whose first scientific contribution of importance was the writing of *The Skeptical Chemist* (1661). In it, he is critical of both the Aristotelian and Paracelsian views of the natural world; he couldn't accept the notions of humors, nor could he believe that matter was simplistically made up of mercury, salt and sulfur. [68] Boyle went on to raise medical chemistry to great prominence, favoring a science that sought more than the formulation of chemical recipes for the treatment of disease. He proposed an elemental or particulate view of matter, hypothesizing the existence of molecules of various sizes, and described the transmutation of substances originating from a single matter he called "Catholick matter, thereby siding, in principle, with the alchemists. [68] His corpuscular model to explain the change in the states of matter gave birth to Iatrachemistry—the study of chemistry in relations to medicine. [52] It is around 1666 that Boyle experiments with blood became critically adventuresome, having unsuccessfully injected broth into the veins of dogs, [47] opening up a field of nutrition that would later be known as intravenous nutritional support. He followed closely Richard Lower's experiments on dog-to-dog blood transfusions, and was the first recipient of an experimental blood transfusion. [47] Boyle's lasting contribution to chemistry, however, was Boyle's Law explaining the inverse relationship between the pressure of gas and its volume. [68] His theory of the corpuscular model of matter led to the belief that reason without experimentation had limitations. As a Natural Philosopher, he believed that scientific experimentation with reason could allow man to uncover the great mysteries of the world. In other words he gave preeminence to controlled experimentation over scholastic syllogistic reasoning—logic and deduction—to uncover truth.[29] Eaton writes: [29]

Boyle argues that the natural world had been not only intentionally designed by God, but had been designed specifically to be understood, at least in part, by rational human minds. He believed that humans equipped with reason could make use of detailed observation, under controlled experimental conditions, to uncover the hidden structure of nature.

The Natural Philosophy embraced by Boyle, did eventually get influenced by the Mechanistic philosophers of the day, notably, Rene Descartes, Francis Bacon and Pierre Gassendi (1592-1655), who proposed that the material world could only be explained by a model of matter in motion. [29] Although Boyle did not acknowledge all propositions of the mechanistic philosophers, he nevertheless was sufficiently influenced to formulate a Philosophy of Science that suggested that all things could be known either by reason or by experimentation.[29] Boyle, despite the atheistic tendencies of most mechanistic philosophers, maintained that God was the author of creation. Eaton writes: [29]

He [Boyle] rejected the view that matter had power beyond its mechanical properties and sought to demonstrate how natural phenomena could be explained in terms of the motion of particles obeying certain laws of motion which he believed God had established.

However, it seemed that the cat was out of bag once science advanced that all things and thus all truths could be known—a dangerous view that fueled the prideful assumption that man had the capacity to know all things—which invariably lead to a slippery slope towards atheism. [62] The scientific revolution had a profound impact as it radically changed man's perception of himself, the world and God. E.M. Adams, a Keenan Professor of philosophy at the University of North Carolina, Chapel Hill developed a philosophical approach he called, **realistic humanism**, in that he perceived the world and universe as being more than a set of scientific facts.[2] Adams advances that ethical codes and religious values can answer the most fundamental questions of life; it is a position contrary to many philosophers who refuse to recognize any kind of deeper meaning in the universe. This **naturalism**-based philosophy contends that reality is strictly limited by scientific facts that define the physical world. As such, science has come to perceive man purely as a physical thing. This is indeed the foundation of the 17th century Scientific Revolution, which set out to objectively know and measure the physical world. Adams, in his papers, "The Meaning of Life" [1] and "Rethinking the Idea of God" [2] attempted to capture the extent to which the nihilistic philosophy that was driving the Scientific Revolution infiltrated the very fabric of the Western world. He writes: [4]

Before the scientific revolution, humankind faced reality asking, what is demanded of me? How do I set myself right with reality? From within the modern scientific worldview, by contrast, we ask: How do I impose my will on the world? How can I control it?

The 17th century Scientific Revolution did however manage to ignite the belief that the once threatening forces of nature could be finally mastered, bringing hope to a population whose ancestors vividly passed on terrifying stories of the plague. Here began the process of Medicine's modernization, a process that wasn't easy as there was resistance to the tendency to reject long held classical beliefs that sustained Medicine for centuries. At last, this Greek classical knowledge was being challenged by the hard empirical evidence that originated from research that generated exact measurements. This meant that conclusions could no longer be derived from "common sense," but rather from very precise calculations.

A mathematical revolution occurred concurrently with a philosophical debate that was to change the practice of Medicine in a very significant manner. René Descartes (1596-1650) was a leader of "mechanistic philosophers;" he believed that all

> Before the scientific revolution, humankind faced reality asking, what is demanded of me? How do I set myself right with reality? From within the modern scientific worldview, by contrast, we ask: How do I impose my will on the world? How can I control it?" [Adams, E.M.]

matter was governed by natural laws that could be decoded mathematically, and that skepticism should be used when considering the validity of something that could not be proven beyond doubt; certainty, he argued, is what the scientific method should ideally achieve. Contrary to his expectations, the scientific method left him with only doubt that was fueled by mathematical models of probability that he was formulating in his research. He concluded that nothing could be shown to be certain except the existence of his mind; he rationalized that because he could think, he could therefore be sure that he existed, and from this realization, transpired the philosophy known as **Cartesianism**, which prized the superiority of the mind over the physical and the corporal world.[38] It was a dualistic philosophy that regarded the mind and body as distinct. Descartes taught that the mind or human consciousness consisted of a non-physical substance, and that it was distinct and detached from the body. In this mindset the intelligence would be physically derived from neurological and biological processes, whereas the consciousness would not. So then, the consciousness, which is ethereal, should thrive to transcend the polluting influences of the physical body. [49]

Descartes was promoting a philosophy that advocated the duality of mind and body, and was in flagrant opposition with the **Idealism** exhorted by Plato (427 357 B.C.), who promoted that only ideas truly existed, thus denying the existence of the material world—the contention being that material had meaning only through the perceptions of the mind. Whereas the Platonic view claimed that only ideas had eternal forms, Cartesianism argued the duality of mind and body, thus creating the **mind-body problem**. This problem exists because if the mind is made up of a substance distinct from the brain's biological matter, and not governed by the laws of physics, then how can consciousness come

> The new spirit of scientific inquiry would eventually move away from the legacy of magical cures toward a better understanding of therapeutic mechanisms of medicine.

into being? The interrelationship between these two realities was critical to the understanding of the human in his fullest. Indeed, how could the mind interact with the body but yet not be physically connected? Descartes had no answer.[3]

From this paradigm of body and mind arose two schools of thought: **Metaphysical Parallelism,** which advocated an independence of the two realms while arguing the existence of a certain synchronicity between them. The second school was called **Epiphenomalism**. It defended the belief that mental activity strictly arose from physical events. In other words, the human person, in his full consciousness, is made up of a total compilation of neuronal networks, fluids and tissues, and nothing else.

The problems with Parallelism and Epiphenomalism arose later when both rationalism and materialism surfaced as offspring, thus dividing western philosophy into two camps. To understand why this division was particularly harmful to the progress of Western Medicine, both must be defined.

Rationalism is an allegiance to the supreme value of reason. For the first time, human reasoning could be considered sound and logical enough to explain the world. To accomplish this, it had to be possible for man to demystify that which was thought to be unknowable, and to explain those things previously thought to be in the realm of Divine mystery.

Materialism also referred to as **Physicalism**, was a belief system that recognized the superior value of scientific inquiry over reason, in that, it could more thoroughly and objectively study the physical world. The Cartesian logic, that advanced the dualism of the mind and the body, fueled a belief system that greatly influenced the split between the psycho-emotional and the biological components of the individual. Consistent with this mind set, it has been argued that Medicine distanced itself from a more holistic view of man by embracing more **Materialism** and **Epiphenomalism**, and less of **Cartesianism**. It became, as it were, focused on a more myopic view of the patient, centrically engrossed with the purely physical reality. The degree to which contemporary Medicine has specialized certainly reflects an interest in physical systems rather than in a human approach to healing.

The impact of the new science was greatly enhanced by the creation of Gutenberg's printing press (1400-1467). It made it possible to compile and systematize information, and disseminate it throughout the continent; published scientific information, in the form of books and scientific periodicals, were issued during the 17th century. The information was used by a broad scientific community as building blocks that would eventually lead to the unraveling of great mysteries.

In the background, the plague was still showing up periodically in Europe. It reinforced by its devastating pestilence that nature could not be trusted, that natural remedies were ineffective, and that chemistry's link to Medicine was mankind's only hope of survival. Chemistry offered the possibility that purified compounds could stop the progress of disease.

One the most famous of the drugs, introduced in 1632, was known as "**quinine**". It was used by the Inca civilization to cure malaria. The Jesuits discovered that it was derived from the bark of a plant called "cinchona." Quinine was the product of a pharmacological breakthrough that produced undeniable therapeutic benefits. Other drugs such as "**antimony**" may not have been effective, but perception sometimes created the illusion of a beneficial impact, and that often times, was enough for a population avid of possessing assured cures. "Antimony" was believed to be effective in treating undernutrition; it appeared to fatten pigs when added to their diet. The alchemist, Johann Tholde decided to administer antimony to a group of undernourished monks as a means of increasing their fat reserves, but caused their death instead. This created a great debate over whether antimony was drug or a poison. [52]

When King Louis XIV was cured of typhus with the administration of antimony, the debate ceased, and this drug became a confirmation of Chemistry's effectiveness at keeping nature in check. The problem was that nobody really questioned whether the king would have eventually recovered without any treatment. It was just good common sense to conclude that antimony cured the typhus, and so it became the panacea of all medical treatments at the time.

The new spirit of scientific inquiry would eventually do away with common sense conclusions, but for a while longer, the lingering legacy of relying on magical cures persisted until research became more precise, and the knowledge of physiology more complete. Understanding the therapeutic mechanisms of the various medicines was perhaps one of the most important endeavors of the day. It became clear that if one could understand how the treatment worked, then remedies could follow a more disease-specific protocol.

Food, elixirs and drugs were three main modes of treatment and, as such, their mechanisms of action were of interest to the doctors. Up until the beginning of the 16th century, alchemy had but two objectives: first, to artificially produce gold and second, to develop an elixir of life which, when drunk, gave life and health. Gold, it was believed, could be produced from the treatment of other metals with the highly coveted philosopher's stone, also called the red elixir.

The transmutation of metals was thought to be quite likely and reasonable, based on practical metallurgic experiences that were well known at the time. For instance, ore galena (PbS) does have a metallic appearance, but when heated in the presence of air, the oxidation reaction resulted in the loss of SO_2 and in the formation of pure lead (Pb).

$$PbS(s) + O_2(g) \rightarrow Pb(l) + SO_2(g)$$

Medicinal chemistry gradually emerged from pursuing the second goal—that of producing an elixir of life—leaving alchemy with the sole objective of gold production. Eastern alchemy contrasted with Western practices in that it persisted solely in trying to formulate the one true elixir of life; it wasn't side tracked by any obsessions with gold. Chinese alchemic pursuits did not influence, in the least, practices in Western Europe, as communications between the two civilizations were non-existent.

European medicinal chemistry did, however, open the door for various abuses to take place, as charlatans of all sorts were peddling their brews and concoctions for a pretty penny, right along the side of apothecaries, who eventually became modern day pharmacists. Consequently regulatory controls were instituted to keep abuses in check. The government established a Medical Royal Commission in 1772 to investigate the activities of the pharmacy profession. From this commission came regulations governing the composition, the preparation and distribution/sale of medicines and preparation patents.[52]

At the time, the inventory of mineral based drugs normally found in the pharmacist's cabinets were not numerous, and generally consisted of magnesium sulfates, sodium and potassium sulfates, silver nitrate, liquor-based arsenic, and potassium chloride. Plants, used for infusions and percolations, were cultivated in hospital gardens. In fact, by 1803, opium was isolated, whereas popular vegetable extracts, such as camphre and quina were imported (**Figure 2.7**). At this point in the science of pharmacy's historical time table, pills and packs were not yet invented, but rather medicine was prescribed as infusions, decoctions, tinctures and syrups. They made the process of medicine-taking more difficult, primarily because of texture and taste.

The prescription of medications and elixirs took on a fascinating new dimension with the 1628 publication of William Harvey's findings on the human vascular system. He in fact disproved Galenic theory that the liver was the center of the circulation, and proposed that arterial blood in the left ventricle of the heart was pumped into the aorta, and distributed throughout the entire body; the venous blood then returned to the heart.

In 1661, Marcello Malpighi completed the work by demonstrating the existence of capillaries. With the understanding of the circulatory system, it became intriguing to study the effect of transfusions (Richard Lower 1631-91) and intravenous injections. Boyle, Hooke, Lower, Mayow and Sir Christopher Wren actually injected food and drugs into the veins of subjects, representing the first reported intravenous feeding and treatment experiments; the outcomes were disastrous as many can now imagine.

Medicine—excluding surgery—was taking on more invasive therapeutic approaches, and distancing itself from the softer therapies of strictly prescribing elixirs and herbal remedies. Iatrochemistry was a science that broke away from the assertion that God is the author of all life, and that suggested that life could be created in a laboratory. Meanwhile, scientists such as Sanctorius, Galileo and Descartes were linking Medicine to physics (iatrophysics); this scientific marriage produced the first thermometer (Sanctorius) and microscope (Galileo and Malpighi (1628-94). The technical innovations were fed by the 17th century preoccupation of wanting to monitor vital signs—this was driven by the scientific community's acceptance of **Physicalism**. Despite the technical innovations, Medicine remained stagnant and ineffective until the Enlightenment Period.

2.7 The Enlightenment Period and Human Health

The eighteenth century opened "the Age of Enlightenment;" it coincided with a time of change driven by new philosophies and new ways of thinking that affected many aspects of life. It challenged traditional establishments, institutions, customs and morals. From it flourished experimentation in the arts, new scientific discoveries, and philosophical discourse and speculation.[49]

It was an age that invited the individual to trust in his own intelligence, and in that sense, was just as much a movement of ideas, as of people. Modern style Medicine began to emerge as the physician was being encouraged to ground his practice on scientific knowledge as oppose to erroneous Galenic principles. Several icons rose from the dust that had settled on the age-old medical traditionalists who persisted in promoting erroneous precepts and inefficacious treatments.

The most illustrious icons that greatly promoted objective scientific research, and forced medical practitioners to abandon phlegmatic treatments and modes of assessment were: Antoine-Laurent Lavoisier (1743-94), Giovanni Battista Morgagni (1682-1771), Herman Boerhaave (1688-1738), William Stark MD (1740-1770) and Edward Jenner (1749-1823). They confidently walked on stage, and the spotlight of the Enlightenment shone on them. Controversy surrounded them until the scientific communities finally relinquished their hold on ancient precepts, and acquiesced to the strength and veracity of their findings.

Paradoxically, it was also a time that favored a wide spread of charlatanism that persisted in offering mystical/magical cures. This is because the therapeutic arsenal of the physician, in the early 18th century, was still very limited. Besides purging and bloodletting, the most frequently prescribed remedies were mostly limited to syrups and tisanes, which were distributed daily by the pharmacy.[49]

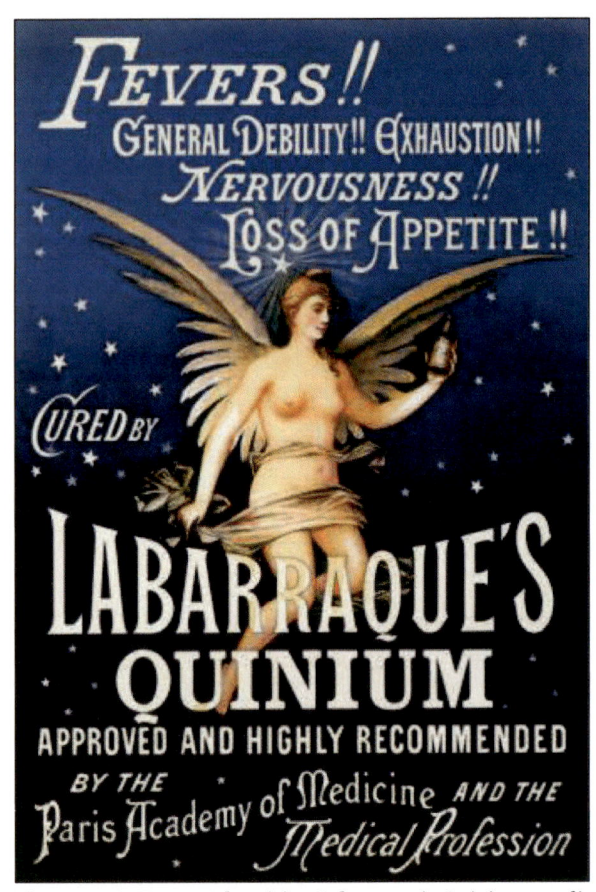

Figure 2.6: Poster Advertising Labarraque's Quinium, medicine with quinine for fevers, general debility, exhaustion, nervousness, loss of appetite. Color lithograph Circa 1889; Source: The Bridgeman Art Gallery. © Getty Images

Organ and excreta-derived substances were also prescribed, but with very uncertain outcomes. This Galenic style of Medicine was not taken seriously by the public; instead of doctors, the public frequently consulted surgeons, astrologers, sorcerers and charlatans for the treatment of illnesses. One of the most famous charlatans of the day was a man named Franz Anton Mesmer (1735-1815). He was one of the most famous Parisian physicians of his day because of his incredible powers to heal and to relieve pain. He put patients into hypnotic trances, revealing the power of suggestion and of the mind. It was from his treatments that the expression "to be mesmerized" became popular.

Hypnotism produced valid findings that suggested that the mind played a great role in healing, and contrasted greatly with tangible medical treatments that used elixirs and tisanes with the intent to treat the physicality of the disease. He recognized the great healing powers of the mind, but also ventured into dubious Medicine. He espoused the powers of magnetic therapy for the treatment of numerous illnesses. It was an approach that grew out of the idea that mysterious fluid in the body he called "animal magnetism" could somehow be influenced.

Inspired by the religious practice of laying-on of hands, Mesmer developed a technique involving physical manipulation of the patients in a manner resembling message therapy or acupressure. He believed that by placing the hands and thumb, in particular locations on the patient, he was facilitating the flow of animal magnetism into the patient, and restoring the body's energies to a natural homeostasis or balance. Today, oriental forms of medicine would use Reiki or other methods to normalize the Chakra energy systems.

The treatments were greatly sought by the rich and famous, and were given in magnificent consulting parlors containing health baths of diluted sulfuric acid. This setting allowed Mesmer to earn fabulous amounts of money. He had as a patient the Queen of France, Marie Antoinette.[49]

Homeopathy also emerged during this period. It offered the patient a more studied and mysterious approach to treatments. The German, Samuel Friedrich Hahnemann (1755-1843), founded the homeopathy movement, based on the principle that the treatment of a disease would be more effective using diluted dosage levels of a substance, which, if administered in a greater dose, would provoke the disease. Homeopathy is still practiced today, and commands a significant following; the principles, however, have not been embraced by the scientific community as not all their treatments have stood up to the rigors of scientific testing.

2.8 The 18th Century Agricultural Revolution

The European population had begun to increase quite significantly since 1740 because of better housing and a greater availability of food. Agricultural output was increasing because of the Agricultural Revolution, which is considered one the great turning points in human history.[49]

The paradox was that even though the food supply increased substantively, the heightened population growth created a greater demand, driving prices upward, but also causing wages to fall, and therefore limiting the purchasing power of the population.

> Even though food supply was increasing, population growth heightened demands, driving food costs upward.

The agricultural revolution lead to the transformation of subsistence farming to commercial agriculture, thereby causing a consolidation of smaller estates into large plantations with better outputs to meet market conditions. Large fields were enclosed and dedicated to increasing the yield of single crop production as opposed to a balance of commodities. This reorganization of the land led to the disintegration of the commons, and then to the buy-out of the middling-sized landholders. The resulting landless agrarian laborer ended up moving from farm to farm looking for work and food.

In the cities the plight of the poor was critically acute (**Figure 2.8**); general hospitals and other charitable organizations came to their aid. Even though widespread famines were no longer wiping out large populations—the last and most devastating famine in European history occurred in 1697, eradicating one third of Finland's population—there was a persistent slow starvation and undernutrition in the population of that time.

It is estimated that between 10-15% of most societies were comprised of the truly starving poor; this represented about 20 million people, mostly situated in towns, who were suffering from hunger. Another 40% included those who were landless and jobless. Large masses were not dying, but the misery of individuals was certainly greater, as the prominence of hunger and of poor quality diets were more rampant at the end of the 18th century than at the beginning.

It has been argued that the nutritional quality of the diet, during that time, may have been the poorest in European history according to Robert Vial.[35] To be well nourished meant that there were enough calories in the form of bread (as in the example of France), and a full cooking pot of soup that usually

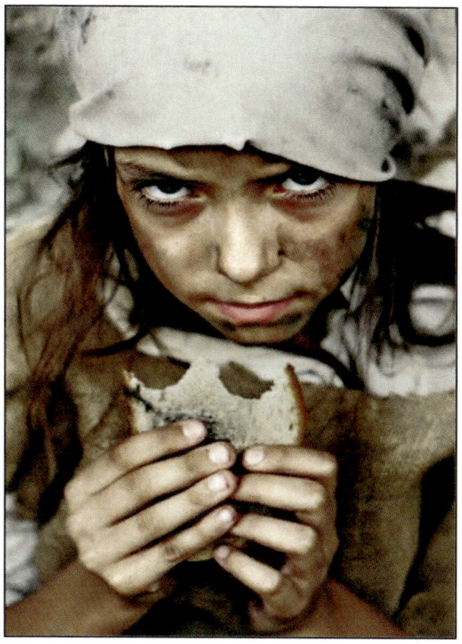

Figure 2.8 A portrait of a poor beggar child with a piece of bread in her hands © NinaMalyna/Shutterstock.com

contained vegetables. The modest families rarely saw excess calories in their diet, and the peasants' diet was even more deprived.[49]

Mark Kishlansky,[49] in his book, Civilization in the West, advances that the peasant usually ate very poorly. His diet consisted of small peas and cabbage during the summer, and turnips, celery and pumpkin during the winter. It was customary to dip the bread into the soup. The bread was usually made from a combination of rye, barley and wheat. If there was work for the father, meat was consumed once a week, and there was generally lard available to enhance the taste of the soup. So it was understood that if the crock was generously filled with soup, and there was enough bread or potatoes, and occasionally some meat, then the people were eating well. This likely meant that the individual and the family could avoid important diseases, but such a diet was more meant as a survival strategy, rather than a means to achieving some kind of optimal health.

2.10 Caring for the Sick and Poor in Hospitals

The 18th century was a period that shed new light on human understanding, leading to an enlightened view of the worth of the individual, and of the innocence children. This was an age that developed an increased awareness of human suffering among the poor and the sick, which led to the creation of many municipal and general hospitals; the latter were large institutions often surrounded by fences or walls, and dedicated to the enclosure of the poor.

They were not as medically oriented as the municipal and Hôtel-Dieu hospitals. In London, during this time, many university teaching hospitals also sprung up including the West Minister (1719), Guy's (1725), St. George's (1733), the London (1740) and the Middlesex (1745).

The sick flooded the hospitals and dispensaries such as l'Hôtel-Dieu de Paris, as the small pox epidemic cyclically swept through Europe during the 18th Century, claiming an estimated 60 million lives by the end of that Century. During these dark times, the Church's mission was primarily dedicated to caring for the sick. Indeed, celibate priests and sisters were clearly the only ones capable of being courageously dedicated to those stricken by various contagions, often at the peril of their own lives—they did not worry about returning home to infect their wives and children.[17] The public clearly perceived that if lives could be whisked away at nature's whim, then surely servants of God would at least ensure the victims' dignified death and the souls' eternal salvation. Both Medicine and charlatanism had nothing of the sort to comfort the sick. In fact, both failed at mitigating the affront of the pestilence, in trying to curb its devastation.

Three events finally broke charlatanism's footing and boosted Medicine's credibility, leaving it with few challengers to its authority until the 20th century: first, Edward Jenner's (1749-1823) discovery of vaccination in 1796, put an abrupt end to the small pox scourge in addition to a variety of life threatening plagues that had relentlessly endangered human life for centuries.

Second, the chemical revolution, near the end of the 18th Century, and specifically Lavoisier's introduction of the scientific method of inquiry; and third, the advent of modern pathology which began with the published research, in 1761, of Giovanni Battista Morgagni (1682-1771), professor of anatomy at the university of Padua, Italy. Modern pathology was critical in unraveling the cause of many diseases, which were still at that time unknown to Medicine. He extensively documented the anatomical differences between the bodies of healthy and unhealthy individuals, making classical descriptions of angina pectoris, myocardial degeneration and tuberculosis to name a few. The practice of Medicine, for the most part, would remain unaffected by the breakthroughs in anatomical pathology up until the 19th century.

> **Although hospitals were available to care for the sick and undernourished, death rates in hospitals were 80%.**

The Church's mission was also to tend to the poor, a mentality observed during the French revolution (1789-1792), during which many famines devastated the population. However, despite the humanitarian attempts at reaching out to the poor, pauperism was too elevated for relief efforts to fully alleviate all of the human suffering.[49] Although the hospitals were built to care for the sick, the death rates in European hospitals at the time were at an alarming 80%.

These statistics on hospital survival rates speak volumes of the quality of hospital care that was being given at the time. The most important shortcoming in some hospitals was the unhygienic conditions: several patients per bed and the preponderance of non-isolated cases of infectious disease and fever were found throughout the hospitals. It wasn't understood then, that contagious patients needed to be kept apart from the general hospital population. Hospital death rates would remain elevated up until the creation of infirmaries dedicated to the seriously ill, and until Joseph Lister (1827-1912) introduced sweeping reforms that promoted disinfection practices in hospital wards.

His findings, initially published in the medical journal Lancet of 1867, spread rapidly throughout the world, thus influencing hospital practices forever. His method involved meticulous cleanliness of hospital wards and patients' dressings with the use of antiseptics in order to cut down on the incidence of gangrene and post-operative infections.[25]

2.9 The Role of Nutrition in Health

At the start of the 18th century, Medicine perceived diet as a significant therapeutic contributor to human health. Food was essential as sustenance, and thus required to ensure basic health and, as such, was prescribed mostly as supplemental feedings to minimize the risk of death or of aggravating illness, and to improve recovery of patients in hospitals.

Doctors and hospital administrators had the reserved right to prescribe supplemental diets to the sick, the elderly and the convalescent patients. And so, the role of nutrition was limited to eating well and in sufficient amounts, at least in France.

Nevertheless, nutrition was central to hospital care, representing 80% of the hospital's operating costs, but was not part of specific medical treatments according to Robert Vial. [81]

The most frequent dietary supplements, given as therapeutic remedies, during the convalescence period were essentially increased portions of the normal diet, wine and bouillons. In fact, rather than therapeutic, these were given as a recompense, a sort of feel good therapy. Today, by contrast, food cost represent 30% of a hospital Nutrition department's budget and less than 2% of a the total operating budget of a hospital.

Dietary restrictions, on the other hand, were hardly ever prescribed by doctors in 18th century France. There were two main reasons: first, obesity was considered a healthy trait that was associated with longevity; women had no problems with rounded hips, fat thighs and protruding bellies. Second, the problem of food scarcity was still persistent in some regions especially near the end of the 18th century. The winter of 1793-94 was particularly difficult for the French who were still caught in the turmoil of the revolution; many towns were without bread, meat, butter and vegetables as represented in this earlier period lithograph (**Figure 2.9**).

The consequences of these famines on human health were all too clear to the doctors in France; they would not have ethically considered diet restrictions as a viable therapeutic approach for the sick, within such a context; the risks were simply too elevated.

The role of nutrition in health was being defined at a most elemental level, grounded in Hippocrates' basic medical precept that hygiene and nutrition could aid the body's natural healing forces. By contrast, the English did support dietary restrictions, having not gone through, to the same extent as the French, chronic starvation. Both England and Holland had advanced agricultural practices that favored greater crop yields, thus ensuring an adequate food supply to the population.

The idea of food restriction and sparse eating was common practice in the English population, and took its roots in the populist thinking that a restrictive diet improved health. In addition, there is evidence that Neapolitan physicians often recommended forty days of fasting to patients with fever. This approach was based on clinical evaluations that were strictly dependent on observable physical characteristics.

And food, rather than being considered as a therapeutic agent of disease, was looked upon as a catalyst of disease. Eating was therefore avoided in some instances, for fear of making the person's illness worse. Dietary restrictions, as a strategy for health management, is still being advocated today for a variety of reasons, but took its roots, so it seems, in 18th century England, without any scientific foundation. It was merely perception that supported the strategy of restrictive diets for optimum health.[49]

The beginning of the 18th century was the epoch of new ideas that espoused a mind-set for a method of "scientific inquiry" involving the direct verification of natural phenomenon, rather than mere observation—a clear offshoot of materialism. It was a daring concept from which spawned the impetus to formulate natural laws that explained many paradigms. It was an approach that clashed with traditionalist views that supported a kind of scientific mysticism and transcendentalism that so typified Paracelsus's time

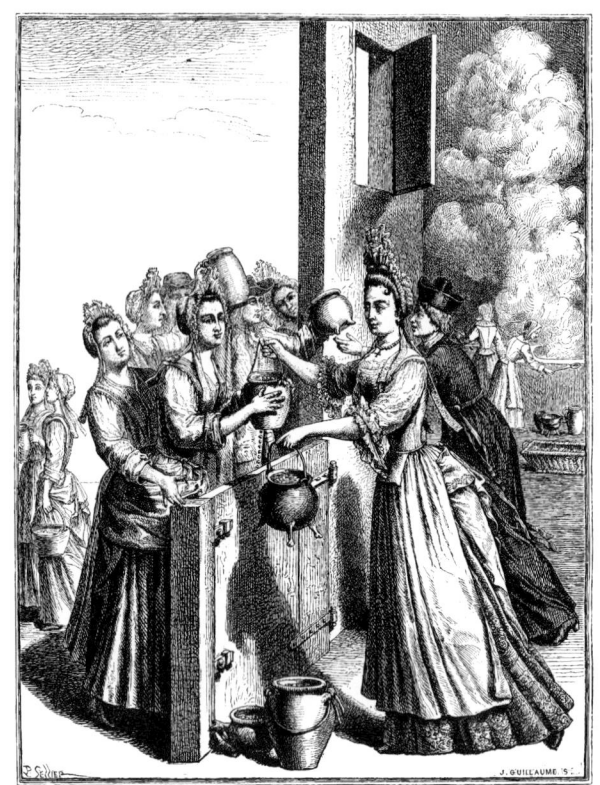

Figure 2.9: Relief soup, in Paris, during the famine of 1709, vintage engraved illustration. Magasin Pittoresque 1875 © Morphart Creation.

It kept alive the philosophical view point that nothing could be known.[49] It is also the time during which a more investigative form of scientific inquiry gradually took the place of the "experimental method" which guided science since the middle of the 17th century.

Science's new mandate and direction was captured by Joseph Francois Magendie when he said:[52]

the aim of science is to substitute facts for appearances and demonstrations for impressions.

Such an impetus was strongly needed if science was to move ahead, if progress was going to take place. And so, the latter period of the eighteenth century, gave birth to the Chemical Revolution, and at the helm were many prominent scientists such as Cavendish (1731-1810), Priestley (1733-1804), but none attained such acclaim as Lavoisier (1743-1794).[52]

Lavoisier revolutionized the discipline of chemistry

> "The aim of science is to substitute facts for appearances and demonstrations for impressions" (Joseph Francois Magendie, 1682-1771)

by disproving old beliefs, most of which originated from the ancient Greek Doctrines. The absence of scientific veracity in the field of Medicine, prompted Lavoisier to write his letter to the French Science Academy. In it, Lavoisier describes the necessity of including controls in various studies. He believed that the methods of scientific inquiry, popularly used at the time, were seriously flawed. His scientific methodologies were, by contrast, highly regarded, and revolutionized chemical thinking. Lavoisier's methods of investigation closely resemble our present day standards of objectively controlled research.[27, 32, 37]

He was presenting a rigorous style of scientific investigation, which contrasted with the heavily biased and scientifically inaccurate methods of study that were seen in chemistry, and among the charlatans of the time. There was a pressing need to quickly disassociate the stringent methods of science from the inaccurate and soft earthly medicines. The sciences—which included Medicine and Chemistry—needed to separate themselves from the earth because the earth was associated with the unpredictable and devastating plagues; they killed large populations while Medicine and charlatans looked on; they were powerless to change the ravaging thrust of the disease.

Within this unpredictable devastation stood the public's mistrust of nature; the memories of the plague were still vividly omnipresent in the minds and psyche of people. Medicine wanted to regain its position of prestige as an authentic field and discipline of health based on credible scientific principles, methodologies and remedies.

Medicine's knowledge-base in the early part of the 18th century was, however, rather slim. But by the second half of the 18th century, a more modern physician began to emerge in so far that his medical practice was better grounded in science rather than in observation. Leopold Auenbrugger (1722-1809), in founding the science of physical diagnosis, was instrumental in standardizing medical diagnostic practices, and providing credibility to Medicine. He did this by describing the technique of percussion to assess air content in the thoracic cavity, and as such, had established a method of determining the extent of lung disease.

Another contribution of notable significance came from the medical teachings of the Dutch physician, Hermann Boerhaave (1688-1738), who espoused the notion that doctors must be present at the bedside of patients and there, he asserts that the physician must...

set aside all academic preconceptions, and assess the situation calmly, for himself.

He began, with his students, the daily practice of conducting medical rounds by first reviewing patients' medical notes, followed by a visit of each patient—a practice that has been maintained until today. Medical students from all over the continent attended his classes.[37]

One of his pupils, the Swiss, Albrecht von Haller (1708-77), became prolific in his writings, publishing 12 books on physiology, four on anatomy and seven on botany. He put out impressive amounts of scientific review articles in addition to several volumes describing the medicinal properties of herbs, surgery, anatomy and medical practices. These writings were essential in setting up a common pool of scientific medical knowledge from which could be established some kind of consensus.[32]

The emergence of this modern physician with concise practices and opinions based on what was known, and less on speculation, was taking place amidst a population that had a great mistrust for the physician. It had consequently turned towards the charlatans for remedies and treatments. Lavoisier was a major critic of Medicine's practices, and a key figure promoting much needed harmony between Chemistry and Medicine.

As science attempted to overtake the herb-prescribing charlatans, and the practices of using earthly medicines, Medicine's poor track record continued to haunt its progress even though its practices were more based on sound scientific knowledge. There is no wonder why public opinion in France, during the end of the eighteenth century, did not recognize the authority and abilities of the physicians to treat and to cure. Instead, their remedies appeared, in many instances, to make the sick, sicker.

It wasn't until the implementation of major medical education reforms at the end of the 18th century that signs of unification, between the Chemistry and Medicine, became visible; Lavoisier was finally heard. The curriculum for medical students no longer included the theories and conventions of the Classical Greek doctrines. Medical education finally embraced contemporary science through courses like the history of Medicine, hygiene, physical medicine, legal medicine, animal chemistry and clinical practice. It is also clear that one of the most important consequences of this distancing from classical Medicine, was the disappearance of nutrition as an important complement of Medicine.

As a chemist, Lavoisier demystified many false precepts; he is most notably remembered for disproving the "phlogiston theory" of combustion. Scientists believed that the combustion of matter was dependent on the presence of a near-weightless compound known as "phlogiston", which was lost from physical matter after it was burned. Lavoisier was able to show this to be a flagrant misconception by introducing the first quantitative chemical measures using very precise balances to measure weights. He demonstrated that some metals, when burned, actually increased rather decreased in weight, thus putting into question the phlogiston theory that had been upheld for so long.[37]

Instead, he proposed that during combustion of some metals, oxygen combined with the metal, thus causing the initial weight to increase; from this observation followed the "*law of conservation of mass*" which stated that the mass of product in a reaction was in fact equal to the weight of the reactants. In other words, nothing was lost and nothing was gained. This was a pivotal enigma to unravel, as combustion was fundamental to the progress of Chemistry.

Although he was a chemist, Lavoisier's work caused medical physiology to progress in leaps and bounds during the eighteenth century; this was seen more specifically in the field of the physiology of respiration. Lavoisier was beginning to understand, through experiments, that respiration and combustion were based on very similar principles. Just as the combustion of matter consumed oxygen and generated heat, so the individual consuming oxygen also generated heat.

More importantly, because his experimental findings could be quantified, he observed that heat generated from the consumption of a given quantity of oxygen, was equal to the heat generated from combusting charcoal with the same amount of oxygen. This finding essentially gave birth to calorimetry—the science of measuring heat flow—which eventually became an area of interest in the nutritional sciences and in the study of human metabolism.

He formulated, after numerous experiments, a theory of respiration that proved to be quite accurate: he hypothesized that from consumed oxygen, carbon dioxide was produced. He worked out the mechanism describing how oxygen enters the blood via the lungs. This was a discovery of great importance that was to have public health ramifications, for indeed, from his finding emerged the understanding that in confined spaces there needed to be a certain amount of available fresh air per person. This fundamental insight brought reforms to patient management in hospitals, thus introducing the idea of restricting the number of patients per bed and per room—5 patients to a bed was common in the 18th century hospital—in order to ensure adequate air circulation in hospitals.

In 1790, in his last letter to the French *Académie des Sciences*, he writes about the need to join forces with the physicians, and to move beyond the mere conjectural causes of disease, and explore the true causes. The need for such a unification originated from the extremely inadequate and limited arsenal of therapeutic agents that were used near the end of the eighteenth century. It was well documented that during this time period, most of these therapeutic agents did not work effectively, and that the clinical instruments, used by the physicians, were primitive and also inaccurate.

The therapeutic methods used by physicians were pretty well limited to "bleeding and anal cleansing" and they relied on syrups and herbal teas as the major remedies according to historian Robert Vial.[35] In his letter, Lavoisier attempts to give a research direction to the Académie and, in doing so, blatantly describes the inaccuracy of Medicine:[32]

...we will attack a revered and Antique Colossus of prejudice and error

Lavoisier was inviting scientists and physicians to use the "scientific method" in investigating and treating diseases. Too many errors based on impressions and poorly controlled experiments had led to the formulation of scientific and physiologic falsities.

Uncovering the mechanism of oxygen exchange in the blood, led Lavoisier to study human blood in relation to digestion. This was, in fact, a concrete example of his desire to unite the fields of Chemistry and Medicine, and one of the strongest indicators that nutrition was possibly going to become a serious player in medical therapy. However, technology was not sufficiently developed to allow such an early alliance with nutrition; the world would have to wait for the 19th and 20th centuries. The metabolic nutrition studies undertaken by Starke, and Lavoisier's advances in calorimetry, had created such opportunity for the progress of nutrition.

> **Lavoisier invited scientists and physicians to use the "scientific method" as too many errors based on impressions and poorly controlled experiments led to false conclusions.**

However, as the chemical revolution began to take hold, nutrition found itself confined to background importance; the therapeutic value of food became limited to the mere recommendation for larger or smaller portions of vegetables and cereals for patients that were ill or undernourished.[81]

The Chemical Revolution that began to take place, as the 18th century was coming to a close, created the opportunity for Lavoisier's call to be finally heard. William Withering (1786) introduced, with his work on digitalis, a more modern therapeutic spin to an otherwise archaic Medicine, causing the Royal College of Physicians in London to discard a number of ancient remedies from their pharmacopoeia. The nineteenth century saw a number of a high potency compounds such as strychnine and morphine introduced into the pharmacopoeia through the work of Joseph Francois Magendie (1783-1855). He was a renowned physiologist of the time who became the founder of modern pharmacology.[52]

One of his pupils, Dr. Claude Bernard (1813-1878), researched every branch of physiology at the time and, based on his own experiments, formulated fundamental physiological doctrines that were instrumental in clarifying metabolic principles of the human body. The first was that the body maintained a constant internal environment. This was a critical concept that supported the physiologic wisdom of an internal homeostasis that meant that any imbalance was naturally counterbalanced by the body.[52]

It seemed clear that Medicine was now preparing to move ahead with the adoption of precise chemical medicinal formulations that were more dependable. It became evident that the return to old earthy notions and beliefs of the curative powers of food, that were peddled by the many charlatans of the time, was not going to benefit the physician who, by now, needed to gain, in the eyes of the public, more credibility.

DISCUSSION QUESTIONS

1. During Lavoisier's reforms in the second half of the 18th Century, describe how the role of nutrition in Medicine changed.

2. Contrast how the practice of dietary restrictions/caloric restrictions differed between France and England, and explain the reasons.

3. Discuss the now popular idea that the Palaeolithic diet may well be the modern man's path to better health

4. Up to the 14th century, the field of Medicine had been relying on the Classical Greek medical theories. Explain why the old Greek theories were falling out of public approval rapidly around the 14th century and afterward.

5. Discuss the historical genesis of why Medicine became more centered on distinct biological systems rather than a more holistic (full person) approach to healing the sick.

References

1. Adams, E.M. (2002) The Meaning of Life," *The International Journal for the Philosophy of Religion,* 51.
2. Adams, E.M. (2001) Rethinking the Idea of God," *The Southern Journal of Philosophy* .
3. Adams, E.M., (1991) *The Metaphysics of Self and World: Toward a Humanistic Philosophy* (Philadelphia, Pennsylvania: Temple University Press
4. Adams, E.M.,(1975) *Philosophy and the Modern Mind, A Philosophical Critique of Modern Western Civilization* (Chapel Hill, N.C.: The University of North Carolina Press,). Reprinted (Lanham, Maryland: University Press of America, 1985).
5. Aeillo, LC & Wheeler, P. (1995) The expensive tissue hypothesis. Current Anthropology 36:199-221
6. Allentoft, M., Sikora, M., Sjögren, K. et al. (2015). Population genomics of Bronze Age Eurasia. *Nature* **522,** 167–172. https://doi.org/10.1038/nature14507
7. Århem, K. (1989). Maasai Food Symbolism: The Cultural Connotations of Milk, Meat, and Blood in the Pastoral Maasai Diet. *Anthropos, 84*(1/3), 1-23. Retrieved July 10, 2020, from www.jstor.org/stable/40461671
8. Arnold D. (2010). British India and the "beriberi problem", 1798-1942. Medical history, 54(3), 295–314. https://doi.org/10.1017/s0025727300004622
9. Barnes, AC. (1964). The Sugar Cane. New York: Interscience Publisher Inc.
10. Berg, I. (2013) Marine Creatures and the Sea in Bronze Age Greece: Ambiguities of Meaning. *J Mari Arch* **8,** 1–27. https://doi.org/10.1007/s11457-012-9105-x
11. Broadhurst, CL., Cunnane, SC, Crawford, MA. (1998) Rift Valley Lake /Fish and Shellfish Provided Brain Specific Nutrition for Early Homo. Br. J. Nutr. 79(1):3-21
12. Brothwell, D and Brothwell, P. (1969) Ancient Peoples and Places Food in Antiquity: A Survey of the Diet of Early People. Thames and Hudson, London 248 pp.
13. Buklijaš T. (2008). Medicine and Society in the Medieval Hospital. *Croatian medical journal*, *49*(2), 151–154. https://doi.org/10.3325/cmj.2008.2.151
14. Carrick, P. (2001) Medical Ethics in the Ancient World. Washington, DC: Georgetown University Press. 108pp.
15. Chamberlain, JG. (1998) Dietary Lipids and evolution of the human brain. Br. J. Nutr. 80:301
16. Charlton, S., Abigail Ramsøe, A., Collins, M., Oliver E. Craig, O.E., Fischer, R., Alexander, M., Camilla F. Speller, CF. (2019). New insights into Neolithic milk consumption through proteomic analysis of dental calculus. *Archaeological and Anthropological Sciences*; DOI: 10.1007/s12520-019-00911-7
17. Corbett, W. (1986) A History of the Protestant Reformation in England and Ireland. New York: Benziger Bros. 406pp
18. Cordain L, Eaton SB, Sebastian A, Mann N, Lindeberg S, Watkins BA, O'Keefe JH, Brand-Miller(2005). J. Am J Clin Nutr; 81(2):341-54.
19. Cordain, L. Boyd Eaton, S. Sebastian, A. Mann, N. Lindeberg, S.,Watkins, BA., O'Keefe, JH.,Brand-Miller, J. (2005). Origins and evolution of the Western diet: health implications for the 21st century, *The American Journal of Clinical Nutrition*, 81 (2):341-354. URL https://doi.org/10.1093/ajcn.81.2.341
22. Cordain, L. et al.(2001) Fatty acid composition and energy density of foods available to African hominids: evolutionary complications for human brain development Wld. Rev. Nut. r. and Dietetics 90:144-161
23. Craik, E. Hippokratic diaita (1995). In: Wilkins, J., Harvey, D., and Dobson, M.(Eds) Food in Antiquity. University of Exeter Press, Exeter UK. p: 353-350
24. Craik, E. (1997)."Diet, Diaita and Dietetics." In: *The Greek World.* A. Powell, (ed.).pp.387-402.London: Routledge.
24b. Daniels, J and Daniels, D. (1988). The origin of the sugarcane roller mill. Technology and Culture; 29(3): 493-535 DOI 10.2307/3105272. URL: http://login.ezproxy.mnsu.edu/login?qurl=https://www.jstor.org/stable/3105272
25. Daynes-Diallo, S.(2011) A touch of France: Theory and Practice: European Renaissance Medicine. Medicographia 33:335-353 Retrieved July 14, 2012 from: http://www.medicographia.com/2011/12/a-touch-of-france-theory-and-practice-european-renaissance-medicine/
26. de Divitiis E, Cappabianca P, de Divitiis O. (2004) The "schola medica salernitana": the forerunner of the modern university medical schools. *Neurosurgery*;55(4):722-745. doi:10.1227/01.neu.0000039458.36781.31
27. Douglas McKie. (1952) Antoine Lavoisier: Scientist, Economist, Social Reformer, New York, H. Schuman.
28. Dowling JE, Wald G. (1958) VITAMIN A DEFICIENCY AND NIGHT BLINDNESS. *Proc Natl Acad Sci U S A*;44(7):648-661. doi:10.1073/pnas.44.7.648
29. Eaton, W. (2010). Robert Boyle (1627-1291). Internet Encyclopedia of Philosophy. Retrieved July 17, 2020 from URL: https://www.iep.utm.edu/boyle/
30. Encycolopedia Brittanica-online (2013) Antoine Laurent Lavoisier update 6-10-2013. Retrieved January 29, 2014 http://www.britannica.com/EBchecked/topic/332700/Antoine-Laurent-Lavoisier
31. Eriksson, G., Lougas, L, and Zagorska, I. (2003). Stone Age Hunter-Gatherers at Zvejnieki, Northern Latvia: Radiocarbon, stable Isotope and Archaeozoology Data. Liverpool University Press Online. 2003(1). DOI: 10.3828/bfarm.2003.1.2
32. Foster, ML. (1926), Life of Lavoisier. North-Hampton, Mass., Smith College. 84pp
33. Galloway, J. (1977). The Mediterranean Sugar Industry. Geographical Review, 67(2), 177-194. doi:10.2307/214019
34. Grandjean P. (2016). Paracelsus Revisited: The Dose Concept in a Complex World. *Basic & clinical pharmacology & toxicology*, *119*(2), 126–132. https://doi.org/10.1111/bcpt.12622
35. Grant, M. (1995) Oribasios and Medical Dietetics or the Three Ps. In: Wilkins, J., Harvey, D., and Dobson, M.(Eds) Food in Antiquity. University of Exeter Press, Exeter UK, p: 371-379.
36. Grimm, V. (1995) Fasting practices in Judaic and Christian Traditions. In: In: Wilkins, J., Harvey, D., and Dobson, M.(Eds) Food in Antiquity. University of Exeter Press, Exeter UK,
37. Guerlac, H (1961) Lavoisier-The Crucial Year: The Background and Origin of his First Experiments on Combustion in 1772, Ithaca NY, Cornell University Press.
38. Hampson, N A (1968) The Enlightenment. Penguin Books pp: 304.
39. History.com editors (2018). Neolithic Revolution. Accessed July 8, 2020 from: URL: https://www.history.com/topics/pre-history/neolithic-revolution
40. Hodgetts, LM et al. (2003). Changing subsistence practices at the Dorsett PaleoEskimo site of Phillip's Garden Newfoundland. Artic Anthropology 40 (1): 106-120
41. Holmes, FL (2020). Voit, Carl Von. Retrieved from encyclopedia.com CENGAGE webpage on July 2, 2020: https://www.encyclopedia.com/people/food-and-drink/food-and-cooking-biographies/carl-von-voit
42. Horard-Herbin, M-P, Tresset, A., Vigne, J-D. (2014) Domestication and uses of the dog in western Europe from the Paleolithic to the Iron Age, *Animal Frontiers;* 4(3): 23-31 https://doi.org/10.2527/af.2014-0018
43. Irwin, JR. (1947) Galen on the temperaments. *J Gen Psychol*; 36:45-64. doi:10.1080/00221309.1947.9918106

44. Keele, KD. (1964). Leonardo da Vinci's influence on Renaissance Anatomy. Med Hist; 8(4): 360–370. doi: 10.1017/s0025727300029835
45. Kelly, J. (2005). The Great Mortality: An intimate history of the black death, the most devastating plague of all time. New York: Harper-Perennial, 364 pp.
46. King, H. (1995) Food and Blood in Hippokratic gynaecology. In: Wilkins, J., Harvey, D., and Dobson, M.(Eds) Food in Antiquity. University of Exeter Press, Exeter UK, p: 351-358.
47. Knight, H., & Hunter, M. (2007). Robert Boyle's memoirs for the natural history of human blood (1684): print, manuscript and the impact of baconianism in seventeenth-century medical science. *Medical history*, *51*(2), 145–164. https://doi.org/10.1017/s0025727300001162
48. Krizan, M. (2013). SUBSTANTIAL CHANGE AND THE LIMITING CASE OF ARISTOTELIAN MATTER. *History of Philosophy Quarterly, 30*(4), 293-310. Retrieved July 3, 2020, from www.jstor.org/stable/43488076
49. Kishlansky, M. Geary, P. and O'Brien, P. (1991) Civilizations in the West. Harper Collins Publ. NY pp:1021.
50. Lippi G, Mattiuzzi C, Cervellin G. (2016). Meat consumption and cancer risk: a critical review of published meta-analyses. *Crit Rev Oncol Hematol*;97:1-14. doi:10.1016/j.critrevonc.2015.11.008
51. Maher, M. (2002) The Odyssey of the Ancient Greek Diet. Totem: The University of Western Ontario Journal of Anthropology 10(1):7-13.
52. Margotta, R. (1996). The Hamlyn History of Medicine. Paul Lewis (Ed) Institute of Neurology. London: Hamlyn Publishing/Reed International Books
53. Mesquita, E. T., Souza Júnior, C. V., & Ferreira, T. R. (2015). Andreas Vesalius 500 years--A Renaissance that revolutionized cardiovascular knowledge. Revista brasileira de cirurgia cardiovascular : orgao oficial da Sociedade Brasileira de Cirurgia Cardiovascular, 30(2), 260–265. https://doi.org/10.5935/1678-9741.20150024
54. Milton, K. (1993) Diet and primate evolution. Sci Amer 269:86-93
55. Molleson, TI. (1994) The Eloquent Bones of Abu-Hureya, Sci. Am. 271:70-75
56. Mithen, S. (1999). The Hunter-Gatherer: Pre-History of Human-animal Interactions. Anthrozoös, 12:4, 195-204, DOI: 10.2752/089279399787000147
57. Nestle, M. (1999) Animal vs plant foods in human diets and health: is the historical record unequivocal? Proc. Nutr Soc. 58: 211-218
58. New World Encyclopedia.(2016). Aztec Civilization. Retrieved June 14, 2020 from URL: https://www.newworldencyclopedia.org/entry/Aztec_Civilization
59. NIH (2013). The Curious History of L'Hotel-Dieu De Paris : I. Its Foundation and Early Days. (1913). *The Hospital*, *53*(1392), 625–626.
60. NIH (2011). The medical chemistry of Paracelsians. Retrieved from the US National Library of Medicine website July 17, 2020: URL: https://www.nlm.nih.gov/exhibition/paracelsus/chemistry.html
61. Nikiforuk, A. (1996) The Fourth Horseman: A Short History of Plagues, Scourges and Emerging Viruses. Toronto: Penguin Group. 262pp
62. Osler, MJ. (2020). Scientific Revolution. Encyclopedia Britannica. Retrieved July 18, 2020: https://www.britannica.com/biography/Robert-Boyle
63. Paroutsa, EL and Manolis, SK (2010). Reconstructing Late Bronze Age Diet in Mainland Greece using Stable Isotope Analysis. J. Of Archeological Sci. 37(3): 614-620
64. Pasca M. (1994) The Salerno School of Medicine. *Am J Nephrol*; 14(4-6):478-482. doi:10.1159/000168770
65. Pendergrast, M. (2000). Uncommon Grounds: The History of Coffee and How it Transformed our World. New York: Basic Books, 554pp.
66. Perri, A. (2016). A wolf in dog's clothing: Initial dog domestication and Pleistocene wolf variation. J. Archeological Science; 68: 1-4. URL: https://doi.org/10.1016/j.jas.2016.02.003
67. Plato. Critias and Timaeus (2005). Chicago: Acheron Press
68. Principe, L (2011). In retrospect: The Sceptical Chymist. *Nature* **469,** 30–31. https://doi.org/10.1038/469030a
69. Purcell, N (2005). Colonization and Mediterranean History. In: Ancient Colonisations: Analogies, Similarity and Differences, H. Hurst and S. Owen (Eds), London: Duckworth: 115-39
70. Reed, CA., (1959). Animal domestication in the prehistoric near East. Science; 130(3389): 1629-1639
71. Richards, M.P. (2002) A Brief Review of the Archeological Evidence for Palaeolithic and Neolithic Subsistence European Journal of Clinical Nutrition 56
72. Richardson, R. (2013). Inflammation, suppuration, putrefaction, fermentation: Joseph Lister's Microbiology. The Royal Society Journal of the History of Science. *Notes Rec.* http://doi.org/10.1098/rsnr.2013.0034. URL: https://royalsocietypublishing.org/doi/full/10.1098/rsnr.2013.0034
73. Rigby, S. (2010). Urban population in late medieval England: The evidence of the lay subsidies. *The Economic History Review,63* (2), new series, 393-417. Retrieved July 15, 2020, from www.jstor.org/stable/27771618
74. Sallam H. N. (2010). Aristotle, godfather of evidence-based medicine. Facts, views & vision in ObGyn, 2(1), 11–19.
75. Sampson, A.A. (2011). The Case of the Cyclops: Mesolithic and Neolithic Networks in the Northern Aegean, Greece. Philadelphia: INSTAP Academic Press, 393 pp.
76. Sandage, T. (2005) History of the World in 6 Glasses. Walter & Co Publishers, New York 311 pp
77. Shi Z. (2019). Gut Microbiota: An Important Link between Western Diet and Chronic Diseases. *Nutrients*, *11*(10), 2287. https://doi.org/10.3390/nu11102287
78. Smith, V. E. (1961). *The General Science of Nature* (Milwaukee 1958). j. gredt, *Elementa Philosophiae Aristotelico-Thomisticae,* 2 v. (13th ed. Freiburg 1961), j. p. anton, *Aristotle's Theory of Contrariety* (New York 1957). g. m. sciacca, *Enciclopedia filosofica* (Venice-Rome 1957) 3:1620–21.
79. Tannahill, R. (1988). Food in History. New York: Three Rivers Press. 424 pp
80. Triggle, C. R., & Triggle, D. J. (2017). From Gutenberg to Open Science: An Unfulfilled Odyssey. *Drug development research*, *78*(1), 3–23. https://doi.org/10.1002/ddr.21369
81. Vial, R. (1989) Moeurs, santé et maladies en 1789; Societe des editions Londreys, Paris, pp.327
82. Vickery, K.F. (1936) Food in Early Greece. University of Illinois, 97 pp.
83. Wilson, H. (2013). Neolithic Medicine: Better than a Hole in the Head. BBC History. Retrieved on Sept 24, 2013 from: http://www.bbc.co.uk/history/ancient/british_prehistory/neolithic_medicine.shtml
84. Wagner DM, Klunk J, Harbeck M, et al. (2014). Yersinia pestis and the plague of Justinian 541-543 AD: a genomic analysis. *Lancet Infect Dis*;14(4):319-326. doi:10.1016/S1473-3099(13)70323-2
85. Wolf, A., Bray, A., and Popkin, BM. A short history of beverages and how our body treats them. (2008). Obesity Reviews 9: 151-164
86. Wong et al. (2012) Gut Microbiota Diet and Heart Disease. Journal of AOA C International 95(1): 24-30
87. Zivkovic, A. M., Telis, N., German, J. B., & Hammock, B. D. (2011). Dietary omega-3 fatty acids aid in the modulation of inflammation and metabolic health. *California agriculture*, *65*(3), 106–111. https://doi.org/10.3733/ca.v065n03p106

CHAPTER 3

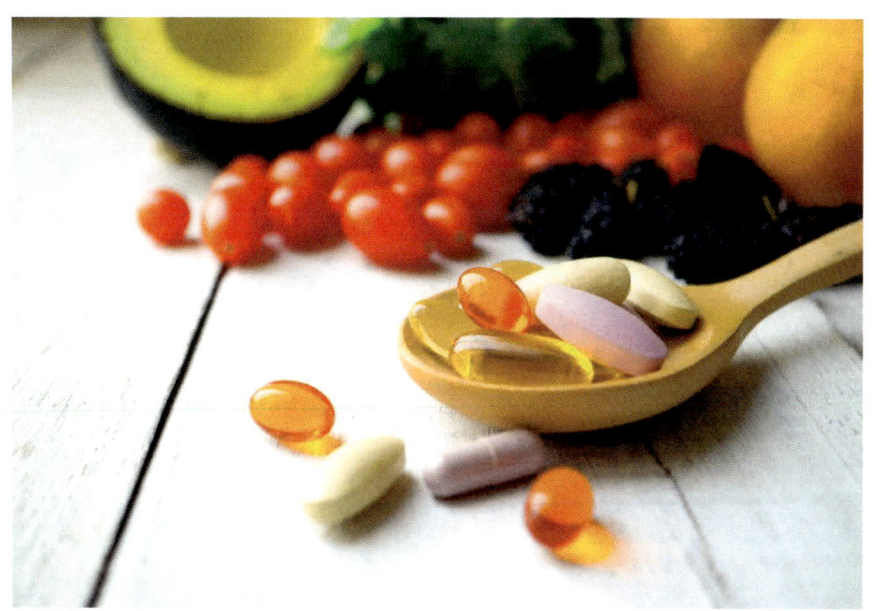

VITAMIN & MINERAL DEFICIENCIES

3.1 Emergence of the Science of Nutrition—

After the period of great French scientific achievements, science—meaning Chemistry—was further matured by Germans such as Justus von Liebig (1803-1873). He became a significant player in the first early phase of the science of nutrition (1850-1950), thus introducing the scientific community to the chemical composition of food. Von Liebig successfully isolated the energy components of food: protein, carbohydrate and fat, thereby advancing the discipline of nutritional biochemistry.[16]

He identified foods substance as either nitrogenous-based, and necessary for growth or non-nitrogenous, and used as fuel in respiration and heat production. [11] His research showed that protein was a master nutrient, necessary for tissue building in plants, animals and humans. [16] In studying metabolism, he recognised the end products of protein as uric acid, urea, carbonic acid and water. [11]

Von Liebig's understanding of nutrition, in terms of distinct chemical transformations taking place in the body, made him the first to comprehend key principles of macronutrient metabolism.

Liebig brought to prominence the idea that sugar and starch can synthesize fat in the body. [11]

> In the 19th century, Justus von Liebig introduced the 3 sources of energy in food: protein, carbohydrate and fat.

Although he inaccurately described protein as the most important fuel source in exercise, [18] the popular belief of the role of protein in building athletic prowess went unchallenged until it was shown to be false by physiologist Adolf Fick (1829-1901) and chemist Johannes Wislicenus (1835-1903) no later than the mid-19th century. This central role of protein did, nevertheless, make its way into the popular literature right up to the twentieth century, popularizing the practice of ingesting large quantities of protein for physical prowess in athletics. [63]

At the end of the eighteenth century, the emergence of technological, cultural, and sociological changes characterized the beginning of the first Industrial Revolution (1760 to 1830)—mostly contained in Britain—and of a second Industrial Revolution with more of a global impact during the late nineteenth to twentieth centuries. [33]

From this period arose technological advances such as the stethoscope, electromagnetism, and new energy sources such as steam, coal, and petroleum; it created the factory system, and more sophisticated chemical assays. It brought Medicine into a new light; public opinion began to slowly change in favor of the physician, a shift that became more pronounced with the introduction of vaccinations in 1796. However, despite these wondrous achievements in Medicine and science, the Industrial Revolution also brought with it a much higher prevalence of disease. Jackson [59] writes:

While industrialization had made Britain rich, it had also made Britain sick. Diseases such as smallpox, typhus, and tuberculosis had dire consequences, and these consequences were intensifying on Britain's increasingly crowded streets.

> Careful investigative work by anesthetist John Snow pinpointed the cause of London's cholera epidemic: Contaminated drinking water

Indeed, industrialization heightened urbanization; agrarian laborers moved to the cities in great numbers, looking for the coveted factory jobs. However, in so doing, agricultural production had to increase to accommodate the working-class' requirements for food in the swelling urban centers. [33] In this setting, Europe was again reminded of the unpredictable and uncontrollable deadly forces of nature; a cholera pandemic began to strike the European continent in the early 1830s, creating terror among its population. [74]

A new generation was witnessing, dumbfounded and bewildered, Medicine's incapacity to halt the scourge that struck both Paris and London between 1832 and 1833, claiming 4000 to 7000 victims in London alone [119] and more than 18,000 in Paris.[118] In a second wave, it hit the district of Soho in London in 1854, claiming 14,000 cases of cholera and causing 618 deaths; [70] there are conflicting reports that the death count may have totalled 12,000. [119] The inefficaciousness of medical treatments and the vulnerability of man had suddenly become obvious once again, spurring riots throughout England, most notably in Liverpool. [13]

It took the relentless investigative work of the anaesthetist, John Snow, to finally demonstrate that the water-borne nature of the disease was afflicting the poorer districts. His thorough epidemiological inquest tied the pandemic to a leaking cesspool that contaminated the drinking water of a well in what is now known as Broadwick Street in London.[70, 43]

The idea that contaminated water could be the source of the cholera outbreak stemmed first, from biblical and Middle Age experiences involving the quarantine of lepers and plague victims; second, confirmation came from the invention of the microscope by Antony van Leeuwenhoek (1632–1723), which clearly detected the existence of microorganisms. This led to the germ theory of disease in 18th century. [118] This theory was in stark opposition to the strongly held belief in the **miasmic theory** of disease that contended that bad air was the main cause of many diseases. [43]

Many believed that the miasma was behind the cholera epidemic, and not even Snow's methodical research could convince health officials otherwise. Only by the mid-19th century, long after Snow's death, would the miasmic theory be disproven. [118] Tulchinsky writes:

Miasmists believed that disease was caused by infectious mists or noxious vapors emanating from filth in the towns and that the method of prevention of infectious diseases was to establish sanitary measures to clean the streets of garbage, sewage, animal carcasses, and wastes that were features of urban living.

In light of Snow's report that the cholera was most virulent among the poorer districts of London, the English government appointed an English reformer by the name of Sir Edwin Chadwick as secretary of the Poor Law Commission in 1838 to investigate more clearly the plight of the poor. [55] His effort led to the British Poor Laws Amendment Act of 1834, which replaced the Elizabethan Poor Laws Act of 1601. In so doing the welfare of the poor transitioned from the local parish's responsibility to that of the central government. [118]

He produced a report titled *The Sanitary Conditions of the Labouring Population* in 1842, which helped dispel the belief that it was the moral fiber of the poor that was making them ill, and clearly demonstrated instead, that it was the impoverished environment, in which the poor were living, that was making them sick. [74] The report findings inspired the English parliament to pass the Health of Towns Act and the **National System of Public Health** in 1848. [74] Consequently, the government began to dedicate funds towards improving the physical environment of the poor in the cities; it enacted legislation directed at the implementation of public hygiene practices which consisted of cleaning up the filth in the streets, repairing the deteriorating houses and improving the working conditions—the main vectors for high death rates and poor health. [118]

Preventative medicine, at a public health level, had suddenly become more meaningful and beneficial to the people than the archaic medical treatments of the time. [74] Morley writes:

...it was through Chadwick's appreciation of the need to promote economic growth and maintain social order that his ideology on health and well-being developed.

The rapid development of large urban centers in England was at the heart of the contagion. Urbanization was so extensive that by 1840, roughly 50% of the population lived in cities. [74] Though the factories brought jobs and some prosperity, they also created unhealthy environments. The cities became dense with dirt, disease, deprivation and death. [74] Morley writes:

So widespread was the presence of disease by about 1840 that the average lifespan was just 26 years if someone lived in a settlement of 100,000 people or more.

Chadwick' Public Health Act of 1848 instituted a set of changes to the public infrastructure that would both improve the living conditions and health of all the population. The Act implemented:[121]
• New street drains and interlocking sewers
• Garbage and refuse collections from homes and streets
• Access to clean drinking water
• The installation of a medical officer for each town

It was specifically the new sewer system that caused the most significant drop in cholera deaths, as it ensured that city dwellers had access to uncontaminated drinking water. Chadwick revolutionized public health in Britain and set the stage for the future implementation of a School Meals program (1906), School Medical Service (1907) and the National Insurance Act (1911), thus providing free medical services to the poorest of the working class. [124] These reforms eventually led to full social security in Britain by 1948.

Working in Medicine's disfavor, was the eventual retreat of the cholera epidemic because of dramatic improvements in public hygiene. The influence of the lower class's greater purchasing power contributed as well in this recovery. The labor class now worked long hours in factories and brought home larger incomes. It was, in truth, the overall improved living conditions of the people that caused disease and death rates to plummet, and not any single medical intervention.[35, 70]

The greater incomes meant that complete families had greater access to milk, potatoes and meats for consumption. The improved availability of food ensured that a broader population base was well fed and resistant to infections.[52]

By the late 19th century, public concern arose over the impoverished miserable living conditions, lack of prenatal care, poor nutrition, and suboptimal general hygiene afflicting women and children specifically.[118] These concerns gave birth to preventive medicine approaches to safeguard the health of children and mothers. One such strategy involved the implementation of Milk Stations in France to ensure children had access to basic nutrition. The combined strategies of milk stations and visiting home nurses was initiated by Lilian Wald (1867-1940) in the US, who coined the term *Public Health Nurse*.[118] Later, efforts were directed at promoting prenatal care, breast feeding and well-child initiatives focused on good nutrition. Tulchinsky[118] writes:

The concept of child health spread to other parts of Europe and the USA with the development of pediatrics as a specialty and an emphasis on appropriate child nutrition. Henry Koplik (1858–1927) in 1889 and Nathan Strauss (1848–1931) in 1893 promoted centers to provide safe milk to pregnant women and children in the slums of New York City in order to combat summer diarrhea. The Henry Street Mission, serving poor immigrant areas, developed the model of visiting nurses and public milk stations.

The notion of a public health intervention aimed at the poor contrasted the pay-for-service concept employed by physicians for those patients who could afford.[118] The strategy of the state and volunteer organizations coming to the aid of vulnerable groups, like pregnant women, paid off, causing a 160-fold decrease maternal mortality rates between 1920 and 1970.[118]

However, before the importance of nutrition in public health could gain some degree of traction, the problem of infectious diseases had to be quelled. The chemist and biologist Louis Pasteur opened the field of bacteriology. His work confirmed the germ theory of disease, contributing to the field of immunology with the development of the rabies vaccine in 1884-85. His research led other European and American treatments for tuberculosis, diphtheria, typhoid, and yellow fever.[55] He studied the effect of heat on the life of bacteria, from which arose the process of pasteurization, or high temperature treatment of foods for preservation. This was momentous for the future development of the food industry. His efforts had an outstanding impact on public health worldwide.[118] Other scientific luminaries of the late nineteenth century such as Julius Cohn, Robert Koch and Joseph Lister contributed to understanding the role of microbes in disease and infections.[118] Indeed, the field of immunology flourished in the late 19th to 20th centuries, creating a considerable drop in childhood deaths. Tulchinsky writes:[118]

The twentieth century produced a flowering of immunology in the prevention of important diseases in animals and in humans based on the pioneering work of Jenner, Pasteur, Koch, and those who followed. Many major childhood infectious diseases have been controlled by immunization, one of the outstanding achievements of twentieth-century public health.

The development of antibiotics soon followed in 1928 with the work of Alexander Fleming. Quickly, different generations of antibiotic followed.[118] The rapid development of vaccines and antibiotics added to the already existing pharmacopeia of therapeutic agents held by the pharmacist [35, 70] and to a tremendous growth of the pharmaceutical industry.[16] This growth empowered modern medicine, especially once the major infections were controlled, but concomitantly diminished interest in public health. It did however, offer opportunity to contemplate and investigate nutritional deficiencies.[118, 16]

3.2 The Identification of the First Vitamins

3.2.1 Ascorbic Acid (Vitamin C). Prior to the identification of vitamins and essential minerals, deficiency diseases such as scurvy, beriberi, and pellagra afflicted various regions of the world, and were classified as infectious.[118] Scurvy—caused by vitamin C deficiency—was almost exclusively associated with extended travel at sea during the discovery of the New World.[20] William Lind discovered in

1747 the protective nature of limes against scurvy in the English navy. Filling the cargo bays with limes extended the time the British navy could remain a sea without incurring scurvy. This made the British navy particularly powerful and was critical in breaking Napoleon's power grip during the Napoleonic wars (1797–1814). [118] It was also mostly linked with the northern climates, which had limited growing seasons. However, scurvy was also associated with the advent of urbanization (Carpenter, 1986).[20]

However, the story of scurvy re-emerges in Ireland during the Great potato famine (1845-1852), which killed over one million people. During the mid-19th century, leading up to the famine, it is estimated that the poor in Ireland—which made up one third of the population—survived on a monotonous diet of potatoes and buttermilk. Medical records from the time confirm the prevalence of scurvy in the Irish population not only during the Great potato blight famine, but there is a likelihood of some level of deficiency during the summer leading up to the fall harvest. [38b] Indeed, the loss of fresh potato over the late spring and summer leading up to the fall harvest, left the poor regularly deficient in vitamin C. Nevertheless scorbutic symptoms such as ecchymoses of the skin (bruises), sore bones, reseeding gums, tooth loss, swelling of feet and legs, and perifollicular hemorrhages—pin-like red dots on the skin—were documented during the blight. [38b] The fresh potato contained close to 30 mg of vitamin C (ascorbic acids), an amount comparable to citrus fruit. Consequently, the Great Famine more thoroughly devastated the poor, who were greatly dependent on the potato for food. [38b]

The story of scurvy is long and torturous as cures had historically been found and then subsequently lost again. Catherine Price [101] writes:

...cures for scurvy continued to be lost and found and lost again. Scurvy appeared among members of the Arctic explorations of the 1820s and miners during the 1848–1850 American Gold Rush. Florence Nightingale reported entire shiploads of cabbage being tossed overboard during the Crimean War of 1853–1856 at the same time that soldiers were perishing from the disease. (The cabbage had been sent specifically to treat scurvy, but thanks to bureaucratic snafus no one had ordered it to be distributed in men's rations.) The disease plagued prisons, refugee camps, and prisoners of war in the 20th century, and emerged among the babies of wealthy and educated Americans and Europeans in the late 1800s and early 1900s because of pasteurized cow's milk. (The heat destroyed the vitamin C.)

Physicians, with their medicines, were powerless at preventing the outbreaks or impeding their progress. The sparse diets, narrowly limited to starch, bread and tinned foods, and the frequent famines that devastated France in 1789, and between 1792 and 1795, caused overt physical manifestations of diseases. Although they were clearly identifiable by the medical doctors, they were nevertheless not preventable. Indeed, it was frequently presumed that the diseases were infectious, as in the cases of pellagra and scurvy. [46]

Sea travel beginning around 1492, often involved more than 45 days at sea, with limited food resources, especially fresh fruits and vegetables. The methods of preserving food involved either drying or brining, which destroyed most of the vitamin C. As the European nations began to more frequently prepare for inter-continental sea exploration, during the early to mid-1600s, the push to uncover the cause of scurvy was being driven with even greater vigor.

Early on, scurvy did not represent a major threat to the sea travellers, since most voyages were rarely longer than 3 months, and remained close to land; it took between 45 to 60 days to deplete human vitamin C reserves and cause scurvy. The extended voyages that were undertaken in the seventeenth century—most of the ships were at sea for months on end—caused the incidence of scurvy to significantly spike. Because many sailors would perish from it at sea, scurvy soon became known as the scourge of the sea.

Scurvy's symptoms were often reported as bleeding gums or clinically referred to as haemorrhagic inflammation, anemia, pronounced general hemorrhaging and general cachexia or wasting of the lean tissue. Such wasting occurred because of a significant fall in appetite.

The countries that were most seriously devastated by scurvy on the high seas were England and Holland. France and Spain, in contrast, often carried onions and leeks as part of their food cargo. These foods were ideal, because their vitamin C concentrations remained relatively stable over time.

There were less frequent reports of scurvy devastating entire French and Spanish crews, although some did exist. This resistance to scurvy may not only be related to the food reserves that were maintained on board, but also to the copious amounts of fruits consumed by the population of these countries; they saturated their body reserves beyond levels normally seen in people of more northern regions.

It wasn't until 1564 that the Dutch physician, Ronsseus recommended oranges in the diet of sailors as an antiscorbutic remedy (**Figure-3.1**). The first Englishman to make a similar recommendation to eat citrus fruits was Dr John Woodall, in 1639. While it had been known for some time that citrus fruits were necessary in order to prevent scurvy, it wasn't until 1753, that Dr William Lind, the first experimental nutritionist, demonstrated beyond a doubt, that something in citrus fruits was effectively preventing the disease (**Figure 3.2**). With his observations, Lind was the first to introduce the concept of **deficiency disease.** He performed a controlled clinical experiment that compared the different remedies that were used in the treatment of scurvy. Lind is renowned for his Salisbury experiment during which he studied the antiscorbutic activity of various acids, notably cider, vinegar, oranges, lemons, sulphuric acid and water. He conducted this study while aboard the warship, Salisbury, which was navigating the English Channel in 1747.

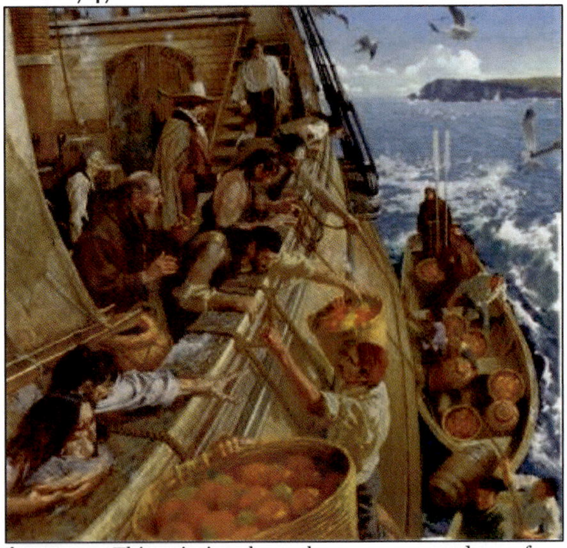

Figure 3.1: This painting shows the passengers and crew from Manila reaching for oranges and lemons, antidotes to scurvy, brought alongside by New Spain, present-day Mexico, friars. Missions planted citrus groves especially to serve the galleon trade. Credit: Robert E. McGinnis © Getty Images

Despite these convincing findings, Lind would have to wait until 1803 for the British navy to implement his recommendation for English ships to carry citrus fruits. The British sailors quickly assumed the nickname of "limeys" because of the regular ingestion of limes for their vitamin C content.[20]

The American navy made similar changes to their sailor's food rations in 1811. The recognition of nutritional deficiency diseases preceded by almost a century the identification of the causes of these disorders. They appeared to be related to accessory food factors later identified as vitamins.

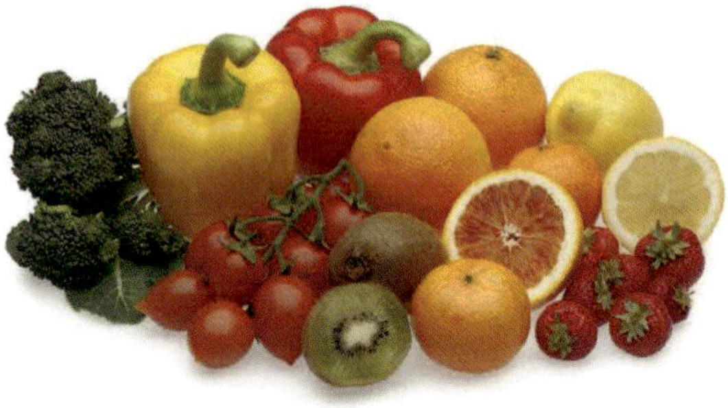

Figure 3.2: Foods Rich in Vitamin C © Effe45/Shutterstock.com

3.2.2 Key Historical Figures in Vitamin Research. It was Dr Nicholas Lunin (1853-1937) who, in his Doctoral thesis, provided the first baseline evidence that purified foodstuff in rats caused an early death. However, Dr Frederick G. Hopkins (1861-1947) is the one who ran with the notion of **accessory food factors**, and promoted the foundation of the vitamin theory, work for which he received, along with Christian Eijkman, the 1929 Nobel Prize in Medicine.[12]

Casimir Funk (1884-1967) was, however, the scientist who proposed the idea of **dietary related disease syndromes**, and further suggested the term "vitamines" to describe the accessory food factor (**Figure 3.3**). The origin of this term came from the understanding of its essentiality to life (vita) and from Funk's work on the disease beriberi, which was present in Polynesians consuming white rice. He showed the vitamin to be an "amine"-based compound; hence **vita amine**. This wording turned out to be a misnomer, as it was later discovered that not all vitamines had an amine component. From the rice husk, Funk had isolated an amine structure that caused a recovery of hand and feet paralysis—a key symptom of beriberi. When fed back to the Japanese sailors, who were suffering from progressive deterioration of the peripheral nerves, the husk caused a reversal of the symptoms. B.C.P. Jansen crystallized the vitamin soon after in 1925, and in 1935.

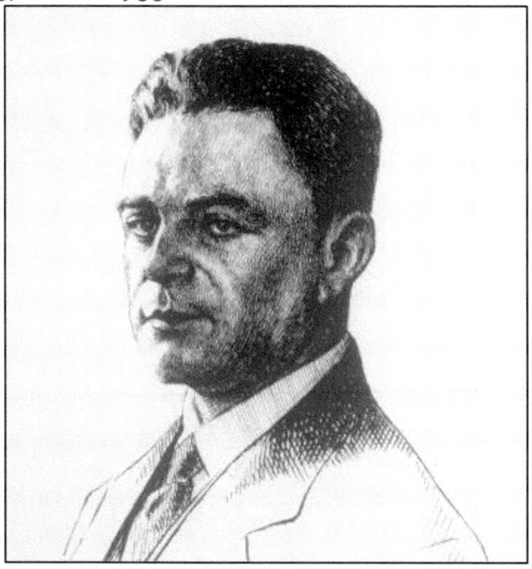

Figure 3.3: Casimir Funk. He was an American biochemist born in Warsaw, Poland, and credited with discovering vitamins. Funk stirred public interest with his 1912 paper on vitamin-deficiency diseases where he coined the term "vitamine". Credit: SCIENCE SOURCE © Getty Images.

The spelling was later changed, by Sir Jack Drummond (1891-1952), to **vitamins**. He also proposed the vitamin alphabetical nomenclature in 1920, which identified the classifications: A, E, K, D, and B.

Robert R. Williams (1886–1965) recognized the molecular structure of thiamin (vitamin B_1), which was a necessary step in its synthetic synthesis in the laboratory. The initial isolation technique facilitated the identification of other vitamins as well. It wasn't, however, until the discovery of vitamin A in 1913 by McCollum and Davis (1879-1967) at the University of Wisconsin, and by a separate team at Yale University, headed by Osborne and Mendel, that the vitamin era of nutrition was launched. They had discovered that vitamin A could be derived from three dietary sources: retinol, carotenoids and carotenes. The teams recognized that retinol was fat-soluble, strictly found in animal products, and was the most biologically active form of vitamin A; retinol was therefore labelled *preformed vitamin A*. The provitamin-A form, which is biologically inactive, is found in the carotenoids. About 67% of vitamin A is derived from the carotenoids. The identification of retinol (vitamin A), confirmed the biological necessity of fat- and water-soluble factors in the diet for the survival of young rats that were being tested.[1]

3.2.3 The Vitamin Era. The excitement around the discovery of vitamins attained a paroxysm between 1930-1940. For the first time, the science of nutrition was taking a firm footing in the domain that once exclusively belonged to Medicine and Chemistry. With the emergence of the vitamin era, in the 1940s, the role of nutrition was no longer going to be assigned to the comforts of kitchen-generated broths and soups for the sick. Rather, it would evolve into a therapeutic domain, which could reverse the process of disease. Such a claim could be tied to the impact of diet as far back as 1564, when Dutch physician, Ronsseus, prescribed oranges as an antiscorbutic agent.

Medicine by contrast, could not make such a claim until the advent of penicillin several centuries later. The sensationalism, surrounding the discovery of vitamins, generated provocative thinking in the fields of Medicine, Chemistry and Nutrition. Nutritionists were most enthusiastic about the possibilities that were linked to vitamins. However, the impact of vitamins truly became evident in the 1940s when malnutrition in the U.S. was running rampant. There were two historical events behind the rise in numerous clusters of nutritional deficiencies around the U.S.: first, president Hoover's food conservation plan of World War-I, habituated the population to white bread; second, the high price of food decreased wholesome food availability to the population during the Great Depression. This prompted a continued population reliance on white bread for calories. Consequently, significant consumption of processed bleached flour led to cases of diagnosable malnutrition throughout the U.S. The Public health strategy of enriching white flour with thiamin, riboflavin, niacin, and later, iron, originated from the governments concerted effort in 1943 to rehabilitate the health of young army recruits, many of whom were not eligible for the US Army because of poor nutrition.[9] A voluntary flour and bread enrichment program soon began throughout the US at the end of WW-II. This single event drew tremendous attention first, to the nutritionally impoverished nature of processed food, and second, to the highly efficacious impact on health of adding synthesized vitamins to food.

> The field of nutrition was gaining prominence as its role in combatting disease was being discovered.

Nutrition gained a great deal of credibility, as it became clear that it was intimately tied with disease. However, the medical and nutrition fields refused to recognize the value of vitamin pills as a treatment modality for either the prevention or the curing of disease. Up until about 20 years ago, vitamin supplements were still cautiously recommended for the prevention of diseases. The fields of Medicine and Nutrition generally advocated, in the mid-1970s and early 80s, the importance of vitamins and minerals, but almost exclusively through wise and broad food selections. Practitioners stayed clear of recommending nutritional supplements.

Yet the public became increasingly eager to purchase vitamin and mineral supplements by the 1970s. Consumer awareness of the potential benefits of vitamin supplements really began with Linus Pauling's bestselling diet book: *Vitamin C and the Common Cold*, which hit the bookstores in 1970. In it, he recommended daily mega-doses of 3,000 milligrams of vitamin C to stop the common cold right in its tracks. Key publications [95, 96, 97] then followed in which he advanced the role of vitamin C in curing the common cold and cancer. Pauling's book and talks wielded quite a powerful impact, principally because he was a two times Nobel Prize laureate. He won the Nobel Prize for Chemistry by the age of 30, and then the Nobel Peace Prize in 1962 for his activism against Japanese American internments during the war, McCarthyism, the Vietnam War, and nuclear proliferation. And so by all accounts, his word was golden.[90]

The problem was that at age 65, Pauling was no longer doing disciplined research, but his book nevertheless became a best seller with reprints in 1971 and then again in 1973. He even published an expanded edition titled: *Vitamin C, the Common Cold and the Flu*. The scientific community was, however, not very impressed as it became evident that Pauling was not diligently reviewing the literature. In truth, the question of whether vitamin C could be used to treat the common cold had, in fact, been more or less settled in 1942, when a team of researchers at the University of Minnesota published a paper in the highly regarded Journal of the American Medical Association. The authors concluded that they found no evidence, among their 980 patients with colds, that vitamin C alone, an antihistamine alone, and a vitamin C plus antihistamine combination, impacted the duration or the severity of colds. [28] In the aftermaths of his best seller, more rigorous studies refuted that vitamin C had any capability to fight off the common cold. One study from the University of Maryland, another from the University of Toronto, and from the Netherlands all concluded that mega-doses of vitamin C had no impact on treating the common cold. Yet, Pauling continued to insist that large doses of vitamin C represented a powerful treatment, not only against colds, but he also advanced in 1977 that cancer death rates could be diminished by 75% using large doses of vitamin C. These claims were subsequently tested by notable research institutions such as the Mayo Clinic in Rochester, Minnesota, and proven to be false. [24] The criticisms directed against Pauling by scientists, did not however, appear to deter vitamin sales. It was specifically the Time magazine cover of April 6, 1992 that became a watershed event for the pharmaceutical industry, according to the National Nutritional Foods Association (NNFA). Time featured colorful pills and capsules with the title: "*The Real Power of Vitamins: New Research Shows they may help Fight Cancer, Heart Disease, and the Ravages of Aging.*" That Time magazine issue became the biggest seller of the entire year. Suddenly, marketing companies began espousing the benefits of organic foods, natural products, and antioxidants.[75] Hoffmann-La Roche, one of the biggest U.S pharmaceutical companies began encapsulating beta-carotene and selling it as an antioxidant supplement in the mid-1990s. The growth in sales was astounding as the highly coveted elixir of life appeared to have finally been created. In 2010 alone, the sale of all carotenoids in capsule-form totalled $1.2 billion. Projected sales of $1.4 billion by 2018 were estimated by BBC Research, a Denver Colorado company specializing in economic, market and policy research.[77] Since the 1990s, carotenoid supplements have evolved to encompass 5 big commercial successes: Beta-carotene, lutein, lycopene, asthaxanthin and zeaxanthin. The explosion of nutraceuticals and functional foods onto the market, in the middle 1990s, changed the conservative tone that had dominated diet therapy. Dietitians, nurse practitioners, P.As, and medical doctors soon began prescribing vitamin and antioxidant supplements, but yet the Dietary Guidelines for American (2010-2020) continued to insist that most nutrients should be acquired from nutrient-dense foods. [91] Nutrition advocates argued that current dietary intake of fruits and vegetables was suboptimal, and left the US population vulnerable to disease. Indeed the NHANES 2007-2010 study found that 75% of Americans eat less than the recommended amount of fruit, and 87% less than ideal vegetable recommendation. [75] It was believed that the free radicals damaged cell membrane integrity, arterial walls, and caused DNA mutations. Conceptually, it was very reasonable to assume that taking these antioxidant supplements would assuredly be beneficial. The reality was actually not as encouraging. In some cases observational studies found a positive association whereas other studies found no impact of multivitamin supplements (MVS) on health outcomes. [91] In several studies, taking MVS increased the risk of disease. The US National Cancer Institute in collaboration with Finland's National Public Health Institute prospectively monitored 29,000 Finnish men who were smokers and over the age of 50. This group of men were at a very high risk of developing heart disease and cancer. Subjects were randomly given vitamin E, beta-carotene, both, or neither, and were followed over 8 years.[51] Researchers had to stop the study prematurely because those taking daily supplements were at a greater risk of dying from lung cancer or heart disease compared to those not taking supplements. Subsequent studies at the Fred Hutchinson Cancer Research Center in 1996, the University of Copenhagen in 2004, Johns Hopkins School of Medicine in 2005, and the National Cancer Institute in 2007, all [74b] that supplement users were more likely to die from cancer and heart disease than non-supplement users. More recently, a research team out of the University of Minnesota followed 39,000 older women and concluded in 2011, that those women who regularly took multivitamins, magnesium, zinc, copper and iron supplements had higher death rates than those who did not. The study concludes: [77]

Based on existing evidence, we see little justification of the general widespread use of dietary supplements.

It appears now that nutrients in foods carry the most potent health effects rather than isolated nutrients in capsule format. It could be that the nutrients act synergistically with one another to deliver powerful health protection. The reality is that there are, for instance, about 600 types of carotenoids in foods, but the pharmaceutical companies only bottled 10 of them for sale.

3.3 Vitamin Deficiencies

3.3.1 Introduction
The goal of this section is not to be exhaustive in the treatment of nutritional deficiencies, but rather to expose the students to the highlights of some of the more important diseases. Since this is an introductory textbook, the author does not want to overwhelm the student with the level of significant detail, normally found in textbooks purposely framed for students in the nutrition or medical majors, but rather desires to briefly introduce students to the more salient and memorable aspects of nutritional diseases. It is the author's hope that the nutrients, covered here, are the most relevant to the students.

3.3.2 Thiamin Deficiency

The vitamin was that extraneous food co-factor considered as essential to life as the calorie, yet it belonged neither to the protein, the carbohydrate nor the fat groups. It provided no energy, yet its role was vital to the normal functioning of metabolism, and of some unknown processes of the biological system. Thiamin exemplifies the central role played by vitamins in human health. Historical records document the devastating blow that a thiamin deficiency can wield. The efforts of tying thiamin with the disease beriberi—the isolation, structural determination and synthesis of the vitamin—were all part of the birth of vitaminology.

The work that evolved around the study of beriberi is an interesting one for two reasons: first, beriberi along with scurvy, were critical in the advancement of the science of nutrition as a credible medical partner; second, the eventual synthesis of thiamin meant that a deficiency disease could be treated without food, but with the isolated vitamin. This brought nutrition into a new era.

Beriberi produces medical symptoms of polyneuritis, which means a degeneration of the peripheral nerves. This essentially caused a paralysis of the hands and feet, and greatly diminished the activity level of the individual. Although it had been documented as far back as 1611 by the first Governor General of the Dutch East Indies, and then in 1642, by the first European physician, Bontius, the cases of beriberi were nothing more than sporadic.[12] The early recorded cases of beriberi were made in what is now called Djakarta in Indonesia, but the number of cases never amounted to any significant threat. It was in the early beginnings of the nineteenth century, a period that coincided with the industrial revolution, that more frequent cases of beriberi began to appear, affecting mostly rice-eating people.

The pathology of the disease fell into three groups affected by changes to: (a) the heart; (b) the nervous system, also called the dry form. There was a (c) wet form characterized by edema or water retention. All three forms could change into the other. The initial belief was that the disease was caused by toxic substances found in carbohydrate-rich foods or because of by-products of natural occurring gut bacteria.

However, one of Eijkman's experiments in 1890, which involved feeding potatoes to hens, produced no visible signs of polyneuritis. It wasn't clear why rice starch would produce beriberi, and potato starch would not in these birds. At the time, Eijkman believed the potato starch was less prone to be fermented in the gut, whereas rice appeared to be more easily fermentable. This interpretation was accepted for a time, allowing him to focus his research on the notion that diet was behind the etiology of this disease.[18]

Looking back on this initial work, he did not understand that the potato contained adequate concentrations of thiamin. He found similar neuropathies in the hens when he fed them raw tapioca and sago, but interestingly reversed the neuropathies when he added rice bran to the starches.[19]

Eijkman found many commonalities between this form of polyneuritis observed in his experimental hens fed rice, and the symptoms typically described in human beriberi. Despite these similarities, he was not yet convinced that diet had as strong a connection with polyneuritis gallinarum. In his opinion, more work needed to be done before the diet connection could be established with certainty. Such a resolution could be found only through human experimentation, a practice considered by Eijkman to be unethical.[19]

Naturally occurring human experiments were, however, taking place in the different penal institutions in Java. Eijkman's friend, Dr A.G. Voderman who medically inspected the jails in Java, observed

> Dr A.G Voderman observed that prisoners fed machine-milled rice had 30 times more cases of beriberi than prisoners fed hand milled rice.

that the prisoners fed hand milled rice were eating a crude form of rice, and therefore not developing beriberi, whereas those prisoners fed mechanically milled polished rice had thirty times more cases of beriberi. Inspired by Eijkman's discoveries, Voderman fed crude rice to those prisoners sick with disease, and found the condition was reversed. From this finding, began a series of investigations attempting to isolate the factor found in the rice bran. With much effort, the antineuritic crystals were isolated in 1926 by Jansen and Donath. It wasn't until 1949 that milled rice was enriched in the U.S, and 1951 before this isolated factor was named thiamin or B_1 according to internationally accepted nomencloture.[17] In modern times, alcoholism can cause a very distinct neurological outcome medically labelled as Wernicke-Korsekoff syndrome.

Although most often diagnosed in chronic alcoholics it can be also found in patients with chronic diarrhea, malignancies, drug abuse and AIDS. If left untreated, up to 20% of cases will die. [85]

The Wernicke encephalopathy is characterized by peripheral neuropathies whereas the Korsekoff psychosis is characteristically recognized by short term memory loss, disorientation and confabulation. [85]

Both the discoveries of ascorbic acid (vitamin C) and finally thiamin opened the flood gates to an enthusiastic community of nutritionists and naturalists who wanted to run with the idea that vitamins could carry broad sweeping health benefits.

3.3.3 Niacin Deficiency—Pellagra in the American South of the Early 1900s

Niacin deficiency appeared in Europe as new world explorers brought back maize from the Americas; it was quickly adopted as a staple in southern Europe during the 17th and 18th centuries. The problem was that the Mexican Indians would typically soak the maize in lime in order to soften the corn and create a more basic environment necessary for the release of niacin; this made it more available for absorption. The southern Europeans did not bring back to Europe the practice of soaking the maize in lime, consequently, the prevalence of pellagra grew significantly. Also, around the 19th century, the maize was reportedly developing toxic molds while in storage. France then banned the maize from the country.[21]

In the Southern US, pellagra began to surface as a problem around 1910 because of the new technology recently adopted in the processing of maize. The procedure involved milling the maize and separating the germ and its oil to derive a cornmeal. This process halved the content of tryptophan, which was already poor and greatly reduced the concentration of niacin.

> **Pellagra, with four classic symptoms – diarrhea, dermatitis, dementia and death, occurs from niacin deficiency.**

This had serious consequences, since the tryptophan—an essential amino acid richly found in meat and dairy products—was not abundantly found in the southern impoverished diet, and therefore could not synthesize niacin. This was a biochemical step normally undertaken through the intermediary action of pyridoxine (vitamin B6). Pellagra became prominent, devastating the populations with the classic 4-D symptoms: diarrhea, dermatitis, dementia and death. Between 1906 and 1940, over 100,000 deaths were attributed to Pellagra. [118]

In 1914, the Surgeon General of the US, Dr Rupert Blue, asked Dr Joseph Goldberger to investigate the pellagra epidemic in the American South—long believed to be infectious in nature. Goldberger was an accomplished physician and epidemiologist, having worked for the US Public Health Service while investigating typhus, yellow, dengue and typhoid fevers between 1902 and 1906. He demonstrated that prisoners fed a diet heavy in maize contracted pellagra; when protein was included and maize removed, the prisoners recovered. He successfully disproved that it was an infectious disease, and confirmed rather, that it was a dietary deficiency. Politically and socially, the findings were unpopular, and thus progress in eradicating this disease advanced slowly until Conrad Elvehjem demonstrated in 1937, that pellagra was tied to niacin and tryptophan deficiencies.[21]

It isn't surprising that a Niacin deficiency would have such serious outcomes, as it is widely utilized as a co-enzyme—nicotinamide adenine dinucleotide (NAD)—in carbohydrate and fat metabolism. [86] Currently in the U.S, synthetic niacin is added back to the flour through a voluntary food industry-based enrichment program, which also includes thiamin and riboflavin.

Interestingly, niacin is used at high concentrations, ranging between 100-1000mg/day, as an alternative to statins to treat hypercholesterolemia. Niacin taken at such high doses exceeds the dietary Tolerable Upper Intake (UL) of 45 mg, resulting in a flushing effect on the face. Nevertheless, its efficacy at reducing blood cholesterol warrants its use as a viable alternative to statins. [86]

Richly found in beef liver, chicken breast, pork, salmon, tuna, enriched breakfast cereals, and rice, niacin requirements can easily be met with a balanced diet. [86]

3.3.4 Vitamin D Deficiency: 1, 25 (OH)$_2$ Vitamin D

The essentiality of vitamin D was first unknowingly documented when English physician, Dr Francis Glisson (1597-1677), in 17th century England, wrote the first treatise on rickets in 1650 titled: "de Rachitide." This was a published work that arose from the initiative of 9 men who began meeting in London in 1645 with the intention of gaining the upper hand on this disease. Glisson was credited for his significant effort in accurately describing, in significant detail, the disease of rickets. He documented how children were clearly affected by disturbing bone deformations during the winter months. It was not clear whether the bone abnormalities were the consequence of the environmental conditions they were living in or some disease process.

In 1919 Edward Mallanby showed that if dogs were kept indoors and fed strict diets, they developed softened bones, which lead to bone deformations similar to rickets in children.[71]

Interestingly, Mallanby showed that the dogs recovered if they were fed cod liver oil. This discovery was significant in instituting the early twentieth century practice of giving one tablespoon of cod liver oil to children living in countries like England, Canada, and the Northern US. This was a practice that greatly diminished the prevalence of the disease because of the elevated concentrations of vitamin D in 1 tablespoon of oil (1360 IU). This amount was more than 3000% greater than the level found in 3oz-wt of beef liver and 200% more concentrated than a 3oz-wt of sockeye salmon. [87]

Indeed, it appears that unless the diet was rich in fish such as salmon, swordfish, tuna and cod liver oil, the diet could not possibly contribute significant amounts of vitamin D, thereby leaving sunlight as the only alternative source of the vitamin. In children, for instance, living in the northern geographical areas, such as Minnesota, North Dakota, Montana, Washington State, Maine, New York and Canada, there is a heightened risk of developing rickets (**Figure 3.4**) between the months of November and March. During the winter months there is unfortunately reduced skin-generated vitamin D, because of diminished skin exposure to ultraviolet light. [87]

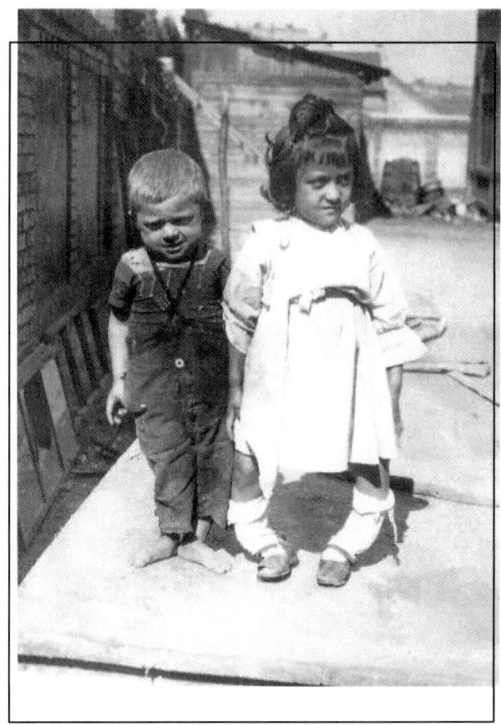

Figure 3.4: Rickets, a vitamin D deficiency, causes human bones to become warped. CREDIT: NYPL/Science Source. © Getty Images

For sun exposure to be a significant contributor of vitamin D, a person would need to have their legs, face, arms or back, exposed to ultraviolet light for between 5 to 30 minutes between 10 AM and 3 PM without the use of any kind of sunscreen.

> 5–30 minutes of sun exposure without sunscreen are needed to produce vitamin D in the skin.

Commercial tanning beds that are used moderately and that emit between 2 to 6% UVB radiation can produce sufficient amounts of vitamin D in the skin as well. Because of the concerns for skin cancers, however, the American Academy of Dermatology strongly advises that sunscreens be used on those parts of the body exposed to sunlight or UV radiation.[67]

There are currently no studies that have determined the minimum skin exposure to sun deemed necessary to safely generate vitamin D with minimal risk of skin cancer. Consequently, the most significant and safe sources of vitamin D can only be from dietary sources.

However, over the last 20 years, there is evidence that the nutritional status of vitamin D in both men and women in the United States has slightly declined because, in part, of increased body weight, more frequent use of sunblock, and decreased milk consumption.[67]

The concern for vitamin D deficiency pertains not only to children who can develop rickets, but also to adults who tend to develop osteomalacia, which is characterized by inadequately calcified bones, and a higher propensity to fracture more easily.

The long-term implication of suboptimal vitamin D intake is the development of osteoporosis. Recent research, has also documented higher prevalence of cardiovascular disease and some cancers in individuals with low serum hydroxyl-vitamin D. Epidemiological data shows lower incidences of colon cancer among individuals with a good vitamin D status. At the moment, the evidence emerging from human studies does not support a protective role against breast and pancreatic cancers (NIH, 2020i).

By contrast, excess intakes of vitamin D can be problematic. Most of the literature supports the toxicity threshold range of between 10,000 to 40,000 international units (I. U) per day. The Food and Nutrition Board (F. N. B.) recommends gauging the adequacy of vitamin D intake based on serum concentration levels of 25(OH)D that do not exceed 125 to 150 nmol/L (50-60 ng/ml). The concern is that concentrations exceeding this range, over the long-term, have been linked to higher overall mortality, and greater incidences of pancreatic cancer and cardiovascular events. [87]

3.3.4.1 Individuals at risk of vitamin D deficiency
There are several groups of individuals who are at risk of vitamin D deficiency today in the U.S. The elderly are at some risk, especially those who are confined to the indoors, those with impoverished diets who do not consume milk, or oily fish, and who have a skin pigment that is less capable of synthesizing vitamin D from UV radiation).[14]

Also, populations with black or dark skin, and those populations that are Asian, Middle Eastern and African are particularly vulnerable to poor vitamin D status. It isn't clear if this diminished D status is the consequence of genetic differences in the efficiency by which the skin synthesizes vitamin D, or if it is because of a behavioral tendency to stay out of the sun. [87]

Another group that is vulnerable to vitamin D deficiency are breast-fed babies. The vitamin D content of breast milk is directly related to the mother's dietary intake of the vitamin according to a recent Canadian study that examined the prevalence of rickets among young Canadian infants that were exclusively breast-fed. [87]

The study reports that mothers who tended to take vitamin D supplements had higher levels of vitamin D in the breast milk. However, those infants with rickets were all exclusively breast-fed. The problem gets compounded because the American Academy of Pediatrics (AAP) recommends that young infants stay out of the sun and wear protective clothing. [87]

Consequently, the AAP also recommends that infants who are exclusively or partially breast-fed receive 400 IUs per day of vitamin D in supplement form. Other groups that are subject to a higher incidence of vitamin D deficiency are homebound individuals, women who wear heavy clothing that covers the entire body including the head, such as religious sisters, and those individuals who use a lot of sunscreen. [87]

Finally, individuals suffering from fat malabsorption or those who have undergone gastric bypass surgery tend to not absorb sufficient fat-soluble vitamins, notably vitamin D. Obese patients are also at risk because of the excess adipose tissue.[14, 87]

3.3.5 Vitamin K Deficiency. Vitamin K is known by two forms of chemical structures: phylloquinone (vitamin K1) and a series of menaquinones (vitamin K2). Phylloquinone is the form in which vitamin K is present in the diet, notably green leafy vegetables, pomegranate, and vegetable oils (**Figure 3.5**). Menaquinones, on the other hand, are the forms synthesized by GI gut bacteria. [80] This is a fat-soluble vitamin, similar to vitamins A, D and E, with very unique characteristics. Consequently, providing a vitamin K injection within a few days of birth is critical to prevent Hemorrhagic Disease of the Newborn. Consequently, the North American Academy of Pediatrics recommends one single dose of vitamin K at birth. [80] In cases of prolonged broad spectrum antibiotic use, vitamin K can become deficient especially when the diet is already poor; the antibiotic kills many of the friendly gut bacteria that produce vitamin K. [22] At the level of bone metabolism, vitamin K plays a significant role via osteocalcin, a protein-hormone involved in bone mineralization. [80]

It acts as a co-enzyme in the synthesis of key proteins, notably involved in blood clotting (hemostasis). Moreover, prothrombin, a protein directly involved in the clotting mechanism, is dependent on vitamin K as part of the clotting mechanism. For newborns vitamin K transport across the placenta can be limited. [53]

Currently, the role of calcium and vitamin D are considered important during childhood, adolescence and early adulthood in the prevention of osteoporosis, [78] however, it is not clear to what extent vitamin K can also reduce the risk of osteoporosis. [80]

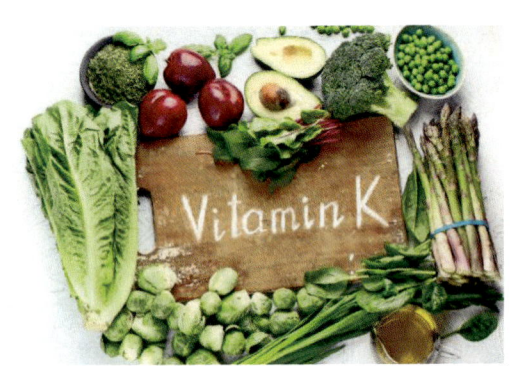

Figure 3.5 Rich sources of Dietary Vitamin K. by Tatjana Baibakova © Shutterstock_ 1389604916/Shutterstock.com

3.4 Micronutrients involved in various types of Anemias

Among hematological defects, anemia is possibly the most common disorder in medical practice. Patients traditionally present with skin pallor, lethargy, dyspnea, poor physical endurance, faintness, nausea, and anorexia. The symptomatic representation of anemia may not always be limited to the classical picture, but tends to be compounded by other pathologies.

Anemia specifically refers to a low hemoglobin concentration in the peripheral blood, which may arise from a number of factors including iron deficiency, B-12 and/or folic acid deficiencies, thalassemic syndromes, sideroblastic anemia and anemia of chronic disease.

The World Health Organization (WHO) has identified three of the most significant nutrient deficiencies in the world and has prioritized them as needing urgent eradication.[120]

First, iron deficiency is the most prevalent form of deficiency worldwide; it is estimated that 80% of the world's population may be deficient in iron, whereas 30% is likely suffering from iron deficiency anemia. Second, vitamin A deficiency is recognized as the most preventable form of blindness, and third, iodine deficiency is now linked to the most preventable cause of mental retardation in the world.

In this section you will discover the key nutrients involved in various forms of anemia. While iron deficiency anemia is commonly recognized as the

> **Dyspnea** – difficulty breathing
> **Anorexia** – diminished appetite

most popular form of anemia, not many are aware

of the fact that even iron deficiency anemia can be caused by copper and pyridoxine deficiencies. There are, however, other types of anemias notably a form of macrocytic anemia called megaloblastic anemia caused by folate and/or B 12 deficiencies.

3.4.1 Iron deficiency anemia

> The WHO identifies iron, vitamin A and iodine deficiencies as urgent health priorities worldwide.

Iron deficiency anemia is identified, by hematologists using a blood smear, as a microcytic anemia because of the smaller size of the red blood cells. This is because iron is an essential component of hemoglobin, the main protein that makes up the red blood cell.[39] This protein carries oxygen throughout the vascular system, delivering it to tissues and cells. In the absence of iron, less hemoglobin is synthesized in the bone marrow, causing the blood cell to be reduced in size; the red blood cell is said to be microcytic. This means that its capacity to transport oxygen to the cells, for aerobic metabolism to take place, becomes reduced and limited. This causes fatigue and a diminished immune system. Those individuals with the lowest risk of developing iron deficiency anemia are adult men and postmenopausal women. Those at highest risk are women of childbearing years especially those with heavy menstrual cycles, pregnant women, low birth weight infants, infants in general, and pre-school toddlers.[25] There is evidence now emerging that up to 50% of children ages 1 to 2 may not being getting adequate amounts of dietary iron.[25]

Most prone to anemia are teenage girls, 12-19 years of age, who are still affected by significant growth and development, [25] and who tend to either practice restrictive dietary behaviors for the purpose of weight control, or who simply have poor dietary habits. In this age group, early exposure to highly addictive fast-foods and snacks create a strong stimulation of the pleasure centers of the brain; often they are unable to change their eating preferences because of taste addiction. When trying to lose weight, young teenage girls tend to not consume breakfast or breakfast cereals fortified with iron. Without breakfast cereals in the morning, it becomes more difficult to meet the requirements for folate, iron and fiber by the end of the day because of the troublesome dietary habits of North Americans.

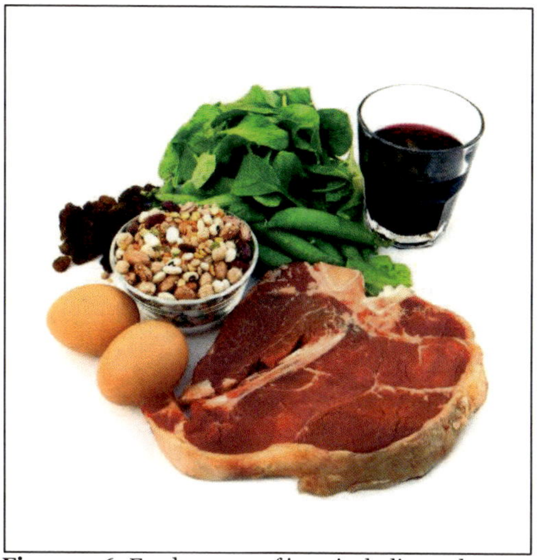

Figure 3.6: Food sources of iron, including red meat, eggs, spinach, peas, beans, raisins and prune juice. © Robyn Mackenzie

Dietary iron can be found in two forms: **heme-iron** and **non-heme iron** (NIH, 2020j) **(Figure 3.6)**. The heme iron is an exclusive constituent of animal products, notably eggs, meats, and organ meats. This form of iron is the most easily absorbed, reaching levels as high as 35% when body iron reserves are low. However, the overall mean absorption of iron in men is about 6%, and 13% in women.[25]

In a North American context, heme iron represents only 20% of our total dietary intake of iron. By contrast, non-heme iron, found in breads, cereals, vegetables and legumes, represents 80% of our total

> **Vascular system** – network of blood vessels that transport blood and nutrients throughout the body

iron intake. This form of iron can reach 20% absorbability when reserves are low and only 2% when body reserves of iron are elevated.[39]

Also at risk are men and women, who engage in intense physical training such as jogging, swimming, and cycling. Lower iron stores can occur because of greater blood loss through the gastrointestinal tract, a higher turnover rate of red blood cells, and the more frequent rupturing of red blood cells in the feet, because of the influence of the high impact of the sport.

Consequently, it has been estimated that athletes may have a 30% greater requirement for iron compared to non-athletes. Most at risk, within the arena sports, are female athletes, distance runners, and vegetarian athletes.[7]

> Athletes may require up to 30% more iron in their diets compared to non-athletes.

There is obviously a balance that needs to be reached between adequate and excessive intakes of iron. This is because the body does not excrete iron very well, but instead it stores it in organs. This means the risk of toxicity can be great.

For instance it has been documented that children who mistakenly consumed 200 mg of iron, died from an iron overload. Also, there are concerns that chronically large intakes of iron can lead to a greater risk of cardiovascular disease. Iron stimulates free radical production in the body, leading to the inflammation or damage of the vascular lining. This is the first step before the development of an atheroma, which either partially or completely blocks the blood circulation in the artery—a symptom of atherosclerosis.

Iron may also increase the likelihood of free radical production [32] and of the resulting oxidation the light-density lipoproteins (LDLs), [92] which precedes cholesterol leaking out into the blood, and being captured by macrophages. From this follows the formation of foam-like compounds that constitute the basic material that form the atheroma.

3.4.2 Pyridoxine (B-6) and Copper (Cu+).

Vitamin B-6 is abundantly found in a mixed diet of meats and fish, and is found in mild concentrations in vegetables and non-enriched grains (NIH, 2020k). In the US, most individuals consume pyridoxine from fortified cereals, beef, poultry, and starchy vegetables. The B vitamin, **pyridoxine** works as a cofactor in the synthesis of haemoglobin. Consequently, a B-6 deficiency can be linked to microcytic anemia—typically seen in iron-deficiency anemia. [89] A B-6 deficiency does not usually occur in isolation but in concert with other B vitamin deficiencies such as folate and B-12. [89] Symptoms can manifest as glossitis, cheilosis, angular stomatitis, depression, and weakened immune system. [54]

Also **Copper** (**Cu**) appears to be involved in the synthesis of haemoglobin though the mechanism has not yet been confirmed. [31] It has been suggested that copper also assists in iron absorption through its incorporation in a metalloenzyme called ceruloplasmin. At this level it is responsible for oxidizing iron from its ferrous Fe^{+2} to its ferric state (Fe^{+3}), a critical step in the binding of iron to the transport protein transferrin. [68] Vitamin C can help in this reduction, thus favoring non-heme iron absorption. [31] Hence in the absence of copper, the body has a diminished capacity to transport iron to the bone marrow, thereby compromising iron reserves in the body and increasing the risk of developing anemia.

When iron deficiency is officially diagnosed, using a combination of diet assessment, and blood biochemistry, it is advisable to prescribe an iron supplement in order to replenish iron reserves. Supplementation is generally recommended when it is clear that the normal diet of the individual is significantly poor in iron.[39]

The prescription most popularly made by physicians is iron fumarate because of the higher level of elemental iron present in the supplement (**Figure-3.7**). Elemental iron refers to the pure form of iron in the supplement. For instance, if the physician prescribes 100 mg of iron fumarate, he knows that his patient will be receiving 33 mg of dietary iron. Contrast that prescription with iron gluconate, which would only contain 12 mg of iron for a 100 mg prescription. [88] Obviously, recovery from iron deficiency anemia would occur more rapidly with iron fumarate. In order to prevent iron supplementation from decreasing zinc absorption, Whittaker [126] recommends that iron supplements be less than 25mg, and be taken between meals.

3.4.3 Riboflavin Deficiency (B-2).

Riboflavin deficiency is not prominent in western societies that have good nutrient enrichment programs, but is the most common deficiency among B vitamin in developing nations where processed white rice is common, and intakes of meat and milk are limited[106] (**Figure 3.8**). In the North American setting, the risk of B-2 deficiency remains a problem however, for the elderly and adolescents whose dietary habits are quite poor.[98]

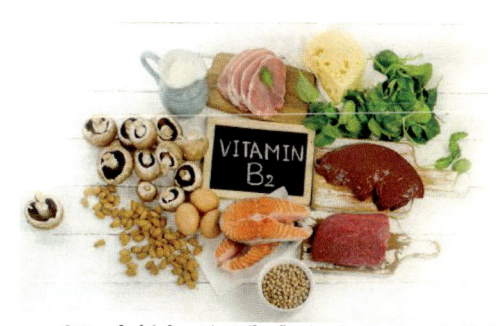

Figure 3.8 Foods highest in Riboflavin. By Tatjana Baibakova © Shutterstock- 519432232/Shutterstock.com

Vitamin B-2 deficiency can lead to iron deficiency anemia by heightening iron loss from the gastrointestinal (GI) level, and it can diminish iron mobilization from the body stores, notably the bone marrow in animals. Additionally, B-2 appears to also enhance iron absorption from the GI tract. In humans riboflavin has been shown to facilitate the recovery of children and adults from microcytic iron deficiency anemia.[106,100, 99] Moreover, B-2 deficiency also causes a set of very recognizable physical symptoms that are quite distinct from other deficiencies, notably edematous lips (cheilosis), sores at the edge of the mouth (angular stomatitis), (**Figures 3.9**) and glossitis (reddened tongue causes by excess blood or hyperemia).[79] Because riboflavin acts as a co-enzyme in metabolism as Flavin Adenine Dinucleotide (FAD), a deficiency can precipitate other B vitamin metabolic deficiencies.[79] Foods that are particularly rich in riboflavin are beef liver, enriched breakfast cereals, yogurt and milk. Additionally, meats such beef and chicken, and fish such as salmon are good sources of the vitamin.[79]

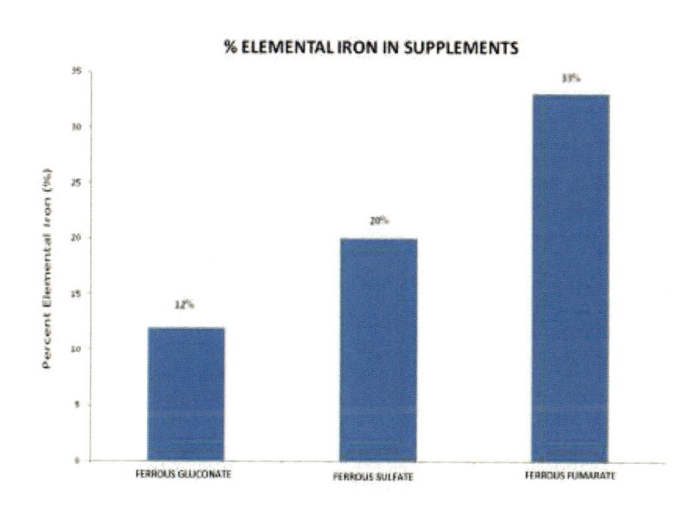

Figure 3.7: The three most common non-heme iron supplements that are recommended; Source: [Iron. Drug Facts and Comparisons.

Facts & Comparisons eAnswers [database online] St. Louis, MO Wolters Kluwer Health Inc; 2013]

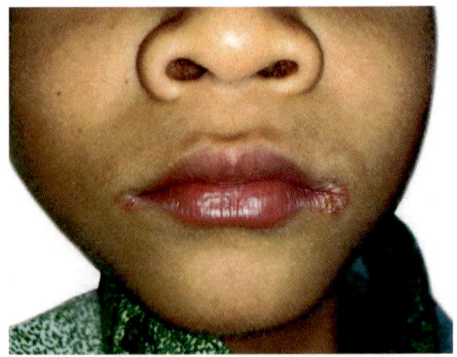

Figure 3.9 Young girl with cheilosis and angular stomatitis by Zay Nyi Nyi © Shutterstock_1451373236/Shutterstock.com

3.4.4 Megaloblastic Anemia (B-12 & Folate)

Megaloblastic anemia refers to an unusually high number of large red blood cells in a standard Blood Smear. These large red blood cells have low hemoglobin contents, and therefore, a diminished capacity to carry oxygen. This results in symptoms of tiredness, weakness, irritability and shortness of breath. These large red blood cells or macrocytic cells are formed because the normal mitotic division of the red blood cell, also called the erythrocyte, is compromised.[34, 39]

Folate is necessary for DNA duplication in the nucleus of the cell to occur. If the nucleus is unable to divide, then the red blood cell simply becomes larger with continued growth, unable to divide into two smaller cells through mitotic division.[49]

It was researcher, Dr Lucy Wills who, in the 1940s, observed that folate was necessary in the prevention of the anemia of pregnancy. From this observation, scientists were able to document the role of folate in cell duplication, and in the production of new cells.

This discovery carried some significance as it allowed scientists to identify folate as a critical component in DNA synthesis and duplication, especially in the periods of rapid growth as seen in infancy, and in pregnancy. Interestingly, folate may also protect DNA from important mutations that could lead to cancer.[34]

Folate is naturally found in dark green leafy vegetables like spinach, broccoli and asparagus, and in citrus fruits like oranges and grapefruits. Legumes like dried peas, beans, seeds and liver are also notable sources. In its natural form, folate needs to be activated by vitamin B-12. Because of this relationship with vitamin B-12, it is possible for an individual to experience folate deficiency evolving from suboptimal B12 intake. In other words, an individual who is consuming sufficient leafy greens and fruits may actually have enough dietary folate in the diet, but because of the B-12 deficiency, that person would be unable to activate the folate found in the green foliage. The result would be megaloblastic anemia or in other words large red blood cells.

Nearly 25 years ago, the National Health and Nutrition Examination Survey (NHANES 1988-1994) reported that folate consumption, in the overall US population, was not adequate because of the notable decline in fruit and vegetable consumption, especially among young women of childbearing years.[103]

Promptly, in 1996, the FDA established regulations requiring the fortification of enriched breads, cereals, flours, cornmeal, pastas and rice with folic acid.

Finally, the fortification program was initiated in 1998, which was an important public health measure intended to correct the suboptimal folate status in the US population, and diminish the prevalence of neural tube defects showing up in newborn American infants.

Neural tube defects are a set of conditions characterized by a defective formation of the spinal cord (Spina Bifida), skull and brain (Anencephaly). Health statistics reported that there were, in the early 1990s, 2500 children born with either Spina Bifida or anencephaly each year in the U.S., with approximately 1500 fetuses aborted yearly. The American diet had become so impoverished, that it was now having an irreversible impact on the progeny of the American people.

As early as the late 1980s, there was a serious shift in the eating habits of Americans; they deviated from regularly consuming fresh produce towards a more abundant selection of ready-to-eat processed dinners, snacks, and fast foods.

The Public Health response to this dietary disaster was to encourage greater fruit and vegetable consumption. The Healthy People 2000 campaign included recommendations for the public to eat 5 or more fruits and vegetables per day.[61]

Also, the National Cancer Institute jointly worked with the Produce for a Better Health Foundation, to implement, between 1991 and 2006, the 5 A DAY for Better Health national program (Johnston et al., 2000).[30] It was an initiative that encouraged a minimum of 5 fruits and vegetable servings per day in order to help decrease cancer rates and other health issues, notably the risks of neural tube defects.

The program was unsuccessful at decreasing neural tube defects (NTDs) sufficiently to align incidence rates with those of other Westernized nations. Hence, the government implemented mandatory fortification of cereals in 1998 in the hope of universally raising blood folate levels in most women of reproductive age.[62]

A study by Honein and colleagues,[51] published in a 2001 issue of the Journal of the American Medical Association, documented that since the initiation of the fortification program, the prevalence of neural tube defects in the U.S. declined significantly. The fortification program was so potent that some fortified breakfast cereals often contain between 50-100% of the RDA in one serving.

Still the percentage of NTDs was higher than it should have been with such a fortification program. The reason for the discrepancy was the sizable number of young girls between the ages of 16 and 25 who did not eat breakfast and who avoided carbohydrates for weight control purposes.

Dr Carole Johnston and colleagues, from the Department of Nutrition at Arizona State University East Meza, investigated in 2000, how effective the 5 A DAY for Better Health program was in causing fruits and vegetable consumption to increase in this young population of women.[61] It was hoped that, in combining the 5 A DAY program with the cereal fortification initiative, perhaps greater numbers of women could be positively affected. They concluded however, in a paper published in the Journal of Nutrition, that while the campaigns did cause a 20% jump in the servings of fruits and vegetables consumed, intake of dark green cruciferous vegetables was still below minimum recommendations.[61] They wrote:

White potato consumption, including the consumption of French fries, remained similar to the earlier survey, and the consumption of dark green or deep yellow vegetables was less than 0.4 serving/d.

Troubled by the rather colorless diet observed in the young women, they go on to write:

Americans are consuming more fruits and vegetables, but they are not regularly consuming the particular fruits and vegetables that are likely to impart robust health effects.

The campaign did not succeed in turning a generation's impoverished eating habits around, but especially, it did not impact those likely to become pregnant. This was significant, as the requirement for folate is significantly higher during pregnancy, as well as during lactation.

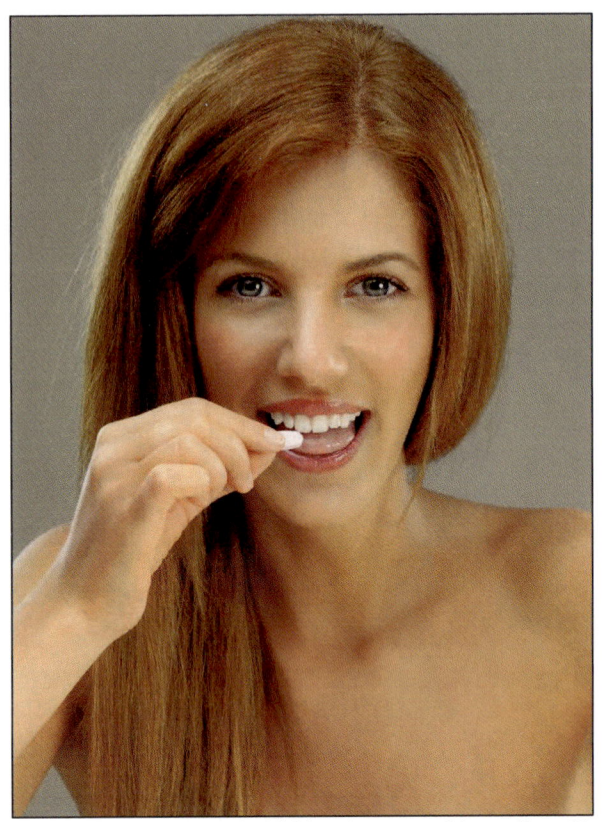

Figure 3.10: Woman of Child-bearing Age Taking Folic Acid Supplement. By Comaniciu Dan © Shutterstock 86966731 /Shutterstock.com

Therefore, in order to optimize pregnancies, it is strongly recommended that young women consume adequate amounts of folate prior to pregnancy even if they have to take folate supplements (**Figure-3.10**).

There are also medical conditions that increase the excretion rate of folate from the biological system, and therefore heighten the risk of deficiency: liver disease, kidney dialysis, malabsorption, and alcohol abuse. And while megaloblastosis remains a specific symptom of folate deficiency, there are other more subtle symptoms that can help in the diagnosis: loss of weight, chronic diarrhea, weakness, sore muscles, and headaches.

Nevertheless, the goal is to increase the intakes of both fruits and vegetables on a daily basis. Failing that, a supplement is highly recommended. The folate in fortified cereals and other grain products has one important difference with the folate in fruits and vegetables: it contains folate that is already biologically active and therefore does not require vitamin B-12 for activation.

Although this seems like a good thing, on the short term, folate fortification created a serious medical screening problem. It turns out that the practice of fortifying cereals and grains with folate, masked B-12 deficiency. In other words, at the screening level, when a physician observed megaloblastosis in a blood smear, they asked three questions: first, is this macrocytosis caused by folate deficiency? Second, is it the result of a vitamin B-12 deficiency? And third, is it from both folate and B-12 deficiencies?

The problem is that with fortification there is a decreased prevalence of macrocytosis because most of the folate consumed is already biologically active. Consequently, B-12 deficiency can now go undetected since the active fortified folate resolves the problem of megaloblastic anemia, but not the neurological disturbances arising from B-12 deficiency.

This is serious enough, because independent of the activation of folate, B-12 plays a very specific function in maintaining the integrity of the myelin sheath. Translated into real medical outcomes, a vitamin B-12 deficiency, if undetected over several years, can lead to irreversible neurological damage characterized by a disturbed gait, tingling in the extremities (parathesias) and a cognitive decline.

Vitamin B-12 is limited to foods containing animal protein. This means milk, cheese, fish, poultry, red meats, pork and eggs are all rich in vitamin B-12.

Historically, it had been taught that pure vegans were more susceptible to B-12 deficiencies because of the absence of animal protein in their diets. However, since many breakfast cereals, soy, rice and almond milks have been fortified with many micronutrients including B-12, the risk of deficiency has greatly diminished in this group.[123]

Moreover, because significant amounts of vitamin B-12 are reabsorbed through the entero-hepatic circulation and reused, it takes appreciable amounts of time for an actual B-12 deficiency to manifest itself; some estimates vary between 5 to 15 years depending on the severity of the B-12 restriction. Nevertheless, between 10-30% of patients, over 50 years of age, eventually become deficient. Interestingly, the parietal cells of the stomach which are responsible for the secretion of both HCl and intrinsic factor (IF), tend to underperform in individuals over the age of 50, but probably more commonly above the age of 70. There is also a tendency to develop the symptom achlorhydria, characterized by the absence of hydrochloric acid (HCl) levels in the stomach or hypochloridia, which means low HCL concentrations. Caused by a condition known as atrophic gastritis, in which the parietal cells of the stomach secrete less or no HCl and intrinsic factor (protein that allows B-12 absorption), the disease leads to a decrease in B-12 being released from animal protein and being absorbed in the ileum of the intestine. The HCl normally activates the pepsin which then hydrolyzes the peptide bonds of the meat protein, releasing B-12. In the absence of sufficient HCl, there is a significant decrease in the amount of B-12 released for absorption.[111]

This decreased acidity may also lead to a heightened proliferation of intestinal bacteria that utilize B-12, thereby further decreasing its availability.

Deficiency of this vitamin is also very likely in patients who have undergone gastric bypass surgery.[16] It is clear that the consequences of a greatly diminished stomach pouch are first, reduced numbers of parietal cells capable of producing sufficient HCl for the release of animal products B-12, and second, suboptimal levels of IF, a necessary glycoprotein for the absorption of B-12.

3.4.5 Vitamin A (Retinol) Deficiency

Worldwide, there are roughly between 250,000 to 500,000 cases of blindness resulting from vitamin A deficiency in young children every year. In fact, vitamin A deficiency is regarded by the WHO as the most preventable cause of blindness in the world.[120]

> **Vitamin A deficiency is virtually unknown in the US because of the abundant protein in the American diet.**

In the United States, by contrast, vitamin A deficiency is virtually non-existent because of the abundant protein in the U.S. diet, and the breakfast cereal fortification program. There are two major sources of vitamin A in the North American diet: first, there are animal sources potentially offering between 500 and 12,000 international units (IUs) per serving, such as beef and chicken liver, milk, butter, cheddar cheese and whole eggs, all providing a preformed-vitamin A known as **retinol**. The most potent animal sources of preformed vitamin A are beef and chicken liver, containing between 11,000 and 22,000 IUs per 3 ounce serving. Milk, cheese and egg, by contrast, contain between 250 and 500 IUs per serving, with non-fat milk containing 500 IU. Over the last 10 years, breakfast cereals have been fortified with retinol to the degree that one serving equals between 10 to 15% of the daily value (DV).

Second, there is a vegetable source of vitamin A known as **pro-vitamin A**, found in the form of carotenoids. Of the hundreds of carotenoids present in our food supply, beta-carotene is the most easily transformed into the active form of vitamin A, called retinol. In the United States, the most abundantly ingested foods rich in beta-carotene are carrots, cantaloupe, sweet potato and spinach.

Nutrient tables indicate that vegetables can contribute sizable levels of the pro-vitamin-A form of beta-carotene. For instance a half a cup of carrot juice or one medium size baked sweet potato with skin, both contain in the area of 22,000 IUs. Also, one half cup of raw carrots or one half cup of cooked kale, contain roughly 9000 IUs per serving.

The rest of the fruits and vegetables, considered excellent sources of pro-vitamin A such as cantaloupe, apricots, mangoes, and papaya, or broccoli, spinach, peas and peppers, contain between 1000 and 2000 IUs per serving. In other words, a diet rich in dairy products, and in dark-colored fruits and vegetables, is always richly supplied with both preformed vitamin A (retinol), and pro-vitamin A (beta–carotene).[39, 53]

A deficiency of vitamin A usually takes place slowly over time. Because it is a fat-soluble vitamin, the body tends to store vitamin A in the liver, and in the adipose tissue, thereby favoring a slow release of retinol into the biological system as it is needed. In practical terms then, a person should not have to ingest significant amounts of vitamin A on a daily basis, but rather on a monthly basis. Indeed when vitamin A deficiency is diagnosed, it is usually the result of chronically low intakes of either dietary retinol or beta-carotene over many months.

There have been subclinical forms of vitamin A deficiency, documented within certain clusters in the U.S., notably among young toddlers and preschool aged children who are living at or below the poverty line. These tend to be recent immigrants or refugee children, coming from developing countries, with a diminished access to healthcare. Finally, deficiencies are documented in individuals suffering from diseases of the liver, pancreas and intestine.[72]

Diseases or conditions of the intestine can make digestion and absorption particularly difficult. For instance, chronic bouts of diarrhea over prolonged periods can greatly increase the risk that the body is absorbing inadequate amounts of fat, and consequently vitamin A. Diarrhea is often documented in diagnosable conditions such as celiac disease and Crohn's disease. Pancreatic disorders greatly disturbs fat absorption since pancreatic lipase, one of the most important enzymes for fat digestion, tends to be significantly compromised.[45]

At the international level, the WHO identified children suffering from measles as being at high risk of vitamin A deficiency, and therefore recommends supplementation.[27] It is noteworthy to point out that when diets are also suboptimal in calories, protein, and zinc, vitamin A deficiencies tend to also be documented. This is because the synthesis of the transport protein, retinol binding protein (R BP), requires proteins, calories and zinc.[27]

Here in the United States, the American Academy of Pediatrics, recommends retinol supplementation for children between the ages of six and 24 months, who were hospitalized with measles, and for hospitalized children over the age of six months.

Vitamin A is not easily secreted from the body, because it is fat-soluble, and therefore potentially represents a source of toxicity if large amounts of retinol are consumed.

Vitamin A is considered the most likely to exceed the tolerable upper intake level (UL) cut-off with normal food and supplement use. This is because the recommended daily allowance (RDA) for women, which equals 900 µg per day, is not far below the 3000 µg per day UL. When the UL is divided by the RDA it becomes clear that a woman would only have to consume approximately 3 times the RDA before reaching levels with high risks of toxicity. Contrast that calculation by dividing the UL for vitamin E by the RDA (1000mg/ 15mg). The answer suggests that for a person to consume toxic levels of vitamin E, he would have to ingest close to 67 times the RDA for vitamin E, a very unlikely practice.

3.4.6 Copper (Cu+) Deficiency.

It is generally agreed that hypocupremia (copper deficiency) is rarely observed in the U.S., however,

> Fat-soluble vitamins like vitamin A are stored in fat cells. Levels can be maintained over time, even during low intake, but the risk of excess and toxicity is possible.

there is ample evidence documenting low levels of dietary copper associated with high blood cholesterol, and higher risks of cardiovascular disease. Additionally, high zinc supplement intake can interfere with copper absorption and lead to deficiency. [81] As part of the antioxidant system in the body called superoxide dismutase (SOD), copper plays an important role, along with zinc, in maintaining the mechanism that keeps oxidative stress in check. In this way it acts as a scavenger of superoxide radicals that are able to cause oxidative damage to cell membranes.[81, 123]

Also, copper is critical in ensuring the proper utilization of iron. In fact, poor copper status can generate iron-deficiency anemia. The protein ceruloplasmin transports more than 95% of the total copper in the body. [48] It oxidizes ferrous iron, located in the lumen of the intestine, bone marrow, liver, and spleen. This is a necessary step before the iron can be transported to the area where erythropoiesis or hemoglobin synthesis occurs.

So then, in the absence of copper, the body remains unable to produce ceruloplasmin, thus preventing the transport of the type of iron (ferric iron) needed to synthesize hemoglobin. Copper also is instrumental in ensuring the quality of the phospholipids forming the myelin sheath that covers nerve fibers. [36, 108] In copper deficiency, there is an inadequate myelination of the nerve fibers, and a resulting necrosis or (death) of nerve cells, possibly causing ataxia. [36, 81] Excellent sources of copper are beef liver, potatoes, mushrooms, cashews and turkey. [81]

3.5 Vitamin E/ alpha-Tocopherol Deficiency

While vitamin E deficiencies, in the U.S. population, remain relatively rare, several nutritional surveys (NHANES 1988-1994 & 2001-2002) report that most of the adult population consumes less than the RDA for vitamin E.[37] In fact, some have advanced that >90% of Americans consume insufficient amounts of alpha-tocopherol, and it seems that children worldwide in particular are vulnerable. [115] When the data is stratified, teenage girls and young women who consume low-fat diets, for weight loss purposes, tend to have very little vitamin E in their diet.

Vitamin E deficiency has been documented among premature babies, patients with malabsorption problems such as Crohn's disease, cystic fibrosis, and in patients with gallbladder or liver disease who produce very little bile. As a consequence, these patients tend to have a greasy stool consistency (steatorrhea) since the fat remains in the stool, and does not get absorbed.[107]

Also, vitamin E intakes tend to be suboptimal when overall fat consumption is low. Oils such as wheat germ oil, sunflower seed oil and safflower seed oil have the highest concentrations of vitamin E. Surprisingly, 1 tablespoon of wheat germ oil contains almost 3 times the amount found in 1 ounce of sunflower seeds, and close to four times the amount found in 1 tablespoon of sunflower seed oil. [23]

Since the refinement of flour, ever since the turn of the 20th century, wheat products and breads no longer contain wheat germ, which, historically has been a very significant contributor of vitamin E in the North American diet.

In order to facilitate mass distribution of bread, across the continental U.S., manufacturers were looking for methods of ensuring shelf stability of bread. The preferred approach was to remove the wheat germ from the wheat kernel. Most shoppers realize that in general, bread tends to remain fresh-looking for several weeks, despite being left on the counter top. This stability allows bread to remain on grocery shelves for longer periods of time without going rancid. Wheat germ oil, found within the wheat germ, is easily oxidized, as it is made up of polyunsaturated fatty acids. The oil, when exposed to air for too long, turns rancid when oxidized; this is an endpoint that imparts an off-taste to the wheat. So then, from a manufacturing perspective, getting rid of the germ and its oil makes sense. Most individuals, consuming processed breads over the last many years, are often perplexed by how quickly fresh-baked bread, if left on the counter,

> There is often too great an emphasis on reducing the total fat in the American diet and not enough emphasis on ensuring an adequate intake of healthy fats.

turns dry and mouldy. The absence of emulsifying and anti-fungal agents, in fresh-baked bread, leads to a rapid deterioration in quality. Moreover, if the wheat has not been refined in any way, or if the baker adds some wheat germ to the refined whole-wheat, the taste of the bread improves noticeably, but certainly becomes unfamiliar to most.

The problem with the highly processed diet, consumed in the U.S., is that the consumer has learned to accommodate foods that don't taste all that good, by smothering them in spicy or hot sauces. However, the concern is not strictly about taste or flavor, but also about the nutrient content of the foods.

Suboptimal levels of vitamin E is a concern, as its primary function is to work as an antioxidant, and protect the integrity of cell membranes from free radical attacks; over time, the constant barrage of these oxidant compounds, can damage the cells. One of the prevailing theories, in cardiovascular research, is that the suboptimal levels of vitamin E, in the diet, make the vascular wall susceptible to injury by free radical attacks.[64, 110] These assaults come in the form of reactive oxygen species (ROS). Alpha-tocopherol (vitamin E) is a fat-soluble vitamin that is imbedded within the cells' lipid layer, lining the vascular wall.[80] It provides an antioxidant balance to the oxidant radicals that are produced by the body, in response to the metabolic processes of converting macronutrients into energy.[60]

Free radicals can also be generated through environmental influences such as smoking, air pollution, and ultra-violet radiation. These radicals can, over prolonged exposure, not only destroy cell membrane integrity, causing cell injury and the build-up of atheromas at the injury site, but also DNA mutations, which lead to some cancers.[58]

The role of antioxidants is to protect the cell against bodily inflammation and stresses, resulting from free radicals that are generated environmentally or endogenously. The present danger of the North American diet is that it aggressively promotes, through the media, the importance of low fat diets for the purpose of weight control. This seems, on the surface, like a reasonable promotion, since over two thirds of North American adults are either overweight or obese, and close to 20% of children and adolescents are obese. And it is certainly correct to identify fat as a significant caloric contributor in the U.S. diet, especially when these calories are stratified into meats, snack foods and fast foods. The vilification of fat, however, is a gross distortion of reality, as we have not been properly educated, as a nation, about the importance of the quality of fat that we eat.

In truth, too much emphasis has been placed on reducing the amount of fat without any kind of discernment regarding the health benefits promoted through healthy oils that contain omega-3 fats, especially the eicosapentaenoic acid (EPA) and docosahexaenoic (DHA) found in fish, and monounsaturated oils, such as olive, peanut or canola.

3.6 The Impact of Fluoride on Health

The interest in fluoride (F) and its impact on human health is linked to studies that show that with the fluoridation of water, prevalence of dental caries tends to decrease. The Center for Disease Control's (CDC), 2001 report on the use of fluoride, concluded that when used appropriately, fluoride could prevent and control dental caries in the United States.[50]

The use of fluoride became so effective—so it appears—that expert scientists have been reporting

> Fluoride sources from food, toothpaste, supplements and water sources add up to increase the risk of reaching toxic levels.

that 60% of children between five and 11 years of age, in the U.S., are cavity-free. This contrasts dramatically with the 1960s records that reported that only 5% in that age group would have been without dental caries.

Very interestingly however, a review by Clarkson in 1991, points out that although it is impressive that 60% of children that age are free of caries—72.4% of the U.S. population consumed fluoridated water according to the 2008 CDC estimate—the United Kingdom, which does not have such widespread fluoridation practice as in the U.S., also showed an important reduction in dental caries.[26]

What is going on? Although the fluoridation of the water supply across the U.S. and Canada was hailed by the Centers for Disease Control and Prevention (CDC) as a public health triumph, there is nevertheless, mounting concern that the effectiveness of fluoride in preventing tooth decay may not actually come from fluoridated water.

Also because of the fluoride content of food, toothpaste, supplements and water, in addition to the dental fluoride treatments administered by dentists, the population is now susceptible to the dangers of fluoride intoxication, albeit with lower prevalence of dental caries.

Investigations into the action of fluoride, shows that the medium is important. Indeed, there are volumes of epidemiological and clinical evidence supporting the use of topical fluoride in the control of dental caries. More specifically, rather than fluoride toothpaste making a significant dent in the prevalence of caries, it appears to be fluoride supplementation and fluoride varnishing treatments that have a greater impact in reducing cavities, but also in causing fluorosis.

Consider that fluoride varnish treatments provide anywhere between 225 ppm to 22,600 ppm of fluoride, a topical application that contains amounts which, when combined with fluoride toothpaste and water, can easily overwhelm a biological system. The important point here is that there is a big difference between the topical versus a systemic application of F on the human biological system.

Unlike previous public health measures, such as fortifying milk with vitamin D or cereals, wheat, and grains with folic acid, it is questionable whether fluoride in water is an efficient distribution medium. This is particularly pertinent in the discussion, given that most of the water in a household is used for flushing toilets, daily showers or clothes washing. Moreover, it is doubtful that fluoride can be considered an essential nutrient since there are no documented deficiencies that arise from poor fluoride intakes except for a higher propensity to develop caries. But this does not occur in everyone with low F intake.

But most importantly, fluoride may be a nutrient that can become toxic very easily, especially if taken systemically. Children and infants are signalled out as most vulnerable to fluoride toxicity because of their lower body weights. There is an apparent consensus in the literature that cautions against prescribing fluoride supplements in children, except in those with high risks of developing dental caries. Fluoridation of water then becomes problematic when framed within the context of this water being used for hydration of adults, children and infants, especially if powdered reconstituted infant formulas are being used in the first year of life.

The position of the American Dental Association is to promote breast feeding for at least six months because of the enormous health benefits to mom and the baby, and also because breast milk contains only between 0.005 to 0.01 parts per million (ppm) fluoride. In other words, tap water levels of 1.2 ppm which are consistent with EPA's health standards are actually 12-fold greater than breast milk. [6]

This comparison should set off alarms and cause more conservative approaches when it comes to using reconstituted infant formula powders with fluoridated tap water. This is especially true, if we accept that breast milk is the gold standard to which infant formulas should be compared to. And yet, the report of the American Dental Association's Council on Scientific Affairs (Berg, 2011) [4] makes the following recommendations to its membership:

The panel suggested that when dentists advise parents and caregivers of infants to consume powdered or liquid concentrate infant formula as the main source of nutrition, they can suggest continued use of powdered or liquid concentrate infant formula reconstituted optimally with fluoridated drinking water while being cognizant of potential risks of enamel fluorosis development.

Practitioners should be aware that children are exposed to multiple sources of fluoride during the tooth development. Reducing fluoride intake from reconstituted infant formula alone will not diminish the risk of fluorosis development.

The panel acknowledges and encourages clinicians to follow the American Academy of Pediatrics guidelines for infant nutrition, which advocate exclusive breast-feeding to age 6 months and continued through at least 12 months unless specifically contraindicated.

The problem from a public health perspective is that although the CDC estimated that 74% of mothers initiated breastfeeding in 2005, only 43% continued to breast feed up to six months and 22% up to one year. Infant formulas are in fact still the most significant form of infant nutrition in the U.S. Moreover, the use of powdered formulas climbed from 43% to 62% in recent years, therefore requiring reconstitution with fluoridated water, a practice that puts greater numbers of infants at risk of fluoride toxicity.

Dr Phyllis Mullenix published a paper on the toxic effects of fluoride on the neurological system in rats in 1995 titled: *Neurotoxicity of sodium fluoride in rats*, which was published in Neurotoxicology and Teratology.[73] They reported that rat behaviors were significantly altered with increasing levels of ingested fluoride, a phenomenon that paralleled increases in the blood.

Another study published by Das and colleagues [30] in the Journal of Clinical Gastroenterology in 1994, reported that 70% of those human subjects treated with 30 mcg of fluoride per day for a period of one year, experienced abdominal pain, vomiting and nausea. Histological examination of the gastrointestinal (GI) tissue showed evidence of atrophic gastritis in all subjects receiving the fluoride, but only one subject in the control. They conclude that long-term use of fluoride is associated with dyspeptic symptoms. It was very concerning that the administered dose was only 0.3% of the tolerable upper intake level (UL) for this element. However, the most troubling studies are coming from countries outside the U.S.

Research conducted in four areas within Anyang and Neihuang Counties in China, showed that those communities with fluoride levels of 2.0 mg/L in the drinking water, had liver and kidney disturbances reported in children—a concentration that is half the recognized as safe level by the EPA.[66] The link to fluoride was powerfully demonstrated in this study because water fluoride concentrations coincided with higher serum and urinary fluoride. Among the 210 children, ages 10 to 12 that were studied, 94% were living in regions with fluoride concentrations in drinking water that varied between 3.1 and 5.69 mg/L. These children suffered from fluorosis of the teeth, and most of them had blood markers indicating liver and kidney damage.[127, 128]

A news release dated March 22, 2006 from the American Water Works Association in Denver Colorado, reassured the American public that typically, fluoride concentrations in community water supplies varied between 0.7 to 1.2 mg/L. This press release came on the heels of an announcement by the National Research Council (NRC) of the National Academy of Science (NAS) also on March 22, 2006. After examining several research papers that studied the impact of various concentrations of fluoride in water on human health, the NRC concluded that fluoride levels that were 4 mg/L or higher pose certain health risks. The NRC's statement caused shock waves since it was essentially identifying the potential toxicity of fluoride. The American Dental Association (ADA) was also quick to minimize the potential public outcry from the NRC's fluoride statement, by issuing a press release that same day intended to appease the populace:

...the report in no way examines or calls into question the safety of community water fluoridation which is the process of adding fluoride to public water supplies to reach an optimal level of .07 to 1.2 ppm in order to protect people against tooth decay. One part per million is the equivalent to about one cent in $10,000. The ADA continues to endorse community water fluoridation as a vital public health measure.

The ADA's press release goes on to suggest that the Environmental Protection Agency's (EPA's) standard recommended maximal cut-off of 4 ppm should be lowered in order to protect the health of Americans. This was a meaningful recommendation given that an estimated 200,000 Americans live in communities where fluoride concentrations are at 4 ppm or greater. The impact on community health can be devastating.

Water fluoride concentrations between 0.6 to 1.2 ppm had been recommended based on studies from the 1950s that advocated fluoridation of the water supply in order to minimize dental caries in the population. This concentration level appears to be safe based on Chinese studies that show that when fluoride concentrations in the water are between 4.3 and 8 ppm, the incidence of bone fractures and hip fractures increased significantly. When the data was stratified, researchers found that when fluoride concentrations were between 1 and 1.06 ppm there was no impact on bone fractures. Recently, however, experts in the field have admitted that the impact of fluoride on kidney and liver had not been studied closely.

3.7 Calcium, Magnesium Deficiencies and Phosphorous Excesses

3.7.1 Calcium Intake Of these three macro-minerals, calcium is undoubtedly one of the most discussed nutrients in the American diet, because of

> Chronic shortage of calcium in the diet makes specific bones such as the wrist, pelvis, vertebrae, hips, and ribs at increased risk for fracture.

its involvement in bone and tooth structures, and the concern over osteoporosis, a bone disease that causes porous and fragile bones. An estimated 10.3% of the older American population suffers from outright osteoporosis, and an estimated 43.9% had low bone mass or are at risk of developing the disease, representing close to 43.4 million older adult Americans. [125]

The problem is that individuals become vulnerable to long-term dietary habits that make specific bones such as the wrist, pelvis, vertebrae, hips and ribs more susceptible to fractures. Indeed, over the short term, individuals do not perceive changes in bone, and therefore receive insufficient feedback to be able to modify the diet appropriately. This is why cultural and family food traditions are so very important. It is these very traditions that establish eating norms or standards within families and societies. If the cultural habits are modified or changed in any dramatic way, there can be long-term health implications. In fact, as soft drinks began to overtake the American landscape, as early as the 50s and 60s, milk gradually was displaced out of the diet, most notably in children and adolescents. The statistics are rather disturbing.[44]

Lisa Harnack and her colleagues[20] reported that 12% of pre-schoolers consumed on average 9 fluid ounces of soda pop per day, whereas 33% of school-aged children consumed 9 fluid ounces. In singling out teenagers, they found that 25% ingested 26 fluid ounces of soft drink on a daily basis, representing about a mean intake of 30 teaspoons of sugar per day or roughly an extra 480 kcal per day. The data supports the suspicion that elevated intake of soft drink consumption, significantly displaces milk out of the diet, and greatly reduces dietary intakes of calcium, vitamin C, riboflavin, vitamin A, phosphorous and folate.

The implications were deemed serious in light of previous studies that documented sub-optimal intakes of calcium among children and adolescents in the US, and in particular among teenage girls.[7] It is well recognized that primary prevention strategies of osteoporosis involve maximizing peak bone mass during childhood, adolescence and early adulthood, leading up to age 30.

> Drinking soda instead of milk in youth represents a large-scale risk to building and maintaining a healthy bone structure into adulthood.

It does currently appear as though the trend in soda consumption, among America's youth, is threatening their bone health on a large scale. National orthopedic data estimate that there are approximately 1.5 million fractures in the US due to osteoporosis. There are some concerns that the growing number of young people, with poor dietary habits, will likely continue to contribute towards higher bone fracture prevalence in the coming years.[44]

The marketing of calcium supplements has been successful in increasing awareness of the critical role played by calcium in long-term bone health. According to NHANES 2003- 2006, 43% of the US population, of which 70% are older women, regularly take supplements containing calcium (Bailey et al., 2010). Men appear less vulnerable to low calcium intake as indicated by the NHANES data, which reported that mean intake varied between 871 and 1266 mg per day. The mean intake of women varied between 748 and 968 mg per day. Adolescent girls and some older women tend to fall short of the healthy daily requirement. The full story of osteoporosis however, is not strictly limited to calcium. There are in fact several lifestyle factors that contribute towards the development of this devastating condition. Epidemiologists have been able to correlate excessive alcohol intake, physical inactivity, smoking, physical thinness and having a family history, with a higher incidence of osteoporosis. [69]

The role of calcium in the development of osteoporosis was seen as significant enough by the Food and Drug Administration (FDA), that it allowed, in 1993, health claims related to calcium on the packages of food rich in calcium. The health claim read: *Adequate calcium throughout life, as part of a well-balanced diet, may reduce the risk of osteoporosis.*

As more long-term prospective studies continued to examine how osteoporosis could be prevented, it became evident that vitamin D also played an important role. The data also are convincing enough that the FDA in 2010 allowed the following health claim: *Adequate calcium and vitamin D as part of a healthful diet, along with physical activity, may reduce the risk of osteoporosis in later life.*

It is noteworthy however, to point out that calcium's role is not strictly limited to bone, because healthy intakes of calcium in the diet are also associated with lower incidences of rectal, colon and prostate cancers, hypertension, kidney disease and obesity.

Calcium is in fact used as a surrogate measure for healthy nutritional practices. In the U.S., for instance, where the population consumes, on average, 35 gallons of soft drinks per person per year, there is also the ingestion of phenomenal amounts of sugar and significantly less calcium overall. It would not be unusual then, to expect the corresponding 33 pounds of sugar per year ingested from sodas, to translate into weight gain, type II diabetes and heart disease.

Very successful marketing campaigns developed by beverage companies are most certainly influencing the elevated consumption of soda in the U.S., and especially among the young. In fact, in 1995, three big companies spent an estimated $400 million that year, to promote soda consumption in the US alone.[44]

This amount of money dedicated to the marketing of a single product line like soft drinks, dwarfs the entire United States Department of Agriculture's (USDA) health promotion program budget for good nutrition, estimated to be around 200 million per year.

Is there any wonder why the dietary habits of the U.S. changed so dramatically in the last three decades? We are, in fact, eating more calories, but lesser nutrients per calorie. In other words, the caloric density of the diet has increased, while the nutrient density decreased. Meeting nutrient requirements should not be such a big deal, if nutritious foods are part of regular food selections. Getting adequate amounts of calcium should normally not be a problem, as long as dairy foods regularly make their way into a daily menu.

Imagine beginning the day with one serving of regular plain yogurt (415 mg calcium) combined with a ½ cup of frozen berry blend, which contains no added sugar. Follow through with one cup of ready-to-eat calcium fortified breakfast cereals (100-1000 mg calcium), and already the calcium requirement for a young teenager has been met thanks to the manufacturing of high potency calcium-fortified cereal that contains a thousand milligrams calcium per serving. Otherwise, 2 cups of milk (594mg calcium) in combination with that yogurt will pretty much meet calcium needs.

While calcium intake of the youth has seriously gone down because of the insidious way soft drinks have greatly altered their diet, other population groups also seem to be susceptible to poor calcium status. [5]

3.7.2 Calcium and Postmenopausal Women

Postmenopausal women are also at risk of low calcium intakes, since they no longer benefit from the protection of circulating estrogen. Consequently, bone loss dramatically increases in the postmenopausal period, unless hormone replacement therapy (HRT), involving estrogen and progesterone treatments, is implemented. The health risks associated with HRT may warrant the alternative use of bisphosphonates which, according to some reports, have the potential of increasing bone density somewhat, especially if milk is regularly consumed.

The goal then is for young women to maximize their calcium intake in their youth leading up to the age of 30, in order to ensure that they reach their full genetic potential for bone density. After the age of 30, it is no longer possible to increase bone density. This invariably means that a progressive loss of bone mass throughout the rest of their lives is inevitable.[41]

3.7.3 Calcium and Amenorrheic Women

> Women have until about age 30 to store calcium in bone. After age 30, bone progressively becomes weaker over time.

There is a relatively high risk that female athletes, who engage in sports where body weight is a key determinant of performance, are chronically overly restricting calories. This practice can lead to significant weight loss, and specifically to an unusually high erosion of body fat.

These conditions can produce amenorrhea, or the temporary loss of the menstrual cycle. The triad that is described in the literature refers to the compounding effects of an eating disorder, amenorrhea and osteoporosis—a very nefarious combination for which the consequences can be devastating on the short and long-term.

This is clearly exemplified in the classic athletic woman with menstrual irregularities, low body weight and bone density, who suffers from frequent bone fractures. The problem arises because of lower calcium absorption and increased urinary calcium excretion. The solution is calcium and vitamin D supplementation and a normalization of calories. [83]

3.7.4 Individuals with Lactose Intolerance and Cow's Milk Allergy

> While cow's milk allergy remains one of the top allergens in infants, 80 – 90% of children recover their tolerance to milk protein by age 5.

In some individuals, there is a susceptibility of not being able to digest milk because of a lactase enzyme deficiency. Lactase is the digestive enzyme secreted by the intestinal epithelial cells to digest the disaccharide lactose, which consists of two monosaccharides: glucose and galactose.[42]

When there is an absence of lactase enzyme or a sub optimal amount secreted with the ingestion of milk, the undigested lactose tends to ferment in the gastrointestinal tract. Short chain fatty acids such as propionate and methane are generated from the bacteria present, leading to abdominal distention, cramps and osmotic diarrhea.

It is estimated that approximately 85% of Asians, 50% of African-Americans and only 10% of Caucasians, living in the United States, experience various degrees of lactose intolerance. [83]

Excluding those rare individuals who have virtually no lactase enzyme, most patients regarded as lactose intolerant, can tolerate up to 1 cup of milk per day without experiencing significant symptoms. The tendency, nevertheless, is for these patients to needlessly avoid all dairy products. This places them at high risk of calcium and vitamin D deficiencies, especially during the dark winter months in the northern states when vitamin D is less available from sun exposure.

Interestingly, these patients can consume aged cheese and most yogurts, as these foods contain fermented lactose, which is transformed into lactic acid, a compound that is perfectly tolerated. Additionally, patients can consume lactose free cow's milk such as Lactaid® and Lacteeze® since they've already been treated with the enzyme lactase, causing the lactose sugar to be already pre-digested to galactose and glucose in the milk. The more numerous free glucose molecules, explains why these milks tend to be more sweet tasting. Patients can therefore consume these milks without any abdominal discomforts, and are therefore able to meet their dietary needs for calcium.

On the other hand, between 0.6% and 0.9% of the U.S. population, and between 2% to 6% of U.S. children specifically, suffer from an allergy to cow's milk. In fact, milk protein is the most frequently encountered allergen in infancy, and can elicit a fairly broad immunological response to different allergenic epitopes found in the proteins of milk. In most cases there are antibodies and cell-mediated immune responses to the proteins. This frequently triggers an inflammatory-mediated response, which causes the recognizable flushing symptoms or other responses. [83]

3.7.5 Calcium and Vegetarians

There are many types of vegetarians, and not all are susceptible to calcium deficiency. Lacto-ovo-vegetarians consume all dairy and eggs, but omit all meats. These vegetarians have easy access to high biological value proteins, vitamin D and calcium.[4] By contrast, the ovo-vegetarians only allow eggs for their source of animal protein, and omit all meats and dairy products. These vegetarians are similar to pure vegans in that they forsake the consumption of dairy products. Consequently, they run a higher risk of consuming suboptimal levels of calcium. [83] Traditionally, vegans, because of the absence of dairy in their diet, had to judiciously ensure that their menu contained foods with reasonable amounts of calcium in order to meet their RDA. They needed to frequently select vegetables such as spinach, kale, turnip greens, Chinese cabbage, and tofu made with calcium. Vegans must also include abundant legumes such as lentils, black and navy beans, chick peas and soybeans, which represent their main source of vegetable protein (**Figure-3.11**).

> Products like soy milk, rice milk and almond milk are now fortified with calcium and have the same nutrient profile as cow's milk.

Cow's milk allergy (CMA) is ranked among the big eight food allergens: soy, eggs, wheat, nuts, tree nuts, shellfish and fish. These patients must avoid, not only cow's milk but all dairy products, a restriction that is far more extensive than a mere lactose intolerance. The long term outlook for these pediatric patients is actually quite good given that 80 to 90% recover their tolerance to milk protein by the age of five.[42]

This recovery is, however, not without consequences, as infants with CMA tend to develop asthma, hay fever or dermatitis in adulthood.
The prevalence of self-diagnosed milk protein allergy is about 10 fold greater than the actual clinical incidence. This causes significant numbers of individuals to unnecessarily restrict dairy products with dire long-term health consequences.

In recent years, orange juice fortified with calcium and fortified soymilks have made it much easier to meet calcium needs. These fortified products make the vegan experience less risky as they no longer have to rely on vegetables alone for significant calcium intake.

Vegetables, as a sole calcium source, were problematic because they contain phytic and oxalic acids, which tend to bind the calcium in the GI tract, making it less available for absorption. With the advent of food fortification, products like soy, rice and almond milks end up having the same nutrient profile as dairy milk. Vegans, if they're knowledgeable shoppers, can now easily ingest adequate amounts of calcium. However, the Oxford cohort, a renowned prospective cohort study in Europe, found that the risk of bone fractures was similar between meat and fish eaters, and the overall vegetarian population. Surprisingly, they report a higher prevalence of bone fractures among pure vegans. The researchers associated this higher risk with the lower overall mean intake of calcium in this group.[4] This finding supports the need for continued nutrition education among vegans.

3.8 Magnesium Intake
The National Health and Nutrition Examination Survey (NHANES), which took place between 1994

and 2000, identified significant segments of American society ingesting suboptimal levels of magnesium—some have estimated that 75% of Americans consume under the recommended levels. African-Americans in particular were vulnerable to lower intakes of magnesium as well as those Caucasians who did not take any calcium supplements.[56]

This is a concern since 50-65% of magnesium is attached to bone and roughly the other 40% associated with lean tissue.[41] There is also additional interest in the association between magnesium intake and hypertension, cardiovascular disease, immune function and diabetes.[2, 3]

There are generally three main reasons behind inadequate intakes of magnesium in the American diet: first, the intake of green leafy vegetables such as spinach has declined significantly in recent decades. This is important since the center element of the chlorophyll molecule that gives the green color to these vegetables is actually magnesium; second, the processing of wheat and cereal products rid the grains of the bran and the germ—a rich sources of oil and of magnesium; third, there has been also a notable decline in the consumption of legumes, nuts and seeds overall in the general population.

Figure 3.11: Colorful mix from different beans, legumes, peas, lentils. © Madlen/Shutterstock.com

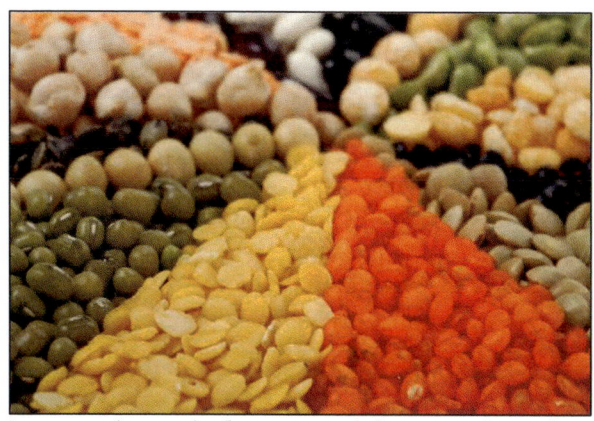

Legumes in particular are much less popular today than they were 40 to 50 years ago, and accordingly because of this change, Americans missed out on a variety of nutrients, notably soluble fibers and magnesium. For instance, just a half cup of soybeans mixed with half cup of cooked brown rice provides a little over one quarter of the magnesium requirements for adult men.

Throw in 3 cups of low-fat milk, half a cup of cooked spinach and a cup of Bran cereal with raisins for breakfast, and suddenly the person is within an acceptable range of the RDA for magnesium. But how many of us today, especially among the youth, fail to eat greens, milk, whole-wheat cereal and brown rice? Very many! And although outright deficiencies of the mineral are not frequently documented in the general population, deficiencies do occur among those suffering from diarrhea, vomiting and gastrointestinal diseases that compromise absorption, such as Crohn's disease.

3.9 Phosphorus Intake

Approximately 80% of phosphorous in found in bone. It is a key component of hydroxyapatite, the main constituent of the bone matrix. In the diet, approximately 50% of phosphorous is ingested through high protein foods such as milk, meats and fish; the most concentrated phosphorous is however found in processed meats and cheeses. Roughly 12% is consumed from cereals. Phosphorous plays a vital role in bone and tooth formation.[25] It is rather critical, for optimal bone calcification, that a 1:1 phosphorous to calcium ratio be maintained in the diet of adults. This helps minimize calcium excretion in the urine, and maximize the formation of hydroxyapatite, a key component of bone that gives it its rigid structure.[105]

Studies have shown that a minor deviance from this ideal ratio causes little disturbance in bone metabolism. Rather, important changes due to excessive phosphorous intake, in combination with significant declines in dietary calcium, appear to contribute to significant losses of calcium in the urine, and threaten bone mass.

With the growing use of calcium supplementation and calcium-fortified foods, in recent years, there is some concern over excessive intakes of calcium versus phosphorous. The main worry is that the calcium supplements (calcium carbonate, calcium gluconate, calcium fumarate, calcium malate) do not contain phosphorus, a much-needed component in the synthesis of hydroxyapatite. Moreover, rat studies have shown recently, that increasing calcium levels in the diet without any changes in phosphorus intake appears to worsen bone conditions by creating greater bone resorption.

By contrast, increasing phosphorus levels in the diet relative to calcium—as long as calcium intakes are adequate—contributes to greater bone mass. And although the Institute of Medicine states very clearly that there are no concerns about phosphorus levels adversely affecting bone health in American society, there is still some suspicion in the scientific community that excessive phosphorous in the diet could be causing some problems. Phosphorous, a main constituent of many additives in food, notably soft drinks, in the form of phosphoric acid, and phosphates in flavor stabilizers are consumed in larger amounts than earlier thought. Tani and colleagues [112] showed that a high intake of phosphorous produced a disruption in phosphorous homeostasis in rats and an increase in parathyroid hormone (PTH), which has been found to produce bone resorption or breakdown.[112] Diets in which abundant meats, processed foods and excessive sodas are regularly consumed, may be affecting bone health in different segments of the population, particularly among low milk and dairy consumers.

There is also a concern that phosphate deficiency may be occurring because of alterations in metabolic processes rather than from poor dietary intake. Some weight-reducing practices, the use of aluminum-based antacids, and vegetarian diet regimes, in which phosphate is primarily found bound to phytic acid, reduce phosphate availability for absorption. In addition population surveys in the United States estimate that 10% of women over the age of 60 and 15% of women over the age of 80 consumed about 70% of their RDA for phosphorus.[56]

3.10 Zinc and Beta-Carotene Deficiencies

3.10.1 Zinc Deficiency

Zinc deficiencies in the United States are fairly uncommon because of the vast assortment of protein foods in the American diet. Nevertheless, there are subgroups of the population that still remain vulnerable to zinc deficiency. Populations affected by zinc deficiency, experience poor growth, skin lesions, delayed sexual maturation, poor appetite and wound healing.[126] The most devastating cases are associated with gastrointestinal diseases such as ulcerative colitis and Crohn's disease, in which inflammation and atrophy of the intestinal mucosa causes malabsorption.

These diseases, in many cases, can become aggressive or persistent enough that they require surgical resection. The consequence is often short bowel syndrome resulting in diarrhea. Chronic forms of diarrhea invariably result in significant loss of zinc. Other conditions like malabsorption syndrome, hepatic and renal diseases, sickle cell disease, diabetes and malignancy, all can cause chronic losses of zinc.

Cross-sectional studies have reported a zinc deficiency in 40% of children with sickle cell disease, whereas 60% to 70% of adults with sickle cell disease suffer from poor zinc status. Alcoholics are likely the next most vulnerable group in western societies. This is because ethanol disturbs the normal absorption of zinc from the gastrointestinal tract, and at the same time it increases urinary zinc excretion. Those alcoholics, most vulnerable to this deficiency, are those who consume a rather narrow diet with little variety or quantity of protein.

And finally the third most vulnerable group are vegetarians, most specifically vegans who consume no meat, but who preferentially ingest protein from wheat, grains and legumes. These foods are high in phytates, which bind significant amounts of zinc. Consequently, it is estimated that vegetarians require approximately 50% more zinc in their diet compared to non-vegetarians.[53]

Zinc intakes also tend to be suboptimal in children who are exclusively breastfed beyond 6 months of age. In these cases, infants exhibit mild to moderate growth failure, which is successfully treated with zinc supplementation.

3.10.2 Beta-Carotene Deficiency

Like copper, and zinc, beta-carotene functions in the body as an antioxidant. Found primarily in fruits and vegetables, beta-carotene is a pro-vitamin-A carotenoid. This means that it is not an active preformed vitamin A, but rather a precursor to vitamin A. The body transforms the pro-vitamin A into a biologically active pre-vitamin A once it is consumed, but only to the degree that vitamin-A is needed in the body. There are other carotenoids that can convert to retinol, but to a lesser extent than beta-carotene. These include alpha-carotene and beta-cryptoxanthin. There is no known deficiency disease that arises from eating deficient intakes of beta-carotene.[72]

However, suboptimal intakes of beta-carotene serve as a proxy for overall fruit and vegetable intake. Hence, chronically low consumption is associated with higher risks of developing heart disease and some cancers (**Figure-3.11**) over the long term.

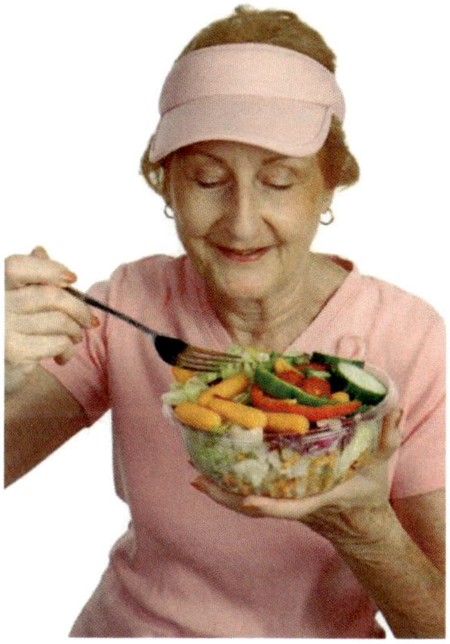

Figure 3.11 A woman dressed for Breast Cancer Awareness, eating a delicious, healthy salad that includes beta-carotene-rich carrots. © Lisa F Young

3.11 Iodine Deficiency

The WHO considers iodine deficiency as the most preventable cause of mental retardation in the world. Approximately 25 countries or 683 million people worldwide are at risk of suboptimal iodine intakes according to the Global Iodine Network statistics,[84] down considerably from 47 countries or 2.2 billion people worldwide last reported around 2008.[130] It still nevertheless remains a problem of such importance that the WHO has prioritized the eradication of this deficiency.[8] Deficiency of iodine is possible when iodine soil concentrations are low. In fact, iodine deficiency is endemic in mountainous regions such as the Andes, the Himalayas, and flood zones like South Asia and South East Asia.[84,94]

Although iodine is needed in microgram amounts in the body, a deficiency can nevertheless be devastating to the biological system.

It was historically endemic in the mountainous areas of the United States and Mexico or in the so called "goiter belt" regions surrounding the Great Lakes.[84] Consequently, the iodine concentrations in vegetables, cultivated in those areas, tended also to be suboptimal in iodine, resulting in goiter in nearby populations. Goiter is characterized by an enlarged thyroid gland that protrudes from the neck like a pouch (**Figure 3.12**).

Thyroid stimulating hormone (TSH), secreted from the pituitary gland, normally causes an increased uptake of iodine by the thyroid, the first step before it can synthesize thyroxin (T4) and triiodothyroxine (T3), which are the key hormones secreted by the thyroid. They regulate biochemical processes, metabolism, skeletal and neurological development in the fetus.[84]

In the absence of iodine, TSH still remains elevated causing the thyroid to become abnormally large. This is a physiological adaptation intended to capture as many iodine atoms as possible. The ramifications of a severe iodine deficiency can however, become significantly more devastating when a pregnant mother's intake is suboptimal, thereby leading to hypothyroidism. This causes cretinism in the newborn, a condition characterized by dwarfism, deaf mutism, and severe mental retardation. The hypothyroidism affects the fetus by causing major neurodevelopmental deficits while in utero, that are irreversible, and growth retardation after birth.[94]

There are, however, instances when a mild deficiency of iodine during pregnancy has been associated with less serious repercussions such as attention deficit hyperactivity disorder (ADHD) in the child.

When an infant is exposed to mild deficits of iodine intake, there are milder intellectual deficits as measured by drops in IQ scores. Public health strategies dating back to the 1950s consisted of iodizing table salt, a practice that continues to this day in the U.S. and in Canada. According to the WHO roughly 70% of the households worldwide consume iodized salt.

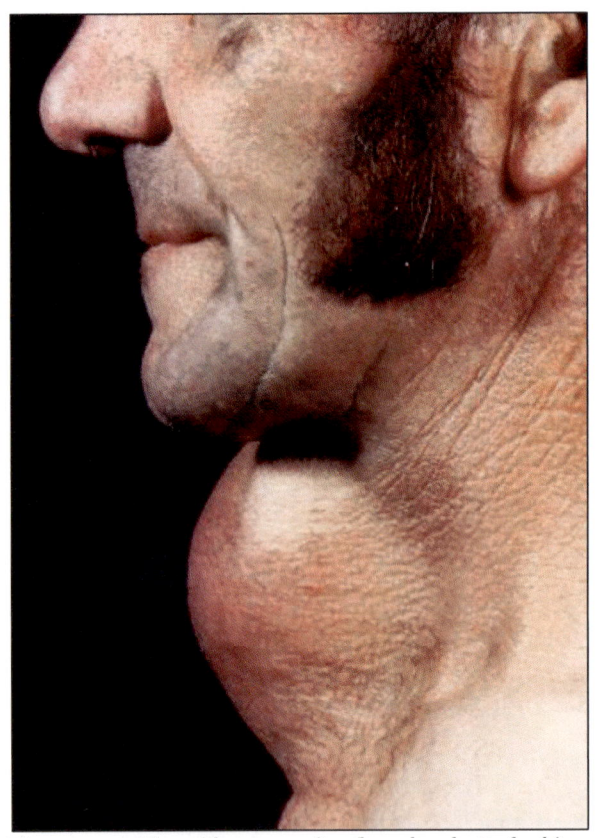

Figure 3.12: Man with severe goiter (bronchocele, Derbyshire neck). A goiter is a swelling of the neck caused by enlargement of the thyroid gland. Simple goiter is an example of an endemic disease caused by drinking water deficient in iodine. Credit: BIOPHOT ASSOCIATES © Getty Images

In Africa, South East Asia and Eastern Mediterranean, regions where iodine insufficiency is prevalent, between 47-67% of the population does not have access to iodized salt. Although the prevalence of iodine insufficiency has significantly declined, since the WHO prioritized this deficiency back in 1990s, it is still troubling that 39% of school-aged children worldwide [58] do not have access to iodized salt.

The problem of goiter stems back to ancient Greece, where manuscripts confirmed the medical use of iodine-rich seaweed to treat goiter. But it was not until 1821 when French Nutritional Chemist, Jean Baptiste Boussingault, discovered that iodized salt could be used to treat goiter, although the idea of using iodine to prevent the disease completely escaped him. Some thirty years later, in the 1850s another French scientist, A. Chatin, proposed that it was specifically iodine deficiency that was responsible for goiters. This idea held some merit, given that a Swiss physician named J.F. Coindet, had already treated goiter patients with iodine therapy. Yet, the **French Académie des Sciences** rejected the notion of a deficiency and essentially squashed the idea of using iodine therapy for another 50 years.

It took a physician from Cleveland Ohio named Dr. David Marine to pick up on the idea in 1907, and begin experimenting with iodine-fortified salts in the prevention of goiter. He made his first attempt at organizing a large-scale clinical trial of iodized salt in the Cleveland Public School system around 1909. His efforts were thwarted, however, by the veto of another doctor who was a member of the school board.

This delayed his efforts substantially, allowing him to only begin the official clinical trial by 1916 in elementary school girls who were afflicted with goiter at more than twice the national average. The trial was a complete success, clearly demonstrating the protective feature of iodine in salt. Discussions were held with the Diamond Crystal Salt Company (now merged into Cargill Salt Company) and the Morton Salt Company to work out the pragmatic steps to fortifying salt for mass consumption and prevention.

By 1924, it was estimated that 90% of the salt consumed in the United States goiter belt was iodized. This was a significant step that single-handedly caused a dramatic drop in the prevalence of goiter in the Detroit area; it went from 9.7% to 1.4% in the first six years of implementing the fortification.[130]

DISCUSSION QUESTIONS

1. Explain the way in which protein became an important macronutrient, early on, and why its role in muscle remained unchallenged until the late 20th century.
2. Explain the impact of the 19th century cholera epidemic on the field of medicine, and further discuss the effectiveness of public health in eradicating the problem.
3. Discuss the two most important vitamins in the development of vitaminology.
4. Describe the role played by Dr William Lind in resolving the cause of scurvy.
5. While scurvy is recognized as the scourge of the sea for obvious reasons, explain how it was also a large problem during the winters in the urban centers of the 18th century.
6. Explain why scurvy became known as the scourge of the sea.
   Discuss the scientific community's position on the use of vitamin supplements in human health.
7. Explain why thiamin and ascorbic acid were so important in the advancement of the field of nutrition.
8. Discuss whether water fluoridation is a useful public health strategy and whether it is comparable in impact to vitamin D fortification of milk.
9. Discuss which nutrient deficiency disease has the most significant human impact, and explain your decision.
10. Suboptimal intakes of vitamin E have been found in some segments of the population. Explain who is susceptible, why they are susceptible and what the long-term repercussions could be.

REFERENCES

1. Ansstas, G. (2012) Vitamin A Deficiency. George T Griffing (ed) e-Medicine Medscape webpage updated March 29. Retrieved October 1, 2013 from:: http://emedicine.medscape.com/article/126004-overview
2. Appel LJ. (1999) Nonpharmacologic therapies that reduce blood pressure: A fresh perspective. Clin Cardiol. 22:1111-5.
3. Appel LJ, Moore TJ, Obarzanek E, Vollmer WM, Svetkey LP, et. al. (1997) A clinical trial of the effects of dietary patterns on blood pressure. N Engl J Med;336:1117-24.
4. Appleby P, Roddam A, Allen N, Key T. (2007) Comparative Fracture Risk In Vegetarians And Nonvegetarians In EPIC-Oxford. Eur J Clin Nutr.61(12):1400-6
5. Bailey, R. L., Dodd, K. W., Goldman, J. A., Gahche, J. J., Dwyer, J. T., Moshfegh, A. J., Sempos, C. T., & Picciano, M. F. (2010). Estimation of total usual calcium and vitamin D intakes in the United States. *The Journal of nutrition*, *140*(4), 817–822. https://doi.org/10.3945/jn.109.118539
6. Berg, J et al. (2011) Evidence Based Clinical Recommendations Regarding Fluoride Intake From Reconstituted Infant Formula And Enamel Fluorosis. Journal Of The American Dental Association; 142(1): 79-87
7. Bialostosky K, Wright JD, Kennedy-Stephenson J, Mcdowell M, Johnson CL. (2002) Dietary Intake Of Macronutrients, Micronutrients And Other Dietary Constituents: United States 1988-94. Vital Heath Stat. 11(245) Ed: National Center For Health Statistics p:168.
8. Biban, B. G., & Lichiardopol, C. (2017). Iodine Deficiency, Still a Global Problem?. Current health sciences journal, 43(2), 103–111. https://doi.org/10.12865/CHSJ.43.02.01
9. Bobrow-Strain, A. (2013). White Bread: A Social History of the Store-Bought Loaf. Boston: Beacon Press, 272pp.
10. Brock, WH. (2020). Justus Baron von Liebig. Encyclopedia Britannica. Retrieved July 20, 2020 from URL: https://www.britannica.com/biography/Justus-Freiherr-von-Liebig
11. Brock, William H. (1997). *Justus von Liebig : the chemical gatekeeper* (1st ed.). Cambridge, U.K.: Cambridge University Press.
12. Bruyn, GW and Poser, CM (2003).The History of Tropical Neurology. Canton, MA: Science History Publications. 149pp
13. Burrell S, Gill G. (2005). The Liverpool cholera epidemic of 1832 and anatomical dissection--medical mistrust and civil unrest. *J Hist Med Allied Sci*;60(4):478-498. https://doi:10.1093/jhmas/jri061
14. Calvo MS, Whiting SJ, Barton CN. (2004) Vitamin D fortification in the United States and Canada: current status and data needs. Am J Clin Nutr.80 (6 Suppl): 1710S-6S.
15. Cameron E, Pauling L. Ascorbic acid and the glycosaminoglycans. An orthomolecular approach to cancer and other diseases. Oncology. 1973;27:181–192.
16. Cannon, G. (2005) the rise and fall of dietetics and nutrition science: 4000 BCE-2000CE. Public Health Nutrition: 8(6A), 701–705 DOI: 10.1079/PHN2005766
17. Carpenter KJ. (2012) The discovery of thiamin. *Ann Nutr Metab.*;61(3):219-223. doi:10.1159/000343109
18. Carpenter, KJ (2003). A short History of Nutritional Science Part-1: 1785-1885. J. Nutr. 133: 638–645
19. Carpenter, KJ (2003b). A short History of Nutritional Science Part-II: 1885-1912. J. Nutr. 133: 975–984
20. Carpenter,K.J (ed).(1986) The History of Scurvy and Vitamin C. Cambridge: Cambridge University Press. 288pp
21. Carpenter, Kenneth J., ed. (1981) *Pellagra*. Stroudsburg, Pa.: Hutchinson Ross Publishing
22. Conly JM, Stein K, Worobetz L, Rutledge-Harding S. (1994) The contribution of vitamin K2 (menaquinones) produced by the intestinal microflora to human nutritional requirements for vitamin K. Am J Gastroenterol;89:915-23.
23. Dietrich M, Traber MG, Jacques PF, Cross CE, Hu Y, Block G. (2006). Does γ-tocopherol play a role in the primary prevention of heart disease and cancer? A review. Am J Coll Nutr;25:292-9.
24. Carr, A. C., & Cook, J. (2018). Intravenous Vitamin C for Cancer Therapy - Identifying the Current Gaps in Our Knowledge. *Frontiers in physiology*, *9*, 1182. https://doi.org/10.3389/fphys.2018.01182
25. CDC (1998) Recommendations To Prevent And Control Iron Deficiency In The United States. Centers for Disease Control and Prevention. MMWR (Recomm Rep. 47:1-29.
26. Clarkson, BH. (1991) Caries Prevention—Fluoride. Adv Dent Research; 5:41-45
27. Committee On Infectious Diseases. (1993) Vitamin A Treatment Of Measles. Pediatrics. 91:1014-5.
28. Cowan, DW. Et al. (1942). Vitamins for the prevention of colds. JAMA;*120(16):1268–1271.* *https://doi:10.1001/jama.1942.02830510006002*
29. Dallman PR.(1986) Biochemical Basis For The Manifestations Of Iron Deficiency. Ann Rev Nutr.6:13-40.
30. Das, TK et al (1994) Toxic Effects of Chronic Fluoride Ingestion on The Upper Gastrointestinal Tract. Journal Of Clinical Gastroenterology 18 (3): 194-199
31. Doguer, C., Ha, J. H., & Collins, J. F. (2018). Intersection of Iron and Copper Metabolism in the Mammalian Intestine and Liver. *Comprehensive Physiology*, *8*(4), 1433–1461. https://doi.org/10.1002/cphy.c170045
32. Emerit J, Beaumont C, Trivin F. (2001) Iron metabolism, free radicals, and oxidative injury. *Biomed Pharmacother*;55(6):333-339. doi:10.1016/s0753-3322(01)00068-3
33. Encyclopedia Britannica (2020). Industrial Revolution. Retrieved July 20, 2020, from URL: https://www.britannica.com/event/Industrial-Revolution
34. Fenech M, Aitken C, Rinaldi J. (1998) Folate, Vitamin B12, Homocysteine Status And DNA Damage In Young Australian Adults. Carcinogenesis.19: 1163-71.
35. Fericks, RR. Broad Street Pump Outbreak. UCLA Department of Epidemiology, School of Public Health website. Retrieved October 1, 2013 from: http://www.ph.ucla.edu/epi/snow/broadstreetpump.html
36. Gaggelli E., Kozlowski H., Valensin D., Valensin G. (2006). Copper homeostasis and neurodegenerative disorders (Alzheimer's, prion, and Parkinson's diseases and amyotrophic lateral sclerosis). Chem. Rev. 106, 1995–204410.1021/cr040410w
37. Gao X, Wilde PE, Lichtenstein AH, Bermudez OI, Tucker KL. (2006) The Maximal Amount Of Dietary Á-Tocopherol Intake In U.S. Adults (NHANES 2001-2002). J utr;136:1021-1026Geber, J., & Murphy, E. (2012). Scurvy in the Great Irish Famine: evidence of vitamin C deficiency from a mid-19th century skeletal population. *American journal of physical anthropology*, *148*(4), 512–524. https://doi.org/10.1002/ajpa.22066
38. Garriga MJ, León AG, Soriguer F. (2004) Intelligence quotient and iodine intake: a cross-sectional study in children. J Clin Endocrinol Metab. Aug. 89(8):3851-3857

38b. Geber, J., & Murphy, E. (2012). Scurvy in the Great Irish Famine: evidence of vitamin C deficiency from a mid-19th century skeletal population. *American journal of physical anthropology*, *148*(4), 512–524. https://doi.org/10.1002/ajpa.22066

39. Gibson, RS. (1990). Principles of Nutritional Assessment. New York: Oxford University Press, 691pp.
40. Glynn RJ, Ridker PM, Goldhaber SZ, Zee RY, Buring JE. (2007) Effects of Random Allocation to Vitamin E Supplementation On The Occurrence of Venous Thromboembolism: Report From The Women's Health Study. Circulation. 116:1497-1503.
41. Goulding. A. and Robinson, M. (1999) Major Minerals: Calcium and Magnesium. In: Essentials of Human Nutrition, Mann, J, and Trustwell, AS (eds), Oxford: Oxford University Press, p: 122-136
42. Grittenden, RG And Bennett, LE. (2005) Cow's Milk Allergy: A Complex Disorder. J Nutrition; 24(6): 582S-591S
43. Halliday S. (2001). Death and miasma in Victorian London: an obstinate belief. *BMJ (Clinical research ed.)*, *323*(7327), 1469–1471. https://doi.org/10.1136/bmj.323.7327.1469
44. Harnack LJ, Stang J, Story M. (1999) Soft drink consumption among U.S. children and adolescents: Nutritional consequences. Journal of the American Dietetic Association 99(4):436-441
45. Harrison EH. (2005) Mechanisms Of Digestion And Absorption Of Dietary Vitamin A. Annu Rev Nutr. 25:5.1-5.18.
46. Harrison M. (2013). Scurvy on sea and land: political economy and natural history, c. 1780-c. 1850. Journal for maritime research, 15(1), 7–25. https://doi.org/10.1080/21533369.2013.783167
47. Heinonen, OP and Huttunen, JK. (1994). The Effect of Vitamin E and Beta-Carotene on the Incidence of Lung Cancer and Other Cancers in Male Smokers. New Engl.J.Med. 330;(15): 1029-1035
48. Hellman NE, Gitlin JD (2002). Ceruloplasmin metabolism and function. Annu Rev Nutr;22:439-58.
49. Herbert V. (1999) Folic Acid. In: Shils M, Olson J, Shike M, Ross AC, Ed. Nutrition In Health And Disease. Baltimore: Williams & Wilkins.
50. Heyroth, FF. (1952) Toxicological Evidence For The Safety Of The Fluoridation Of Public Water Supplies Am J Public Health Nations Health 42; (12) 1568-1575
51. Honein, MA, Paulozzi LJ, Mathews TJ, Erickson JD, Wong LC. (2001) Impact of Folic Acid Fortification on the US Food Supply On The Occurrence Of Neural Tube Defects. J Am Med Assoc. 285:2981-6.
52. Hueston W, McLeod A. OVERVIEW OF THE GLOBAL FOOD SYSTEM: CHANGES OVER TIME/SPACE AND LESSONS FOR FUTURE FOOD SAFETY. In: Institute of Medicine (US). Improving Food Safety Through a One Health Approach: Workshop Summary. Washington (DC): National Academies Press (US); 2012. A5. Available from: https://www.ncbi.nlm.nih.gov/books/NBK114491/
53. I.O.M (2001) Institute of Medicine. Dietary reference intakes for vitamin A, vitamin K, arsenic, boron, chromium, copper, iodine, iron, manganese, molybdenum, nickel, silicon, vanadium, and zinc. Washington, DC: National Academy Press; 2001.
54. IOM (1998). Institute of Medicine. Food and Nutrition Board. Dietary Reference Intakes: Thiamin, Riboflavin, Niacin, Vitamin B6, Folate, Vitamin B12, Pantothenic Acid, Biotin, and Choline. Washington, DC: National Academy Press; 1998.
55. I.O.M (1988) Institute of Medicine (US) Committee for the Study of the Future of Public Health. The Future of Public Health. Washington (DC): National Academies Press (US); 1988. 3, A History of the Public Health System. Available from: https://www.ncbi.nlm.nih.gov/books/NBK218224/
56. IOM (1997) Institute of Medicine. Food and Nutrition Board. Dietary Reference Intakes for Calcium, Phosphorous, Magnesium, Vitamin D and Fluoride. Washington, DC: National Academy Press,.
57. Interagency Board for Nutrition Monitoring And Related Research. (1995) Third Report On Nutrition Monitoring In The United States. Washington, DC: U.S. Government Printing Office,
58. Jacobs EJ, Henion AK, Briggs PJ, Connell CJ, Mccullough ML, Jonas CR, et al. (2002) Vitamin C And Vitamin E Supplement Use And Bladder Cancer Mortality In A Large Cohort Of US Men And Women. Am J Epidemiol;156:1002-10.
59. Jackson, T. (2003). What the industrial revolution did for us: Modern Medicine. BMJ; 327(7422): 1056. URL: https://www.ncbi.nlm.nih.gov/pmc/articles/PMC261680/
60. Jialal I, Devaraj S. (2000) Vitamin E Supplementation And Cardiovascular Events In High-Risk Patients. N Engl J Med. 352:154-60.
61. Johnston, CS. et al (2000). More Americans are eating 5 A DAY, but Intakes of Dark Green Cruciferous Vegetables Remain Low. J. Nutrition 130(12):3063-3067 web Article Retrieved July 17, 2012: http://jn.nutrition.org/content/130/12/3063.full
62. Kamen B. (1997) Folate And Antifolate Pharmacology. Semin Oncol;24:S18-30-S18-39.
63. Katch, FI. (1998). Justus von Liebig (1803-1873). Retrieved from History Makers July 20, 2020 at: URL: https://www.sportsci.org/news/history/liebig/liebig.html
64. Knekt P, Reunanen A, Jarvinen R, Seppanen R, Heliovaara M, Aromaa A. (1994) Antioxidant Vitamin Intake And Coronary Mortality In A Longitudinal Population Study. Am J Epidemiol. 139:1180-9.
65. Lewis CJ, Crane NT, Wilson DB, Yetley EA. (1999) Estimated Folate Intakes: Data Updated To Reflect Food Fortification, Increased Bioavailability, and Dietary Supplement Use. Am J Clin Nutr. 70:198-207.
66. Li, YY et. al. (200) Effect Of Long Term Exposure To Fluoride In Drinking Water On Risk Of Bone Fracture. J. Amer. Soc. Bone & Mineral Research 16(5): 932-939
67. Looker AC, Pfeiffer CM, Lacher DA, Schleicher RL, Picciano MF, Yetley EA. (2008) Serum 25-hydroxyvitamin D status of the US population: 1988-1994 compared with 2000-2004. Am J Clin Nutr. 88:1519-27.
68. Lopez MJ, Royer A, Shah NJ. Biochemistry, Ceruloplasmin. [Updated 2020 Feb 5]. In: StatPearls [Internet]. Treasure Island (FL): StatPearls Publishing; 2020 Jan-. Available from: https://www.ncbi.nlm.nih.gov/books/NBK554422/
69. Mangano, K. M., Walsh, S. J., Insogna, K. L., Kenny, A. M., & Kerstetter, J. E. (2011). Calcium intake in the United States from dietary and supplemental sources across adult age groups: new estimates from the National Health and Nutrition Examination Survey 2003-2006. *Journal of the American Dietetic Association*, *111*(5), 687–695. https://doi.org/10.1016/j.jada.2011.02.014
70. Margotta, R. (1996). The Hamlyn History of Medicine. Paul Lewis (ed). London: Institute of Neurology, 192 pp.
71. Martins e Silva J. (2007) Brief History of Rickets and of the discovery of vitamin D. Acta Reumatol Port. 32(3):205-29.
72. McDowell, L. R. (2000) Vitamins in Human and Animal Nutrition. Ames: Iowa State, University Press.

73. Mullenix, P. et. al. (1995) Neurotoxicity Of Sodium Fluoride In Rats. Neurotoxicology And Tetatology; 17(2): 169-177
74. Morley I. (2007). City chaos, contagion, Chadwick, and social justice. The Yale journal of biology and medicine, 80(2), 61–72. URL: https://www.ncbi.nlm.nih.gov/pmc/articles/PMC2140185/
74b. NCI (2014). Antioxidants and Cancer Prevention. Retrieved February 18, 2014 from: https://cancer.gov/cancertopics/factsheet/prevention/antioxidants#r8
75. NCI (2015). National Cancer Institute. Usual Dietary Intakes: Food Intakes, US Population, 2007–10. National Cancer Institute, Division of Cancer Control and Population Sciences, Epidemiology and Genomics Research Program; 2015. [Accessed July 25, 2020] .http://epi.grants.cancer.gov/diet/usualintakes/pop/2007-10/
76. National Research Council (2005) Committee to Assess the Health Implications of Perchlorate Ingestion. Health Implications of Perchlorate Ingestion. Washington, DC: The National Academies Press.
77. Natural Products Insider (2011). Beta-Carotene leads Carotenoid Sales. Retrieved October 2, 2013 from:http://www.naturalproductsinsider.com/news/2011/10/beta-carotene-leads-carotenoid-sales.aspx
78. NIH (2000) National Institutes of Health. Osteoporosis prevention, diagnosis, and therapy. NIH consensus statement;17:1-45.
79. NIH (2020). Riboflavin. Retrieved from the NIH's Office of Dietary Supplements website July 24, 2020. URL: https://ods.od.nih.gov/factsheets/Riboflavin-HealthProfessional/
80. NIH (2020b). Vitamin K. Retrieved from the NIH's Office of Dietary Supplements website July 24, 2020. URL: https://ods.od.nih.gov/factsheets/vitaminK-HealthProfessional/
81. NIH (2020c). Copper. Retrieved from the NIH's Office of Dietary Supplements website July 24, 2020. URL: https://ods.od.nih.gov/factsheets/Copper-HealthProfessional/
82. NIH (2020d). Vitamin E. retrieved from the NIH's Office of Dietary Supplements website July 24, 2020. URL: https://ods.od.nih.gov/factsheets/VitaminE-HealthProfessional/
83. NIH (2020e). Calcium. Retrieved from the NIH's Office of Dietary Supplements website July 24, 2020. URL: https://ods.od.nih.gov/factsheets/Calcium-HealthProfessional/
84. NIH (2020f). Iodine. Retrieved from the NIH's Office of Dietary Supplements website July 25, 2020. URL: https://ods.od.nih.gov/factsheets/Iodine-HealthProfessional/
85. NIH (2020g). Thiamin. Retrieved from the NIH's Office of Dietary Supplements website July 25, 2020. URL: https://ods.od.nih.gov/factsheets/Thiamin-HealthProfessional/
86. NIH (202h). Niacin. Retrieved from the NIH's Office of Dietary Supplement website July 25, 2020. URL: https://ods.od.nih.gov/factsheets/Niacin-HealthProfessional/
87. NIH (2020i). Vitamin D. Retrieved from the NIH's Office of Dietary Supplement website July 25, 2020. URL: https://ods.od.nih.gov/factsheets/VitaminD-HealthProfessional/
88. NIH (2020j). Iron. Retrieved from the NIH's Office of Dietary Supplement website, July 25, 2020. URL: https://ods.od.nih.gov/factsheets/Iron-HealthProfessional/
89. NIH (2020k). Vitamin B-6. Retrieved from the NIH's Office of Dietary Supplement website July 26, 2020. URL: https://ods.od.nih.gov/factsheets/VitaminB6-HealthProfessional/
90. NIH (2019). Nobel Prize Laureates. Retrieved from the NIH Amanac webpage on July 23, 2020. URL: https://www.nih.gov/about-nih/what-we-do/nih-almanac/nobel-laureates
91. NIH (2019b). Multivitamin/Mineral Supplements. Retrieved from the NIH's Office of Dietary Supplement website July 25, 2020. URL: https://ods.od.nih.gov/factsheets/MVMS-HealthProfessional/
92. Niki E. (2011). Do free radicals play causal role in atherosclerosis? Low density lipoprotein oxidation and vitamin E revisited. Journal of clinical biochemistry and nutrition, 48(1), 3–7. https://doi.org/10.3164/jcbn.11-007FR
93. Offitt, P. (2013) The Vitamin Myth: Why we Think We Need supplements. The Atlantic, Jul 19. Retrieved October 1, 2013 from: http://www.theatlantic.com/health/archive/2013/07/the-vitamin-myth-why-we-think-we-need-supplements/277947/
94. Patrick L. (2008) Iodine: deficiency and therapeutic considerations. Altern Med Rev. 13(2): 116-127.
95. Pauling L (1980). Vitamin C therapy of advanced cancer. N Engl J Med.;302:694–695.[PubMed] [Google Scholar]
96. Pauling L (1977). Diet, nutrition, and cancer. Am J Clin Nutr.;30:661–663. [PubMed] [Google Scholar]
97. Pauling L (1971). Vitamin C and common cold. JAMA.;216:332. [PubMed] [Google Scholar]
98. Powers HJ. (2003). Riboflavin (vitamin B-2) and health. *Am J Clin Nutr*;77(6):1352-1360. https://doi:10.1093/ajcn/77.6.1352
99. Powers, HJ., Weaver, LT., Austin, S., Wright, AJ., and Fairweather-Tait, SJ (1991). Riboflavin deficiency in the rat: effects on iron utilization and loss. Br. J. Nutr; 65(3): 487-96
100. Powers HJ, Bates CJ, Prentice AM, Lamb WH, Jepson M, et al. (1983) The relative effectiveness of iron and iron with riboflavin in correcting a microcytic anemia in men and children in rural gambia. Human Nutrition-Clinical Nutrition 37: 413–425
101. Price, C. (2017). The Age of Scurvy. Retrieved from the Science History Institute webpage July 23, 2020. URL: https://www.sciencehistory.org/distillations/the-age-of-scurvy
102. Produce for Better Health Foundation. http://www.pbhfoundation.org/about/res/general/health_ben/references.php Retrieved July 17, 2012
103. Raiten DJ and Fisher KD. (1995) Assessment of Folate Methodology Used In The Third National Health And Nutrition Examination Survey (NHANES III, 1988-1994). J Nutr. 125: 1371S-98S.
104. Rigmont Barber, L and Wilkins EM. (2002) Evidence-Based Prevention, Management, And Monitoring Of Dental Caries Journal Of Dental Hygiene. 76(4): 270-275
105. Shapiro, R and Heaney, RP. (2003) Co-dependence of calcium and phosphorus for growth and bone development under conditions of varying deficiency. Bone. 32(5): 532-540
106. Shi, Z., Zhen, S., Wittert, G. A., Yuan, B., Zuo, H., & Taylor, A. W. (2014). Inadequate riboflavin intake and anemia risk in a Chinese population: five-year follow up of the Jiangsu Nutrition Study. *PloS one*, *9*(2), e88862. https://doi.org/10.1371/journal.pone.0088862

107. Skeaff, M. Vitamins C and E. (1999) In: Essentials of Human Nutrition, Mann, J, and Trustwell, AS (eds), Oxford: Oxford University Press, p: 217-233
108. Skjørringe, T., Møller, L. B., & Moos, T. (2012). Impairment of interrelated iron- and copper homeostatic mechanisms in brain contributes to the pathogenesis of neurodegenerative disorders. *Frontiers in pharmacology*, 3, 169. https://doi.org/10.3389/fphar.2012.00169
109. Simopoulos AP. The nutritional aspects of hypertension. Compr Ther 1999;25:95-100.
110. Santiago-Fernandez P, Torres-Barahona R, Muela-Martínez JA, Rojo-Martínez G, García-Fuentes E, Stampfer MJ, Hennekens CH, Manson JE, Colditz GA, Rosner B, Willett WC. (1993) Vitamin E Consumption And The Risk Of Coronary Disease In Women. N Engl J Med. 328:1444-9.
111. Suter PM, Golner BB, Goldin BR, Morrow FD, Russel RM. (1991) Reversal Of Protein-Bound Vitamin B12 Malabsorption With Antibiotics In Atrophic Gastritis. Gastroenterology. 101:1039-45.
112. Tani, Y et al. (2007) Effects of a prolonged high phosphorous diet on phosphorous and calcium balance in rats. J Clin Biochem Nutr. 40(3): 221–228.
113. The International Council for the Control of Iodine Deficiency Disorders (ICCIDD); Accessed April 27 2012:http:// www.iccidd.org/pages/protecting-children/fortifying-salt/history-of-salt-iodization.php
114. The Office of Dietary Supplements of the National Institute of Health. Accessed Feb 29, 2012 from: http://ods.od.nih.gov/factsheets/VitaminD-HealthProfessional.
115. Traber M. G. (2014). Vitamin E inadequacy in humans: causes and consequences. *Advances in nutrition (Bethesda, Md.)*, 5(5), 503–514. https://doi.org/10.3945/an.114.006254
116. Traber MG. Heart Disease And Single-Vitamin Supplementation. Am J Clin Nutr 2007;85:293S-9S.
117. Trustwell, S and Milne, R. The B Vitamins. In: Essentials of Human Nutrition, Mann, J, and Trustwell, AS (eds), Oxford: Oxford University Press, p: 197-216
118. Tulchinsky, T. H., & Varavikova, E. A. (2014). A History of Public Health. *The New Public Health*, 1–42. https://doi.org/10.1016/B978-0-12-415766-8.00001-X
119. Tynkkynen, K. (1995) Lontoon neljä 1800-luvun koleraepidemiaa [Four cholera epidemics in nineteenth century London.]. Hippokrates (Helsinki); 12:62-88
120. U.N.I.C.E.F. (2003) Micronutrients Iodine, Iron and Vitamin A. Retrieved November 18, 2013 from: http://www.unicef.org/nutrition/index_iodine.html
121. UK Parliament (2020). The 1848 Public Health Act. Retrieved July 21, 2020 from parliament.uk website: URL: https://www.parliament.uk/about/living-heritage/transformingsociety/towncountry/towns/tyne-and-wear-case-study/about-the-group/public-administration/the-1848-public-health-act/
122. U.S. Department of Agriculture, Agricultural Research Service. 2011. USDA National Nutrient Database for Standard Reference, Release 24. Nutrient Data Laboratory Home Page; Retrieved October 10, 2012 http://www.ars.usda.gov/ba/bhnrc/ndl
123. Verhagen H, Buijsse B, Jansen E, Bueno-De-Mesquita B. (2006) The State Of Anoxidant Affairs. Nutr Today. 41:244-50.
124. Wash. B (n.d). Britain: 1906-1918: Achievements of Liberal Reforms. Taken from the National Archives on July 22, 2020. URL: https://www.nationalarchives.gov.uk/education/britain1906to1918/g2/background.htm
125. Wright, N. C., Looker, A. C., Saag, K. G., Curtis, J. R., Delzell, E. S., Randall, S., & Dawson-Hughes, B. (2014). The recent prevalence of osteoporosis and low bone mass in the United States based on bone mineral density at the femoral neck or lumbar spine. *Journal of bone and mineral research : the official journal of the American Society for Bone and Mineral Research*, 29(11), 2520–2526. https://doi.org/10.1002/jbmr.2269
126. Whittaker P. (1998) Iron and zinc interactions in humans. Am J Clin Nutr. 68:442S-6S.
127. World Health Organization. (2007) United Nations Children's Fund & International Council for the Control of Iodine Deficiency Disorders. Assessment of iodine deficiency disorders and monitoring their elimination. 3rd ed. Geneva, Switzerland: WHO.
128. Xianzhi Xiong et. al. (2007) Dose–Effect Relationship between Drinking Water Fluoride Levels and Damage to Liver and Kidney Functions in Children. Environmental Research; 103(1):112-116
129. Xiong, X. et al. (2007) Fluoride related to liver, kidney effects in children? Environ Res. 103(1): 112-6
130. Zimmermann MB. (2009) Iodine deficiency. Endocr Rev. 30(4):376-408.

CHAPTER 4

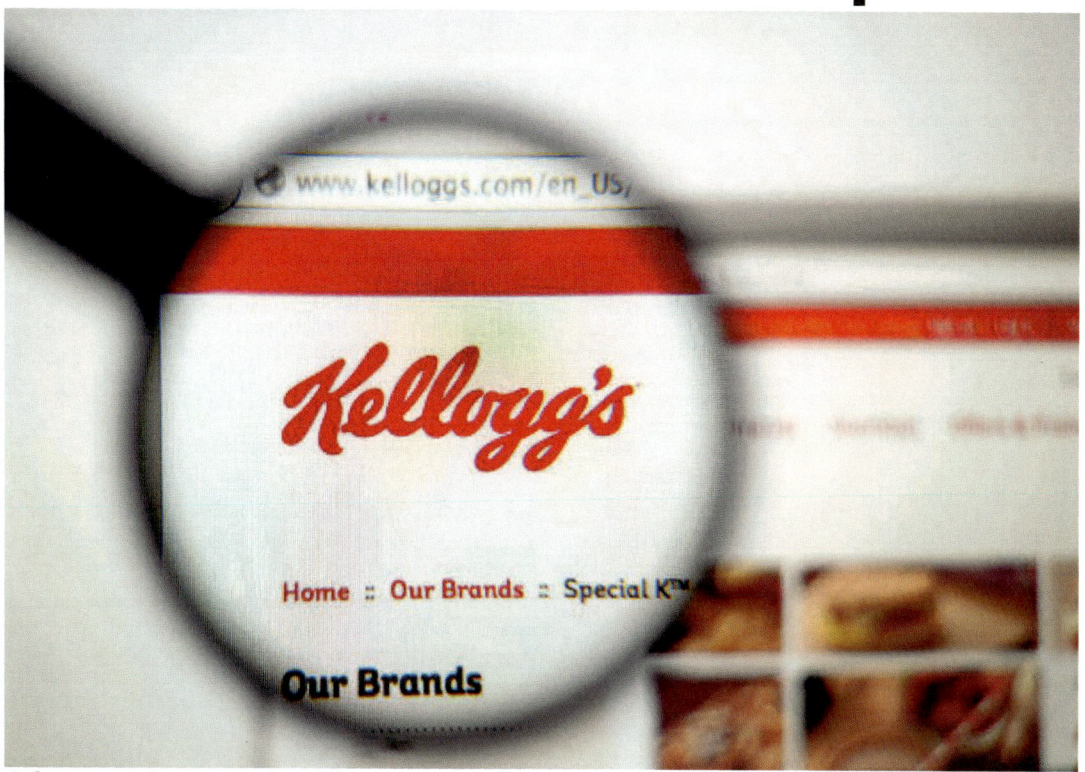

©Gil C / shutterstock_293225849/Shutterstock.com

EMERGENCE OF THE FOOD INDUSTRY

4.1 The Birth of Manufactured Foods

In Europe, between 1880 and 1914, the food supply and food production were undergoing important changes that were concentrically driven by the nutrient paradigm and the hope for safe food. In the late 19th century, the discovery of vitamins fuelled a new and deeper understanding of food, first, from the scientific perspective, second, in terms of the business of manufacturing and marketing foods, and third, at the political level. It is here that legally binding government regulatory systems were set up to ensure consumer health and prevent fraud.[23]

The nutrient paradigm propelled efforts toward nutrient-based standardizations, and regaining the consumer's trust, which had been lost since the food adulteration scandals of the early 1800s (see chapter 7 for more information on U.S. food adulteration).

In Europe, there was a strong push to establish a codification system of foods called Codex Alimentarius; its purpose was to classify foods on the basis of food identification, quality grades, and food production, all in order to preserve the health of the population. The first food codex was called *Codex Alimentarius Austriacus*—the result of an Austrian-Hungarian cooperation in 1898.[27]

By 1908, revisions to the codex included a nutrient-based inventory, which minimally attempted to quantify a very narrow range of nutrients. The public's mistrust of the food industry continued up to 1914, because of the codex's redefinition of food in terms of chemical structures which some have argued, was quite distant from the consumer's palate. In the end, for Europeans, it was about the taste of the food and the food traditions. Dr. Uwe Spiekermann, Deputy Director at the German Historical Institute, in Washington, DC writes:

Consequently, science-based standardization is an integral element of public distrust and health concerns—although there are no real alternatives.[32]

In the U.S., by contrast, the drive to standardize food was squelched by the U.S. Board of Trade, which argued against strict obligatory standards for food. They were concerned about setting up a highly rigid system that offered no flexibility. Spiekermann concludes:

Obligatory food standards were not really discussed, but the idea of pure, unmixed foodstuffs without any substitutes or additives was generally accepted.[34]

Despite attempts at legislating food controls to protect the health of the American public from food adulteration, only weak legislation emerged in the 1880s. Afterwards, the Bureau of Chemistry, which came under the control of the Department of Agriculture, investigated suspicions of possible fraud. Moreover, in the U.S., there was no initiative for a food codex system. Hence, by 1908, nutrient-based food standardization had not taken place in the United States.

Nonetheless, cheap food was now being produced at an industrial scale all through Europe and the U.S., and the standards of quality were being defined at the level of analytical chemistry. The quest for food purity—especially in the U.S.—was the new vision, and science had become the gatekeeper of that vision.

The idea of achieving a pure food supply was generally the impetus of the food laws that were being written in the U.S. at the time. This pure food vision was intolerant of the notion that foodstuffs could be mixed and diluted down; however, the vision did not address whether it was permissible to use substitutes or additives in food. However, the new science and technology that were emerging from the chemical revolution of the late 18th century, provided business with the ability to develop a wider assortment of cheaper foods in the U.S. and abroad.

The nutrient paradigm, in Europe, had opened the door to the possibilities of manipulating ingredients, while still maintaining food composition standards. And so, ingredients of lesser quality replaced those of high quality. With respect to the German chocolate industry, Spiekermann writes:

Expensive cocoa butter was replaced by cheaper animal fats; some producers even added starch or farina. Their producers argued that a combination of cocoa, starch, flours, and cheap fat was not unhealthy and would allow a 'democratization' of the consumption of former luxuries.[34]

In the U.S., there was a delayed awakening to the reality that a pure food supply could not be the complete answer to population health. By the late 1800s, food manufacturing had attained such a sophisticated level of processing—most of it aimed at feeding a large population base—that many food ingredients were devoid of nutrients.

Three things were occurring that hinted that this pure American food was scandalously compromised nutritionally. First, by the 1930s and 40s, as the U.S. continued to manufacture and market cheap processed foods, food chemists were identifying sizable amounts of food products that were nutritionally deficient. At the same time, some nutritionists and dietitians stood on their soap boxes promoting the idea that the nutritional quality of the food was paramount for individual and population health. Meanwhile numerous cases of malnutrition were popping up everywhere as the U.S. reliance on bleached white bread continued to grow.[3]

Second, the FDA in the United States and Health and Welfare Canada, began proposing a number of bills that would somewhat regulate the food industry, which by the 30s had begun to increasingly refine food, and in so doing, removed important concentrations of nutrients and non-nutrients. One of the bills was intended to force the food industry to add some of those nutrients back or in other words to "enrich" the foods they were producing. However, the bill was defeated in the U.S.; the enrichment of flour and cereals, however, eventually became voluntary after World War-II. Even today, enrichment is not forced. In Canada, regulatory policies for the enrichment of processed flour were first past in 1964, requiring that all flour be enriched with thiamin, riboflavin, niacin, and iron.

Third, as the 50s, 60s and 70s began to unfold, there was a sense that synthesized vitamins could be used by the food and pharmaceutical industries to mimic and surpass the quality of breast milk and food in general.

> With Tang™, General foods created a drink made from mainly sugar to simulate natural orange juice.

A classic example is General Foods' attempt to imitate orange juice by creating synthetic flavoured crystals called: Tang™ in 1959. Its main ingredients were sugar, a coloring agent and a whopping amount of vitamin C. An 8fl-oz volume of this crystal drink, mixed to the recommended concentration, contained sufficient vitamin C to meet 100% of the recommended daily allowance (RDA) in the U.S and 133% of the recommended nutrient intake (RNI) in Canada. It was a synthetic product, loaded with sugar and with one vitamin, and marketed as a healthy way to begin the morning, despite not containing a single once of orange. There was nevertheless a strong insinuation that these crystals were not just the equivalent of an orange but, because NASA's Mercury and Gemini missions had adopted it for their astronauts, were indeed superior to the natural orange. And to create the illusion that it was an actual food product, General Foods added vitamin C. More importantly, this product's targeted audience was children, and consequently several generations of young people, regularly consumed Tang™ without even a single parental concern about the impact on children's health. If it was good for the astronauts, it had to also be good for our children. This was a golden endorsement that caused sales of Tang® to skyrocket by the early 1960s.

4.1.1 The Breakfast Cereal Revolution. General Foods was not alone in generating foods that impoverished rather than enrich the American food supply. In the U.S., breakfast cereals represented a relevant example of over processing. The Kellogg's company was among the early pioneers in breakfast cereal technology. Here's a company whose founder, William Keith Kellogg (1860-1951), believed that every American should have access to a nutritious and convenient breakfast. This is the story of a young high school drop out with entrepreneurial skills, teaming up with his brother, Dr John H. Kellogg, who may have been one of the first physicians to have pioneered and popularized the concept of "sound nutrition" being critical for human health. J.H. Kellogg wrote: *"Practical Manual of Hygiene and Temperance"* in 1877 as part of the U.S. Health Reform Movement's attempt at reforming modern dietary practices. He identified several foods and eating practices that singled out Americans as the unhealthiest people in the world. He writes:

America is known abroad as a nation of dyspeptics. This unfortunate condition is the result of the universal disregard of dietetic rules for which our countrymen are notorious.[13]

The most impoverished food was identified as fine-flour bread, from which he claimed the milling process removed the best nutrition. Second, he recommended consuming an abundance of vegetables and significantly less animal foods; the idea here was that meat was inconsistent with longevity. Third, being a Seventh Day Adventist, it is not surprising that he vilified alcohol consumption. Fourth, he discouraged tea and coffee ingestion as they were known stimulants. Fifth, Kellogg advised against eating between meals and recommended limiting daily meals to two per day: a hardy breakfast at 7:00 a.m, and a dinner at 2 pm. And finally, sixth, he advised against eating in haste, something Americans are still known for today.

A Seventh Day Adventist, John Kellogg joined the Battle Creek Michigan Western Health Reform Institute, which was later renamed the Battle Creek Sanatorium. He acted as the Sanatorium's physician and nutritionist, and promoted his own health food, which included "Granose"—a type of granola—and wheat flakes which was his answer to Henry Perhy's creation of "Shredded Wheat" in 1892.

C.W. Post, while experiencing heart trouble, sought relief at the Battle Creek Sanatorium, known also as the "San". During his stay, he found little relief, and left dissatisfied. In response, he founded his own health home called "*La Vita Inn*" and proceeded to restrict coffee, tea and physicians from its premises. This drastic approach of eliminating the medical doctor was reminiscent of practices often seen during the 15th to the beginning of the late 18th centuries. It was, in a sense, a forewarning of what was to come again in the late twentieth century as soft natural therapies began to surface in protest to Medicines harsh drug therapies.

Post went on to produce significant market sensations like the all-natural coffee substitute by 1895, made up of bran, wheat, molasses, and still known today as "Postum. The cold cereal called "Grape-Nuts", was later introduced in 1898, followed by the first corn flake in 1906, which Post initially called " Elijah's Manna", but was later persuaded by religious authorities, to change to "Post Toasties".

Meanwhile, both Kellogg brothers experimented with different ways of transforming cereal grains into roasted flakes. These flakes were first introduced to the menu of the Battle Creek sanatorium, in Michigan. The cereal was then marketed by a mail order company named "Sanitas Food Company" beginning in 1900. The consumers of these cereals were mostly upper class health food users who were exercising a unique prerogative, that of healthy eating.

By 1906, the Kellogg brothers developed and perfected the famous corn flake (**Figure-4.1**); it was a more difficult process because corn is a less flexible and a more difficult grain to manipulate. The roasted corn flake was Kellogg's response to Post's Toasties, and gave birth to what was initially called: "The Battle Creek Toasted Corn Flake Company".

This name was quickly changed to the "W.K. Kellogg Company". The marketing scheme of the Kellogg's company revolved around four basic concepts that described the way they hoped the public would perceive their cereal:
(a) Health food cereal
(b) Healthful cereal
(c) Enjoyable cereal
(d) Convenient breakfast for everyone

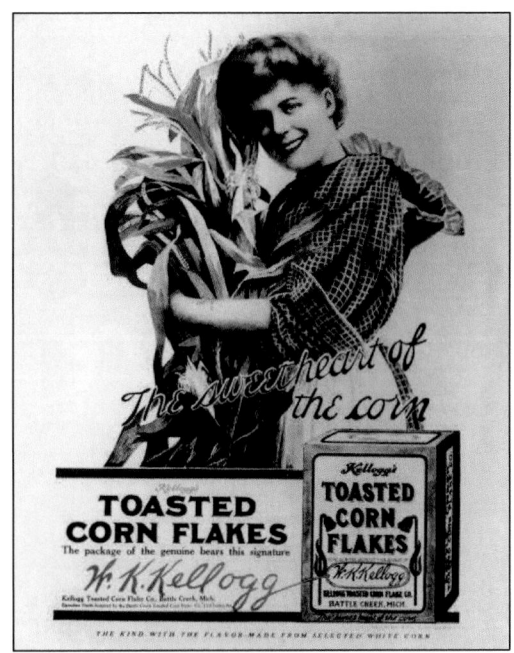

Figure 4.1: Retouched image of the first print advertisement placed by W. K. Kellogg to sell his corn cereal shows a hearty American peasant woman in a dress as she embraces a collection of corn stalks; a box of the cereal is also displayed at lower right, 1906. Text of the advertisement reads in part 'The sweetheart of the corn' and 'The package of the genuine bears this signature W. K. Kellogg' and 'The kind with the flavor made from selected white corn.' (Photo by Frederic Lewis/Getty Images)

W.K. Kellogg and C.W. Post effectively set in motion a breakfast revolution in North America, and in doing so, the roasted flake cereal displaced hot cereal consumption from the American breakfast table.

The significance of this revolution can be observed at two levels: First, in the mechanical manipulation of the cereal grain, which was a technical achievement that rid the grain of most of its nutrients, but ensured taste, texture and convenience; second, the disappearance of the hot cereal meant a less labor-intensive morning for the housewife.

It also, by contrast, carried the serious implication of a less nutritious breakfast. This meant that insufficient calories and vitamins were possibly going to be ingested at the critical morning period—A significant change that would affect North American breakfast eaters.

The problems faced by the cereal manufacturer were in the areas of processing, shipping, and length of storage in warehouses and stores. To leave the cereal grain untouched, unprocessed, meant that the wheat germ, which contained the nutritious wheat germ oil, would go rancid if storage time or turnover of the product in the stores was too long. Given the vastness of the distribution area, this was likely to happen. The quality of the product would

> Processing wheat removed both the bran and the germ from the grain, resulting in a loss of important vitamins, minerals and fiber.

greatly suffer and, naturally, the companies could not afford such a mistake. The bran had to also be separated from the endosperm (the white corn flour) for two main reasons: First, there was a tendency for little bugs to lodge in the bran layer; second the bran mixed into the endosperm made the flour more difficult to manipulate.

Extensive food processing of the kind proposed by the Kellogg brothers required that the bran and the germ be removed, and with them, extensive amounts of vitamins and minerals. The loss of the bran was initially perceived as an unimportant event. Little did they know that cereal companies would be scrambling, years later, to put the fiber back into the breakfast cereals.

Although, initially W.K Kellogg was hoping to provide the consumer with a healthful product, he was probably not aware of the fact that the cereal had little nutritional value, save for the milk that was added. During World War II, practices of enrichment were encouraged because clusters of malnutrition were found peppered throughout the country by 1942. In order to strengthen the health of the new military recruits in 1943, the U.S. military had orders to only purchase enriched flour and bread. This meant that certain nutrients had to be added back to the product in concentrations equal to those found in the food before the processing. Many mills and bakeries voluntarily enriched their bread, wheat flour, cornmeal, corn grits, ready to eat and uncooked cereals, and macaroni products, with thiamin, riboflavin, niacin and the mineral iron by 1949. In some rare instances, vitamin D and calcium were added as well.

> Whole or unprocessed wheat contains wheat germ. Wheat germ is high in nutritious oil, but more prone to spoilage.

The intent of these measures was to safeguard the population from specific nutritional deficiencies, and to rehabilitate those individuals already malnourished, who had been greatly dependent on wheat flour. This is because the mechanical milling process of wheat, and other flours, impoverished their nutrient content.

So in the end, Mr Kellogg provided the public with a nutrient-impoverished food convenience, which some government food scientists and dietitians tried to counter; their warnings fell on death ears. This is because the population, for the most part, was still overjoyed by the advent of a technology that was making food much safer by the early twentieth century. There is no doubt that the development of temperature-controlled storage, rail transportation, and refrigeration systems were critical for the production of safe and healthy food in the U.S. and Canada. The 40s and 50s saw the expansion of that food technology as the baby boomer phenomena hit the North American landscape, and as the structure of the North American family began to change.

Breakfast cereal companies, in the 50s and 60s, created some of the most sugary and highly profitable cereals at that time. They were engaged in a fierce battle for the dominant market share of the American breakfast table. Slick advertising campaigns, along with loveable cartoon mascots helped drive the desire for the highly sugared products, especially among children. Kellogg's Froot Loops®, became the company's most profitable cereal of all time, and was instrumental at displacing healthier choices out of the menu of the youth.

4.1.2 Sugar and the American Diet.
During the 60s and 70s, average sugar intake was estimated at 125Lbs/person/year in the U.S. And while health professionals claimed that there were no serious health side effects associated with such levels of sugar intake, doubts were being raised that such sugar loads were causing behavioral problems among young delinquents. Barbara J. Reed, Chief

probation officer at the Municipal Court of Cuyahoga Falls, Ohio, advanced that elevated sugar and more specifically, sucrose, was responsible for the aggressive and impulsive behaviors of delinquent adolescents. She testified before the U.S. Senate Select Committee on Nutrition and Human Needs in 1977, that eliminating high sugar doses and junk food, from the diet of her parolees, caused a significant reduction in delinquent relapses. She claimed that eliminating sugar from the diet of parolees' also significantly improved their hypoglycaemia, and eased their readjustment to living harmoniously and violence-free. After 20 years as a probation officer, Barbara Reed Stitt went on to earn a doctoral degree in nutrition, and continued to study the impact of diet quality on behavior. More recent work by Schoenthaler in 1997 showed, in a controlled study, that when good nutrition was included in the diet of incarcerated juvenile detainees, violent outbursts significantly dropped concurrently with notable changes in specific brain activity patterns and improved serum vitamin concentrations.[31]

Around that same time period, a then not so famous researcher, Dr Ben Feingold, suggested that naturally occurring salicylates in food may be the cause of childhood hyperactivity (attention deficit hyperactivity disorder, ADHD). His findings took the scientific community, as well as the public by surprise. The ramifications of such a finding were that food additives derived from salicylates could be responsible for as much as 50 to 70% of childhood hyperactivity. Shock waves of seismic proportion went through the food industry, and caused aggressive rebuttals with teams of researchers tearing Feingold's methodology apart. For one thing, they accused him of not correcting for dietary sugar concentrations, and for using anecdotal reports; critics advanced that instead of the artificial colors and flavors, present in the experimental diets, that it was sugar causing the hyperactivity. His research was completely dismissed as poor science. Nagging concerns over the safety of the American food supply were quickly rejected, allowing food companies to forge ahead in the development of cheap, tasty and affordable foods.

No other products than General Foods' Jell-O-brand of puddings and gelatine desserts, better illustrates the artificiality of the U.S. diet in the 1960s and 70s. Created in 1897 by Mr Pearle Wait, a carpenter in LeRoy, New York, he founded the Jell-O Company Inc. twenty six years later, in 1923. It was subsequently purchased by the Postum Cereal Company in 1925, which was soon renamed General Foods. It did not take long before Jell-O was known as "America's Most Famous Dessert". By the 1960's it was widely distributed around the world, and became such a familiar household dessert that

> Food and diet are now considered by scientists on the impact that food components have to either promote or diminish health status.

every hospital served it on their "Clear Fluid" diet, as well as on their regular menu as a dessert option. Yet, it became apparent, by reading the ingredient list, that the raspberry Jell-O dessert contained no raspberries, but only:

Sugar, Gelatin, Adipic Acid (For Tartness), Contains Less Than 2% of Artificial Flavor, Disodium Phosphate and Sodium Citrate (Control Acidity), Fumaric Acid (For Tartness), Red 40.

Indeed the ingredient list clearly suggested that Jell-O may not have been even rightfully classified as an actual food, and continued to fuel suspicions that we shouldn't be feeding these products to our children.

Yet despite alarm bells, food companies continued to market questionable products. Kool-Aid is possibly the third most significant 20th century perversion of the food supply. It was created in 1927 by Edwin Perkins, who was inspired by the success of Jell-O. He was an entrepreneurial inventor and businessman, who, by working with a chemist, devised a method of producing fruit pectin powders that consisted of dextrose, citric acid, tartaric acid, flavoring and food coloring. During the Great Depression of 1929, Kool-Aid crystals were manufactured as 6 flavors, and sold for 5¢ a package. It became an affordable treat in the midst of economic hardship and prolonged droughts. The product became so successful, that the Perkins Products Company was producing 325 million packets of Kool-Aid annually by 1950.[1] It was purchase by General Foods in 1953, and marketed with the now famous smiling face pitcher.[14]

Since the 1920s, the FDA has maintained a growing inventory of food additives that is currently estimated at 3000 accepted compounds, some of which include sugar, salt, baking soda, vanilla and yeast.[6] The issue of human health, as it relates to nutrition, has attained a far greater complexity than the mere availability of food, which was the problem that historically threatened the health of populations during the great famines. Now health professionals are faced with a population that has been raised on such elevated sugar loads and disturbing amounts of additives, that it puts into question the nutritional quality of a sizable proportion of the food supply.

The isolation of vitamins, in addition to a more complete understanding of their functions in the human body, created a certain scientific mystique. It wasn't so much around food itself, but increasingly around the vitamin pill. As baby boomers began to come of age in the early to mid-1970s, nutritional supplements became their vehicle to optimal health and productivity.

At the same time that vitamin pills hit the shelves in an ever-growing assortment, the food industry was being accused of impoverishing the food supply through excessive food processing. Cursory reviews of several issues of the health magazine "Prevention" dated back to the mid-70s, attests to the climate of mistrust, by natural food proponents, that existed towards the food industry.

The abundance of white bread in supermarket shelves barely caused any kind of concern, as most consumers were simply unaware that the loss of fibre from the diet represented a health risk. Not only was brown bread difficult to find, but you couldn't find canned fruit anywhere that didn't have added sugar or that wasn't laced with either heavy or mild syrup.

Canned vegetable soups, so it seemed, contained as many stabilizers, emulsifiers and flavor enhancers, than actual vegetables. In the U.S., pastas were not required by law to be enriched with vitamins and nor were rice and flours.

The public of the early 1970s was awakening to an alarming reality about the integrity of the food supply, the recklessness of food manufacturers in producing worthless junk for the sake of profit, and the clear lack of government protection in the area of stiff nutrition regulations. In the 1980's the "*Shareholder Value Movement*" caused the growth of the food industry to mushroom, thus allowing maximal return on investments for Wall Street shareholders who had stakes in the food industry. Americans began snacking everywhere: in bookstores, hair salons, gyms and gas stations because food was cheap and widely available. Indeed, the U.S. had the cheapest food supply in the world, but it was also poor in quality. Derek Thompson captured the essence of the problem in an article published in the January 11, 2010 issue of The Atlantic. He wrote:

The cheap food revolution hasn't just given low-income families cheaper options. It's come at the expense of healthier food. A dollar today buys 1,200 calories of potato chips and 250 calories of vegetables or 170 calories of fresh fruit. Walsh gets it right: it simply costs too much to be thin.[38]

Concurrently with the massive explosion of the fast and snack food industries, in the 80s and 90s, there was a relatively impressive customer shift towards natural foods. The food industry was caught off guard, and so moved swiftly to recapture customer allegiance: it began marketing no sugar, low salt and low fat food products that were tailor made to match customer concerns.

Today, the scientific community is increasingly aware that food components can affect health on the short and long term. Very clearly, frequent and abundant meat consumption has been tied to heart disease and cancer.[2,5,] There are now increasing numbers of companies that produce healthy foods with minimal artificial preservatives, sugar, salt, sodium, and fat. Cheap and impoverished foods, however, still stock significant grocery store shelf space.

4.1.3 The Soft Drink Revolution

IT'S THE REAL THING—No product exemplifies the impact of flavor and taste manipulation, on driving mass population consumption, more than Coca-Cola. Invented in May 1886, by the pharmacist John Styth Pemberton, Coke went on to become the most popular soda of all time. The 36 year old Pemberton combined the coca leaf with the kola nut, and blended in copious amounts of sugar, flavors, and caffeine. Initially patented as a medicinal tonic used for headaches, hysteria, and melancholy, it gained popularity quite rapidly as a picker-upper, and for good reason. The kola nut contained a good dose of caffeine, and the cocaine extracted from the coca leaf had an amazing soothing quality and a slightly addictive edge. The amount of cocaine was never officially established, but Coca-Cola officials were quick to reassure critics that the amount was negligible. The soda was served for the very first time from Willis Venable's *"Soda Water King of the South's"* fountain concession stand located on the ground floor of Jacob's Pharmacy in Atlanta, in May of 1886. Pemberton died two years later, having sold the secret formula and the company for a mere $2,300 US to businessman, Asa G Candler. In 1889, Candler formed the Coca-Cola Corporation and proceeded to develop a very sophisticated marketing campaign that galvanized sales of the soda throughout the U.S and its territories. One year later, in 1890, a New Bern, North Carolina pharmacist by the name of Caleb Bradham, created Pepsi-Cola, which was eventually going to become Coca-Cola's main rival by the 1960s. In order to clearly distinguish Coke from copycat imitators who were trying to edge into the cola market, Coca-Cola developed the new contour bottle, in 1916, which made this cola very recognizable and distinct from Pepsi Cola and other competitors. By 1917, the company was recording 3 million Coke sales per day, which was a dramatic jump up from the 9 sodas per day sold at the Atlanta fountain shop in 1886. Then in 1919, Candler sold the Coca-Cola Corporation to Ernest Woodruff and a group of investors for $25 million, and immediately Woodruff opened bottling plants in Paris, Bordeaux and a few other European countries. It was under Woodruff's leadership that Coca-Cola pioneered the 6 bottle carton in 1923 which was designed with a handle for more convenient and easy purchases; it also created opportunity to increase availability to consumers and significantly impacting sales. [35c] In 1923, Ernest Woodruff's son, Robert became the first president of the Coca Cola Corporation, a position he successfully held for the next 60 years. By 1929, the "A PAUSE THAT REFRESHES" campaign was launched in the U.S and internationally in an attempt to distance Coke from its earlier portrayal as a medicinal tonic, and repaint its image as a wholesome and good product. Under his stewardship, the company experienced incredible growth internationally with the creation of The Coca-Cola Export Corporation in 1930. Though he achieved modest success initially—28 countries by 1939 had bottling plants—international growth did not begin to soar until World War-II with the opening of an additional 36 bottling franchises by 1945 that were mostly government-financed. In the meantime, leading up to the second world war, Pepsi-Cola—having gone bankrupt twice: once in 1928 and a second time in 1931—launched one of its most impressive comeback attempt in 1933 with the marketing of the 12Fluid-Oz bottle for only 5¢. It locked horns with Coca-Cola on the principle of value or in other words, on how much product the consumer could acquire for the lowest price. Pepsi's value strategy won over many converts from Coke, and created the first illusion in food commercialism: **Big is better**! This was a blow to Coke who sold the 6 ½ Fluid-Oz bottle for the same price, but it also further awakened, what was to become by the late 1970s, a national problem of excessive calorie consumption. Once the second World War began, Coca-Cola's marketing strategy was strictly focused on ensuring the availability of Coke to the US troops for only 5 cents—a commitment Woodruff maintained despite some financial loss. It was considered a morale booster for the soldiers in that the bottle of Coke provided them with a little taste of home. But Coca-Cola's commitment to ensure that the American soldiers got their Coke, no matter what the cost to the company was, created a very big consumer allegiance after the war. But at the same, time Coca-Cola symbolized freedom, and thus was intimately tied to the wartime cause. Symbolically, having a Coke was patriotic, a very American thing to do. This is one of the first examples of a food product being so culturally tied to a nation's identity, and to a powerful feeling of hope in the midst of such tragic war-time disarray. The European bottling plants were also strategically positioned to ensure Coke was available for American soldiers during the war, but also to facilitate widespread distribution of the cola throughout Europe after the war. The Ally victory came in 1945 and freed Europe from the Nazi oppressors, but post-war Europe was left devastated with bombed cities, bridges and roads; national despondency prevailed as the overwhelming prospects of rebuilding Europe weighed down on the spirit and resolve of the people. The 1947 United States Marshall Plan brought American financial aid, material resources, manpower, and significant hope that European infrastructures and economies could be rebuilt, and prosper once again. The prevailing fear, at that time however, was that an unconstrained Americanization would sweep through Europe, writes historian Richard Kuisel, professor of history at the State University of New York at Stony Book. American culture could be seen through so many prisms, and it really came down to which one people chose to look through. For certain, the U.S carried with its flag and popular culture, a strong message rooted in freedom and tolerance, but also consumerism. It was the commercial stronghold the US was trying to achieve in Europe that caused some hesitancy and resentment. It was quite a conundrum: Western Europe needed the money and economic credits from the Marshall Plan, and did not want to insult the American people, but Europe also felt the importance of maintaining its cultural sovereignty and identity, and was resistant to the prospects of cheapening European lifestyle and values through commercialism and unabated consumerism. Hidden beneath this protectionist philosophy, aimed at safeguarding the main tenets of its people's culture, was this daunting European fear of becoming subservient to the United States, something France's government especially struggled with during the Cold War era, writes Kuisel, [16b] in "Coca-Cola and the Cold-War". The French National Assembly clearly was resistant to Coca-Cola's attempts at entering the French market place with its high profile Coke logos and advertising. The Communist Party—the main opposition party—was clearly against the Coca-Cola Corporation, and was desperately trying to drum up popular support for the resistance against Coca-Cola's infiltration, as it was clear from their perspective that American economic dominance was forthcoming, and so Kuisel writes:" [16b]

Coca-Cola was only one feature of a multifaceted American "invasion" that included Hollywood films, the Reader's Digest, and tractors."

To more fully understand the disparaging manner in which French culture perceived the unsophisticated nature of America, three images, used in magazines at the time, to capture the essence of Americanization, boiled down to hot dogs, baseball and Coke. And so hidden within the long outstretched tentacles of US imperialism, was the Coca-Cola Corporation, leading the cultural invasion or what the French Communist Party coined as the *Coca-Colonization of Europe*. The Communist party had a particular problem with Coke, as it embodied everything American; capitalism was somehow mysteriously seen as contained within the Coke bottle, and the communists hated it. The symbolism was so extensive in post-war Europe, that drinking Coke was indeed the equivalent of embracing those American ideals of individual freedom, free enterprise and popular culture; and so Coca-Cola became one of the most recognized companies in the world. This set the stage for an incredible boost in worldwide sales of the infamous cola in the aftermaths of the war. In France, the opposition Communist Party was fighting tooth and nail to halt Coca-colonization. They chose the disingenuous strategy of resisting Coca-Cola's attempt at building a syrup production plant in Marseille on the basis of protecting the health of the French public; they accused Coca-Cola of producing a product that did not respect public health standards. They utilized many other tactics, but this one stands out because there was some truth to this. European standards forbade the use of chemicals of any kind in food. In reading Kuisel's analysis,[16b] it seems that Coca-Cola's attorneys were arguing that the accusations were baseless, however, a closer look indicates that a number of top Coca-Cola executives were very nervous about the content of phosphoric acid in Coke as it appeared to be in flagrant violation of the 1905 French Health Code. Meanwhile, the wine, fruit juice and mineral water lobbyists were clawing away at Coca-Cola's plan to begin a production facility in France, arguing that it would compromise their own sales of healthy nutritious drinks, and diminish the nutritional quality of the people's diet. Interestingly, they never drew from a 1942 position paper by American Medical Association's (AMA's) Council on Food and Nutrition—one of the most authoritative medical bodies in the US—on the use of carbonated soft drinks. At that time Americans were consuming 5.6 gallons per person per year, an amount that was drastically smaller than the current 54 gallons per person per year. The Council stated with authority the main concerns behind the use of such products especially among the youth:
"From the health point of view it is desirable especially to have restriction of such use of sugar as is represented by consumption of sweetened carbonated beverages and forms of candy which are of low nutritional value. The Council believes it would be in the interest of the public health for all practical means to be taken to limit consumption of sugar in any form in which it fails to be combined with significant proportions of other foods of high nutritive quality."

It is rather amazing that the AMA's Council had already saw health problems arising early on when average per day consumption was the equivalent of only 2 fluid-Oz per person per day. In the end, Coca-Cola's formidable legal team in concert with US political maneuvering and posturing, wore and tore on the French resolve to exclude Coke from the market place for whatever reason. By 1953, all legal actions directed at Coca-Cola were dropped; the wrangling had gone on for 7 years, but never could the opponents of Coke prove that the product was bad for the public's health. This opened the doors for a very ambitious Coke marketing campaign that was unleashed throughout Europe, using billboards, magazines and television ads, so that by 1959, Coke was bottled in over 100 countries. [16b]

In 1963 it launched its "THINGS GO BETTER WITH COKE" campaign. It was an innocuous enough jingle but it carried a surprisingly strong punch, as it was attempting to move Coke several notches up from a mere "Refreshing Pause"–the theme of its 1929 campaign—to a meal complement. At this point it was clear that Coke was vying for a seat at the dinner table. And sure enough, visually attractive marketing depicted a glass of Coke right beside either a hamburger or hotdog (**Figure-4.2**) with fries. Here was, possibly the image that most accurately captured the early perversion of the American diet.

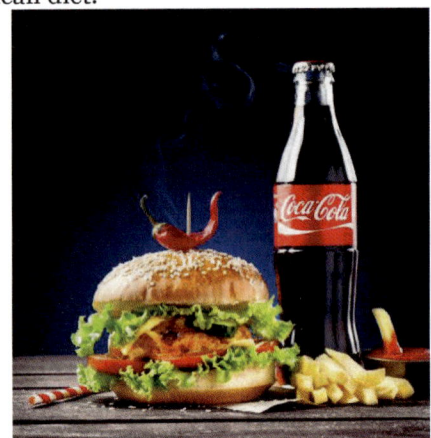

Figure-4.2 A 1950s restaurant menu display By Pikoso.kz © Shutterstock___314676233/Shutterstock.com

Very gradually Coke was depicted as a wholesome product, shedding as it were, its earlier image as a medicinal tonic. Meanwhile, Pepsi-Cola latched on to that whole new baby boomer generation that was entering the teenage years with its 1961 campaign: "COME ALIVE! YOU'RE IN THE PEPSI GENERATION". This was a bold and aggressive attempt by the Pepsi-Cola Corporation to define itself as the drink of an entire generation. By 1964, Pepsi bid to integrate the pop-culture through music, with the recording of the jingle: "Girl Watchers" which hit the top 40 on the pop charts. But it was officially the merger of the Pepsi-Cola Corporation with Frito-Lay, in and around 1965, that made the newly formed PepsiCo a formidable challenger to Coca-Cola's dominance in the cola market. That year, PepsiCo posted $510 million in sales and employed 19, 000 people. PepsiCo was, in 1965, the sole distributor of Pepsi-Cola, Mountain Dew, and Diet Pepsi.

Coca-Cola responded to PepsiCo's market challenge, in 1969, by launching its newest and perhaps most successful slogan: "IT'S THE REAL THING". In the midst of a flower power revolution, headed by a hippie movement that opposed the artificiality of the business and financial establishments, and the corrupt war-mongering strategies of government, many baby-boomers embraced Coke as "The Real Thing," or in other words the real emblem of peace and love. Coke is promoted as that one" real thing" the young could depend on at the time of an interminable and unpopular Vietnamese war. By July 1971, Coca-Cola followed up with its most successful promotion of all time: the "I'D LIKE TO BUY THE WORLD A COKE" TV campaign.[29b] The jingle was so successful, that it hit number 13 on the pop charts, and was rewritten and re-recorded into the top 10 pop hit: "*I'd Like to Teach the World to Sing*" by The New Seekers. In the Coke jingle, the song states "...it's what the world wants today. It's the Real Thing". A midst a generational movement looking for truth—having been disillusioned by the business establishment and the Vietnam War—Coke positions itself as "The Real Thing" the world is looking for. The multi-ethnic makeup of the hundreds of singers in the TV commercial, confirms Coca-Cola as a true international entity that unites the globe and its peoples who are searching for authentic truth. Coca-Cola was all too ready to reassure the world that COKE WAS IT! As if to consolidate the wholesome and authentic image of the corporation, Coca-Cola committed to donating the first $80,000 of royalties from the hit song to UNICEF. Slam-dunk! The company hit the nail on the head and saw a whole new post-war generation embrace a carbonated beverage as a common emblematic banner that united an entire generation that was looking for a common symbol they could all agree on: it was Coke. [29b] Since its inception, in the late 19th century, the Coca Cola Corporation saw its sales of soda dramatically increase from nine 6 fluid-Oz bottles per day in 1886 to 44,000 8Fl-oz drinks per day in 1904, to finally reaching 1.3 billion drinks /day worldwide in 2004. Presently, the Coca-Cola Corporation distributes over 800 food products, and posted annual net revenues of $48.017 billion in 2012, representing a 50.32% increase since 2008. [35c] Soda consumption has become a very difficult problem worldwide, but especially here in the United States, because of the high prevalence of obesity. According to the USDA's Economic Research Service, the growth of soda production (**Figure-4.3**) has been extensive since the 1940s, especially with both big players—Coca-Cola and Pepsi—battling it out in the market place. Indeed between 1947 and the year 2000 total soda production—diet and regular combined—increased 6-fold.

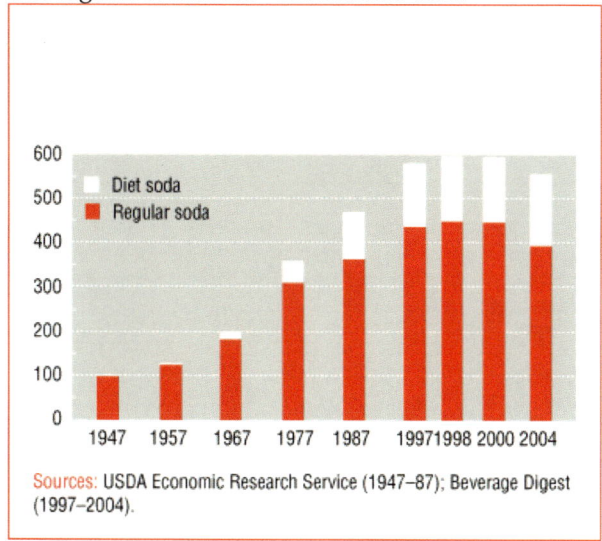

Figure 4.3 Annual Soft Drink Productions in the US. (12-oz cans/person). Source: USDA Research Service 1947-87)

PepsiCo now holds the lion's share of the market with combined sales of chips, cola, 7up and nachos, plus it peddles Tropicana. In 2011, PepsiCo posted net revenues of over $65 billion. Combined together, these two giant corporations rake in over $100 billion in net revenues from the sale of predominantly junk and highly processed foods. Most consumers would be surprised by what companies are owned either by Coca-Cola or PepsiCo. Let's take a peek at PepsiCo's annual report for 2012. For starters, the company features the following 5 brands: Pepsi-Cola, Tropicana, Frito-Lay, Quaker and Gatorade. Without trying to be exhaustive in the breakdown, allow me to highlight the main recent acquisitions by the corporation: Sierra Mist Natural, Ocean-Spray, Mountain Dew, AMP Energy, Seattle's Best Coffee, SoBe energy drinks, Aquafina, Lipton's vast selection of teas. In a typical grocery store, in between 25-30% of the shelf space is occupied by either PepsiCo or Coca-Cola Products. [21c, 21d]

The dominance of both PepsiCo and Coca-Cola in the US and internationally should surprise nobody, given that their ability to move product is intimately tied to the combined $3.1 billion per year spent on advertising—value taken from their 2012 financial statements. This is phenomenally large compared to the mere $90 million tagged by the USDA's Agricultural Marketing Service (AMS) in 2012 to promote healthy eating in underserved US urban and rural areas. Is there any wonder that we are losing the battle to obesity? Government simply cannot compete against these giant corporations that wield an advertising budget that is 3444% greater than what the Federal government can muster. Coca-Cola and PepsiCo have such a powerful grip on the media and advertising in the US, that they can single-handedly control the eating behaviors of the young and adults alike. The Coke and Pepsi-sponsored events and programs in high schools and universities make it almost impossible to break away from their iron grip—their products are in school hallways, locker rooms, cafeterias, and gyms. Even the Academy of Nutrition and Dietetics (A.N.D) kowtows to PepsiCo and Coca-Cola who financially support their monthly professional journal and most, if not all, obesity research conferences organized by the Academy. The A.N.D. is the largest professional body of nutrition and dietetic professionals in the world. This organization regulates the professional dietitians that are therapeutically managing the obese in medical out-patient clinics and in hospitals. They are taught that carbonated beverages can fit into a well-balanced diet, as long as the patients avoid consuming them regularly. The reality however, is that soft drinks are so addictive that nothing less than a complete avoidance will help the patient to vanquish the addiction—this is especially true for children. There should be zero tolerance for carbonated beverages in the human diet, especially the young, and dietitians should be leading the charge to put these guys out of business. The problem is that they can't since they depend so heavily on the financial support provided by these corporations in order to run part of their professional operations.

Here lays the problem: One 12fl-oz soda, like Coke, contains 10 teaspoons (40g) of sugar in the form of high fructose corn-syrup; similarly, one 12fl-oz Mountain Dew, has close to 12 teaspoons (47g) of sugar. When consumed regularly, at a conservative rate of two Mountain Dews per day, a person ingests a total of 75 ½ lbs of sugar at the end of one year. This represents a surplus intake of 137,108 calories; these are extra calories that can contribute towards 39 lbs of fat deposit in a typical consumer after one year. So this kind of extrapolative calculation does not always work out exactly, but assuming that the Coke is only ingested as surplus calories, and does not displace other foods out of the diet, then 39 lbs. of fat would be added on.

Examined through this lens, it is truly not surprising that Americans, and especially its youth, are becoming overweight and obese, in addition to undernourished. But in truth the obesity paradigm is never that simple because of the complex mechanism that drives our appetite and hunger. One thing though that all researchers in the field do agree on, is that empty calorie products such as carbonated beverages—I refuse to call them foods, because they are not—can displace other wholesome and nutritious foods out of the diet, causing in some cases irreparable damage to the health of the adult, the youth or the fetus.

The United States Department of Agriculture's (U.S.D.A's) Economic Research Service has as a mission to track the foods consumed every year based on food disappearance data. In other words, it tracks how much food there is in the national inventory at the end of the year, and subtracts that amount from the food recorded at the beginning of the year. The subtraction provides the amount of food that disappeared from that inventory. The USDA must make some calculation adjustments such as how much food was exported, imported, and wasted, before they get a pretty good idea, at the population level, of the quantity of food consumed. The Economic Research Service's 2012 report compared food consumption between the 1950s and the year 2000. [38c] In that time span, total milk consumption dropped 37.9 percent—the most acute decline occurred throughout the 1970s—while total regular-sweetened soda intake rose 5-fold. The findings of this report show very clearly that the dietary displacement effect of soda took place during the 70s when soda consumption and the prevalence of obesity were increasing noticeably. This same report reveals that the use of salad dressings and cooking oils jumped 259 percent between the 1950s and 2000, greatly contributing to the obesogenic environment. Again, the most dramatic increase was during the 70s and 80s. [38c] In addition, Americans consumed, in that same time period, 41 percent more red meat and 224 percent more poultry. These increases are astounding as they paint such a troubling picture that depicts the origins of the US obesity crisis. We have become more of a meat consuming society than our predecessors, and the abundant fast food we ingest conspires with the junk food, to boost our total caloric load. The USDA's Economic Research Service's 2000-report, reveals that the current market place has 800 more calories available per individual compared to the 1950s and 500 more calories than the 1970s, and that when adjusted for waste and loss, Americans consume an additional 530 calories per day since the 1970s. When those extra calories are broken down, it turns out that the excess calories come mostly from refined grains (white flour), fats and oils, and finally sugar—the main ingredients of food processing.

4.1.4 Extrusion: Making Food that Needs No Chewing—Chewing food is part of the normal process of breaking down foodstuff in order to help release flavor, facilitate swallowing, and digestion. Another method to magnify mouthfeel and great taste sensation is to minimize chewing. The food industry achieves this through a process called extrusion, whereby cereal products are cooked and then formed into specific shapes. The geometry of the die hole, the extrusion speed and the cutting mode establishes the shape and texture of the cereal. A thermal treatment step is also applied for the browning process, controlled expansion and surface structure to name a few purposes. At the same time, the mechanical manipulations of the ingredients and severe heat treatments of the proteins, impoverish the nutritional quality of the foods. Indeed, the nutrients found in our grains are decimated through the extraction process. Both extrusion and high temperature heat treatments impoverish the food in addition to producing pro-oxidant compounds that can cause cell destruction in places like the intravascular lining and along the enterocytes of the small intestine, and colonic cells of the large intestine. [1b] The consequence of a continuous onslaught of pro-oxidant compounds is the eventual progression towards disease. Many of the foods we now purchase from grocery stores have been manufactured by a food industry bent on sales bolstered by a marketing plan that makes big promises of imparting optimal health.

In other words, the cheaper these foods are to make, the greater the profit margin, and the happier the shareholders. Here is the problem though: the purer the ingredients the more costly the food. This reality incentivizes food production companies to create foods that look, smell and taste real, but that are made up of the cheapest and most highly processed ingredients possible. These nonfoods are cheap to produce and are generally very shelf stable. This means companies can mass produce these nonfoods, and ship them to grocery stores, assured of their long shelf life.

Foods with a short shelf life generally translate into financial losses that result mainly from higher numbers of products discarded, and from the high cost associated with expensive atmospheric-controlled transportation in order to control freshness. The industry is clearly working to limit costly losses of this kind. So what are we left with? Next time you are in the grocery store, pay more attention to the proportion of the grocery store layout that is dedicated to these foods with unrealistically long shelf lives.

You will find that one complete grocery aisle is dedicated to sodas, and power drinks of various types; a second aisle is made up only of junk and snack foods. Here, multiple flavored potato chips, salty pretzels, cookies of all sorts, candies, sweets, gums, tarts, and ready-to-eat cakes line the shelves at eye-level for maximum sales. The third aisle is committed to baking products. Except for the whole wheat, durum, rye, rice and oat flours, in addition to the yeast, baking powder, baking soda and sugar for baking, almost everything else should be avoided, including the numerous cake mixes, cake and pie fillings, puddings, fake maple and chocolate syrups.

The fourth aisle is made up of breakfast cereals that are entirely processed, high in sugar, sodium, and low in fiber except for the whole natural oats, and few select quality cereals. The processed cereals for children should be almost entirely avoided because of the sugar load in addition to the high taste sensations experienced by children who eat them; it habituates them to seek more highly flavorful foods. This is where the conditioning to food preferences actually begins. Aisles 1 to 4 contain the foods that have impoverished the health of our youths.

Food sensitivity is often referred to as hypersensitivity reactions, which suggest immunological involvement. This is what is traditionally called a true antibody-mediated reaction. Food sensitivities of this type have become a frightening reality for food producers, manufacturers and processors, since the 80s and 90s.

The reactions tied to immune system hyperactivity can fall into a broad range, and can be as innocuous as mild skin reactions, and as serious as anaphylactic shock, leading to death in some cases.

The case of the young child allergic to peanuts has been heard many times; the child avoids the peanuts and the peanut butter that is frequently passed around at summer camp, but somehow the counsellor and the cook do not pick up on the nut-based breakfast cereal. The child's air passages become so constricted that he suffocates.

The field of immunotoxicology is particularly interested in the phenomenon of allergic reactions such as these. Proteins and other compounds of similar dimensions are generally recognized as responsible for eliciting such immunological responses.

The sodas and a sugar sweetened beverages have been shown, in a review of 88 longitudinal studies, to be directly related to energy intake and increases in body weight in children and adolescents. These are no longer debatable findings; sugar intakes from sugary beverages are so elevated among the young, especially, that they are displacing dairy products out of the diet and compromising long term health.

The Bogalusa Heart study has shown that between 1973 and 1994, milk intake has dropped 13.8%. During that time vegetable intake also declined nearly 9%. Despite the study showing a decrease in total fat intake, a more careful look at the data, reveals that as many as 75% of the children were still consuming total fat and saturated fat that exceeded national recommended cut-offs, and that adiposity in the children had dramatically increased. Other studies have also shown that when milk intake declines in adolescents, specifically, body weight increases.

The impoverishment of the diet has had serious implications on the overall health of the nation, as evidenced by an astounding rise in the proportion of the population that has become chronically ill over the last 36 years.

4.2 Food Intolerances and Sensitivities

The foods that are most often associated with a greater hyper-allergenecity (greater probability of creating an allergic reaction), are listed here: nuts, eggs, wheat, milk, bananas and tomatoes. There are others, of course, but these more specifically seem to be removed more often from the diets of people suffering from possible food allergies.[35]

So the quest for optimal nutrition becomes one centered on removing all foods that can potentially cause allergic reactions. It turns out of course, that almost any food can precipitate an immune response, but reassuringly, allergic reactions amongst consumers occur very infrequently. The term allergy is loosely used here to refer to what Steve L. Taylor describes as the:

... *individualistic adverse reactions to foods....*[35]

This is, in fact, a quote used to describe what many allergists call "food sensitivities". This term carries a much broader significance than allergy, because it does not exclusively assume that an immunological reaction is occurring. Rather, its significance suggests four possible biological reactions.

> Food allergies and sensitivities are categorized from I to IV based on the severity of the reaction.

First of all a "food sensitivity" can suggest an outright allergic reaction that elicits an immunological response. As a food allergy reaction, it can fall under category-I, which entails a very rapid immune response that is mediated by immunoglobulin E (IgE). It is specifically this kind of reaction that is referred to as either "acute hypersensitivity" reaction or "anaphylactic" reaction, which occur within 15 to 30 minutes of exposure. The ingestion of even one small piece of nut or egg, in a highly allergic person, would be sufficient to cause hives followed by anaphylactic shock within minutes.

Category II hypersensitivity is referred to as cytotoxic, and will tend, through an antibody-mediated reaction, to affect multiple organs anywhere between minutes to hours.

A category III allergic reaction occurs between 4-6 hours after the ingestion of an allergenic food. Such an effect is mediated by immune complexes. There is some controversy, because of the 4-6 hour delay, about the strength of the relationship existing between the food and the allergic reaction.

Category IV reactions involve a delayed response that is greater than 6 hours following the intake of the offending food. The typical symptom, that characterizes such reactions, is delayed dermatitis, and it can affect the body generally in localized areas.

The second kind of food sensitivity is referred to as "food intolerance" or "metabolic disorder". A food sensitivity of this type is often seen in cases of lactose intolerance. This means the individual cannot digest milk because he or she is missing or is deficient in the digestive enzyme called "lactase". The problem here is that the disaccharide, lactose, is not hydrolysed into its simple mono-saccharides glucose and galactose, thereby causing a fermentation of the sugar by bacteria in the small intestine. This invariably leads to gas formation and a very uncomfortable bloating in the intestine. This produces an osmotic draw of water from the extracellular environment into the intestine, where the fermenting sugars are localized. This result is an osmotic form of diarrhea that causes some distress to the patient. There appears to be a strong genetic tendency, in some families or cultures, towards having suboptimal levels of the lactase enzyme. This is why Asians and African Americans tend to have a higher prevalence of lactose intolerance. There is, however, no immune response occurring in these people.

There are individuals suffering as well from intolerances to sucrose, a disorder which is rarely found. In some individuals, there are also metabolic abnormalities that prevent the metabolism certain amino acids, which are the building blocks of protein. One such disorder is referred to as "Phenylketonuria" and describes patients that cannot metabolize the amino acid "phenylanine".

Drugs can also cause some patients to react to certain key nutrients. The most notable cases are patients on monoamine-oxidase-inhibiting drugs who develop tyramine sensitivity, an amino acid that is abundant in the diet.

There are also those patients that are on the drug "Isoniazid" who can, in some cases develop "histamine" sensitivities. This is not a good thing, since histamine secretions usually occur in response to "allergens" or compounds that cause allergic reactions. If a person develops sensitivity to histamine, he can become very ill, as in the case of a ragweed allergy, for instance.

A third kind of hypersensitivity to foods is called an "idiosyncratic reaction". This is a sophisticated way to say that the reaction occurring between the food and the body is not understood. It could also mean that the physician does not believe that the food is responsible for the physiological reaction that is quite obviously taking place.

There are a few examples that illustrate these cases. For instance, there was allegedly some relationship between food coloring and hyperkenesis (hyperactivity) reported several decades ago. When some children would ingest foods that contained certain coloring agents, they would exhibit hyperactive behaviors according to concerned parents. Yet, controlled studies done on similar children, in which one dye is placed on the tongue of several children—a direct challenge study design—could not find any relationship between the dye and the behavior.

However, there are substances like sulfite and tetrazine (yellow dye #5) which can clearly induce asthma in some individuals, but the reaction in such cases is not well understood.

What about the role of sugar in behavioral changes? Presently, there is no evidence that moderate amounts of sugar intake can significantly alter the behavior of people in general.

> There is no evidence to demonstrate that moderate amounts of sugar can significantly alter behavior.

However, sugar may play some role in specific groups of people as suggested by Reed in the 1970's. In addition, the role of food in the etiology of migraines and of irritable bowel syndrome (IBS) also demands clarification.

People suffering from IBS appear to be sensitive to many foods one week, and different kinds of foods the next week. Again there is no immune response associated with this physical malaise, yet the physical pain is most certainly an acute reality. Try saying to people suffering from IBS that this is idiosyncratic, and that there may be no relations to food. It's not likely to go over well. This disease is real and has true symptoms. The problem is we cannot explain why certain foods appear to cause such intense discomfort.

However, there is a strong tendency for the patient to try the old trial and error approach to alleviating symptoms; it is a reasonable and logical strategy. Perhaps the person eats an apple and then experiences pain followed by some diarrhea. The apple is then eliminated from the diet. Another attempt is made with a carrot; an adverse reaction is also experienced and carrots are removed from the diet.

In the end, the patient's inventory of allowable foods is greatly diminished, making her life extremely difficult from several fronts: First, the family who must eat with or around this individual is troubled by these restrictions. This necessitates special cooking practices and restricting many foods. Second, it means an awkward social life, and third, a seriously compromised dietary intake, that can likely jeopardize the nutritional status of the individual. IBS could be the consequence of leading a life that is unusually stressful, in as much as it is dominated by guilt and unchannelled stress.

Finally, the fourth type of food insensitivity is termed "anaphylactoid". Such reactions are often difficult to distinguish from true allergies. It is associated with the internal release of histamines unaccompanied however, by any release of immunoglobulin E (IgE) or other immune responses. This is seen with the ingestion of strawberries; histamines are abundantly released into the system, causing a severe reaction. However, the specific component in the strawberry, that is responsible for the reaction, has not been identified. The physiological response is, nevertheless, severe and appears to require very little time to develop.

Food sensitivities encompass a broad meaning that often escapes the full understanding of the consumer. What does appear to be clear to the informed population is that people react to food in ways and in frequencies never seen previously. Does this suggest that our food is contaminated with additives, toxins, and environmental contaminants to a much greater degree than previous decades?

4.3 Science and the Food Industry

Science and the food industry have not been best of friends almost from the beginning. In fact, food technology did not form an alliance with science until the 1800s. Prior to that time, any development in food processes was overseen by those uneducated in science. This is because technology did not closely follow the "Great scientific awakening" of the 17th century. By contrast, engineering seemed to follow more on the heels of the progress of science. For instance, the invention of the first steam engine prototype was spearheaded by Denis Papin and Thomas Newcomen. These men were engineers but also artisans; one was a mechanic and the other an iron monger, and they based the development of their invention on principles of steam dynamics that had been documented during the 17th century. This also led them to the invention of the first autoclave or "digester" in 1679. Peterson[22] calls them one of the earliest of the "industrial engineers".

A common interest between food, technology and science was fermentation, because it was a process centered on cheese, wine and beer production. These were without question, important and significant elements of the diet.

In 1680, a Dutch naturalist by the name of Anton van Leeuwenhoek conducted some early microscopic work on beer. He identified yeast cells but could not understand their involvement in fermentation, nor could he get any sense that they were alive. The famous chemist, Stahl in 1697, was convinced that fermentation was a chemical process. It took a series of respectable scientists like Tour and Kutzing in 1837, Schwann in 1839, Berzelius and Liebig in 1843, to finally document what they identified as the spore-forming ability of the yeast.

However, it was the work of Louis Pasteur in 1876 that authenticated yeast as a living plant. Fischer and Buckner determined that yeast synthesized enzymes, thereby providing further credence to the notion that fermentation was a biochemical process.

Before the emergence of Pasteur onto the scientific scene, the food industry was not progressing very rapidly, especially if one compares its rate of innovation to areas like transportation and textiles. The literature tells us that food preparation practices like curing, drying, pickling and fermentation, were essentially home practices that met the family needs. There was, in fact, little need for a food industry prior to the middle of the 19th century. Furthermore, there was no universally based industrial society to be found in any country, worldwide. It took important advances in steam technology, refrigeration, rapid freezing and canning before modernization of food technology could begin to move forward.

Even then, progress did not move rapidly. For example, even though the prototype for the steam-powered-mill was established on the Thames in England by 1786, and that similar models soon appeared throughout Europe and in the United States, the production of milled flour did not significantly increase.

There were still some problems to contend with: first, there were insufficient storage areas; second, the transport systems for distribution of the flour were not quite established; and third, many of these steam-dependent flour mills were built in close proximity to cities, since feeding the urban population was of greatest priority.

The automated flour mills were not, initially at least, working at full potential. Near the end of the 18th century, the process of industrialization began to expand vigorously with the support of food technology and engineering. Flour milling is considered an important gauge of the progress of food technology because of the many engineering steps or problems that had to be overcome, in the process of transforming the wheat kernels or raw material into white flour.

Inventors were studying the process of production, and began creating inventions to solve some of the engineering problems associated with food manufacturing. Oliver Evans became so interested in Watt's steam engine, that he adapted steam technology to power his screw conveyor. This facilitated the movement of grain and meal horizontally around the mill, and was a major breakthrough in reducing labour intensity and increasing cost effectiveness.

The raw grains entered the mill from the top, and from gravitational pull, underwent a vertical, and then a horizontal distribution process. The automated conveyor system, developed by Oliver Evans, brought to prominence the importance of considering the labor costs linked to material handling (**Figure 4.4**). It was primarily an issue of cost and time efficiency, as the cost accounting figures of the day estimated that food material handling mobilized 30% of total labor cost. It took up until the 1920's and 30's before the handling of plant food, and animal products became more mechanized and sophisticated.

Evans' screw conveyor, although still considered the baseline technology for the movement of grains, has been adapted into pneumatic conveyors for the transportation of powdered food, and hydro-conveyors to ensure the movement of water-conveyed solid foods, like peas and beans, through a system of pipes. In addition, the application of vacuum pumps was a significant innovation in the transportation of milk and fruit juices.

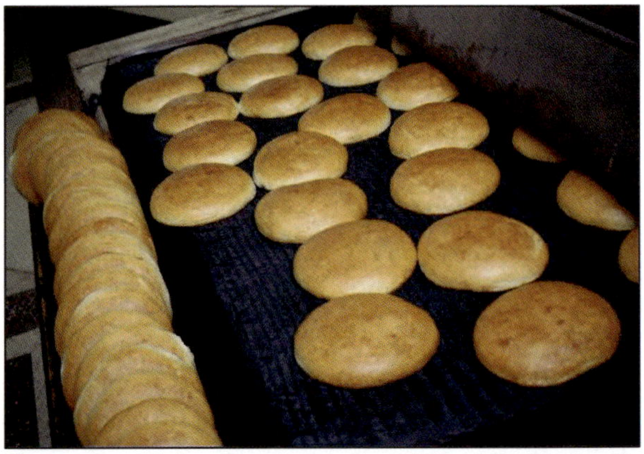

Figure 4.4: Modern Day Automation of Bread Production © Evru.

The automated method of conveying food product throughout the plant, although primarily motivated by time efficiency and lower labor costs, also carried important ramifications from the stand point of hygiene or public health. The enclosed food was shielded from manhandling and protected from external contamination.

More importantly, the issue of public health also revolved around the science of microbiology. The spoilage of food became another problem that the industry had to contend with. The putrefaction of the foodstuff, occurring after a relatively short time, meant considerable loss of inventory and of dollars, and represented a threat to the safety of the consumer. There was strong impetus to resolve this problem rapidly. In particular, the research conducted by Pasteur had direct and significant applications in the dairy industry. High temperature treatments conserved the quality of the milk for longer periods of time, by destroying critical pathogens that could be deadly to humans. Prior to Pasteur's work, Nicolas Appert, who observed putrefaction in food, had done some experiments with a sort of pressure cooker in 1810, and was able to halt it with heat treatment and a hermetic seal. It wasn't, however, until the late 19th century, following Pasteur findings, that science and technology led the canning industry to a successful launch. Canning allowed vegetables and fruits to leave the large centers, and reach geographically isolated regions. From a nutritional standpoint, food accessibility was being addressed, and isolated populations, as well as those individuals in the lower income bracket, could now afford vegetables and fruits year around.

Although heavily criticized today by natural food advocates, canned food originally had an impressive impact by facilitating food distribution, primarily because of the stability of the food product. The thermal treatment of the autoclave raised the internal temperature to such an extent that bacteria and pathogens were killed.

> Canning of goods allowed not only for increased storage time for fruits and vegetables but also wider distribution of products.

Today canning is widespread; an impressive variety of possible foods, from fruits through to soups, stews and beans, and on to fish and meats are sold in cans. Peterson[22] argues that there is very little doubt that the canning industry took on, in its origins, a leadership role in establishing the foundation of a food industry system. The stocking of canned food product was, in fact, one of the first indices that "convenience foods" had hit the kitchens of the North American household.

The food processing industry unofficially declared war with the American housewife. It subtly conveyed the message, that cooking was drudgery, and that manufactured bread, canned foods and other products, were labor saving. Moreover, food processing promoted the emancipation of the North American woman. Who would dare attempt to abrogate such a socially sensitive issue?

It's surprising to think of canned food as having any worth, but its impact was not limited to the empowerment of women, but in addition, the automation of canning favored the mass production of food to feed an ever-growing population.

Even back in the mid-60s, the loss of essential nutrients such as vitamins from the foods that were thermally treated at high temperatures, or bleached, as in the case of specialized flours, drew some attention. However, the problem received little press, as the marketing departments of the stakeholder companies took over the reins, and explained that lost nutrients were added back to foods through enrichment and fortification. Somehow, this provided reassurance to a population, that technology could still be trusted. But there was a problem that was beginning to rear its ugly head in the form of contaminants derived from the automation of food processing. No longer were the issues simply vitamin losses and biological filth on the food, but in addition, concerns were being raised, in the early 50s, about traces of chemicals detected on food, that were coming from conveyer belts contaminants, trays, valves, lubricants, storage containers, cleaning fluids as well as anti-rust compounds used in the upkeep of the machinery.

These difficulties, did not however, appear to slow the growth of the food industry. Don't believe for an instant that the food industry, as a whole, was benevolent and altruistic in its corporate goals. Far from it; the 1950's and 60's were decades of tremendous growth for the food industry. It wasn't surprising since throughout the post-war period, industrial growth was also at a peak.

The modern household was slowly being conceived, and the industrial complex was employing millions of Americans and Canadians. They, in turn, began to experience higher incomes and therefore a substantially greater purchasing power. And through all these rapidly occurring societal changes, convenience foods made their way into the kitchens of the North American family.

The changes that took place were dramatic, starting with the dry cereals, soft drinks, packaged puddings, and the ubiquitous Jell-O that seeped into every household. We saw boxed cookies, potato flakes and the potato chip, in addition to TV dinners or that famous macaroni & cheese, all rise to prominence on grocery store shelves.

The public dependence on processed food rapidly increased as two income families became the norm, and the management of homemade meals a virtual impossibility because of the ever growing time crunch. Between the 1960s and 2000, reliance on flaked potatoes increased from 5lbs to 15.7lbs/person/year, representing a 214% increase.[5] In addition, Americans currently consume 22% of high temperature-treated processed meat preserved with:

Sodium nitrite, BHA, BHT, sodium erythorbate, MSG, hydrolyzed milk and vegetable proteins, sugar, corn syrup....

Likewise, the macaroni & cheese contained a plethora of compounds that sounded more like the ingredients of a chemical concoction than of a food. The ingredients listed on the label read as follow: *wheat flour, powdered sauce: whey (milk protein), milk protein concentrate, milk, milk fat, cheese culture, salt, sodium tri-polyphosphate, sodium phosphate, calcium phosphate, yellow 5, yellow 6, citric acid, lactic acid, and enzymes.*

4.4 Food Additives and Contaminant
Food became not only convenient, but also appealing and tasty. To meet that important challenge, the science of sensory evaluation was also growing. An important portion of most food companies' R&D (research and development) budget was allocated to what is technically called organoleptic or sensory evaluation research. This kind of research essentially tests the flavor, texture and aroma of foods, with the goal of maximizing their acceptability in the marketplace. There are numerous examples that illustrate how foods got manipulated to such an alarming extent that, rather than get rejected by the

Did it ever occur to the convenience-starved public that the bag of cheddar cheese sauce mix, inside the macaroni and cheese box, may not have contained any cheese?

Did it ever cross anybody's mind that the flaked potatoes were perhaps no longer a vegetable? It is doubtful. The general public gradually regarded manufactured food was acceptable, probably because it was so accessible and convenient. The need to educate the public about wise food selections was already beginning to be felt in the mid-50s. The concepts of "good and bad" foods were being pushed by the health professionals. They did not have powerful voices, nor did they form strong lobby groups. They were up against no small time adversary; the advertising industry was becoming a powerful manipulator of the masses. The messages of the food industry became far reaching, using magazines, newspapers, radio and television as their medium of communication. There were also the weekly flyers, and the roadway billboards, which captured the attention of the public and significantly influenced their food selections. Joan Gussow is Mary Swartz Rose Professor emerita and former chair of the Nutrition Education Program at Teachers College, Columbia University. In a speech given several years ago she said[24]:

In the thirty four years I've been in the field of nutrition, I have watched real food disappear from large areas of the supermarket and from much of the rest of the eating world.

This was truly and indictment of the U.S. food supply, a prophetic cry in the arena of public opinion that resonated only with the few who were able to hear through the noisy background or American corporatism.

consumer, they were marvelously received; a sort of paradox that isn't easily explained.

An example of food manipulation is the maraschino cherry; close the lights and don't be surprised if it begins to glow in the dark. Here is a perfectly natural product that grows on trees and that Mother Nature saw fit to give a pigment different from that which we observe in the clear jar. There is a similar cherry found in canned mixed fruit. Why couldn't the industry just leave Mother Nature alone? The heat treatment used on the cherries during the canning process, causes severe damage to the color pigment, precipitating a breakdown of not only the pigment but also the texture. In such a state, the cherries could not be marketed.

Through various laboratory sensory evaluations that considered the size, the color and the natural look of the food, the company came up with an ideal color and texture. The most desirable color pigment was obtained using red dye no.4. It is however alarming that this dye, along with red dye number no. 1 were delisted from the FDA's registry of acceptable food additives, by passage of the Color Additives Amendments of the Food, Drug & Cosmetic Act. Despite this restriction, red dye no.4 was given provisional status because of its popular use in some foods such as maraschino cherries, syrup and some drugs prescribed on a short term basis. The dye was given a quantitative limit of 150 ppm.

Ever notice that the cherry remains firm following the processing? Why isn't it soft and mushy as one would expect following a heat treatment that uses processes of agitation and pressurized steam, which rise the temperature up to 260 F for anywhere between 2 and 20 minutes? With more conventional commercial sterilization processes the time range could vary between 15 and 80 minutes at 240 F°.

The use of calcium salts, like calcium chloride, appear able to ensure the firmness of the cherry as well as other fruits and vegetables such as beans, tomatoes, apricots, and cucumbers. The process, by which the calcium salts act is not totally clear, however, it seems the calcium chloride binds with the pectic substances, found in the outer layer of the fruit and preserves the firmness.

This is an essential step in food acceptability that focuses on food texture. We should also be comforted by the thought that since the mid-60s, the U.S. Department of Agriculture had conducted extensive studies in the area of sensory food evaluation, particularly in the fields of flavor and quality. Although the manipulation of flavors is possible with the practice of artificial and natural flavor substitutes, it is less clear how food quality is defined by the industry, and to what extent it can be manipulated.

Using coloring agents and mostly artificial flavors, food was manipulated to such an extent that products like colored breakfast cereals (**Figure 4.5**) and margarines began appearing. Margarines were synthesized to resemble butter in appearance, taste,

and in some cases texture. Another example is the vast array of very appetizing cakes covered in a white creamy topping with multi-layered fillings, as well as a tender and moist crumb. The first unusual observation that becomes striking is the length of time these cakes can remain on store shelves before they no longer look fresh. It is the food industry's goal to create cakes that maintain a fresh appearance thanks to the use of thickeners, stabilizers and artificial colors.

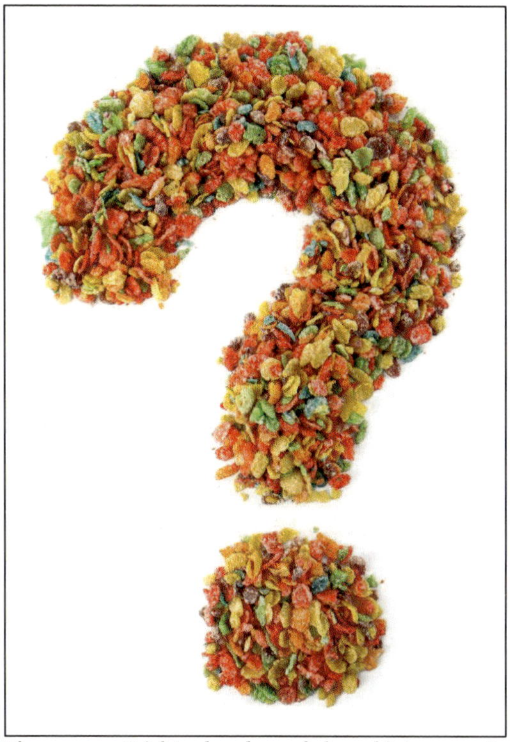

Figure 4.5: Bright colored cereal shaped into a question mark. © Suzi Nelson.

For example, the glazes and icings must not melt nor stick to the wrapper under normal transportation and storage conditions. Product acceptability would be compromised, and of course sales would decline. The icing must keep its just-made-fresh appearance. Icings and glazes are basically composed of sugar and water. Their appearance varies depending on whether the producer desires (a) flat icings, as observed on sweet goods; (b) fudge icings, as used on cakes; (c) cream icings, used as well on cakes; or (d) coating icings, as observed on candies. The stable fresh look is preserved by preventing, in the case of flat icing, the icing from melting in hot humid weather. Chemical compounds are not always necessary, but tend to be preferred as they tend to work more efficaciously. Flat icing can, in fact, be preserved by minimizing moisture build up under the cellophane wrapper. This moisture, which is found in the icing and cake, turns the icing to liquid by solubilizing the sugar. The solution is to heat-treat the icing, and remove most of the moisture, and then add a gum like agar, locust bean, carrageenan, pectin or karaya, therefore binding any residual moisture coming from the cake. These are natural sounding products that have a high acceptability rating with the consumer. Contrast this icing with a 1954 patented icing preparation made up of: egg albumin, calcium sulfate, sodium aluminum sulfate, starch, sugar and sodium carboxy-methyl-cellulose (CMC). Why would a manufacturer introduce such an artificially sounding mixture? Because icings made with CMC are able to prevent the loss of moisture from the cakes. This approach differs from binding the water once it is lost from the cake. In fact, sealing the water in the cake is far more effective. It prevents the transformation of icing into syrup and maintains the moistness of the cakes.[15]

Most importantly, in the 1950's, the ingredients used in food were not at the top of the public's agenda; the Cold and Korean wars, were eating away at the North American psyche. Instead, Americans were more interested in creating a society of convenience and brotherhood, rich in family values, condoning material wealth, and an overall American way of life that offered unlimited opportunities. The public was not paying attention, and food manipulation was increasing at a fantastic rate. In fact, by 1965 Luckey's review of the field reported 661 million pounds of food additives utilized in the United States per year.[18]

> By 1965, Americans were consuming 3 pounds of additives per person per year.

This represented 3 pounds of additives per person per year. By 2009, that percent rose to between 8-10lbs per person per year, indicating a progressive acceptance of additives rather than an increasing public reticence. So then, as the variety of foods available to the public increased, so did the yearly consumption of additives.

The most abundantly used food additives, by the food industry in the 20th century, were the artificial flavors in addition to the coloring agents. There has been, however, an irrational fear of food colorants in the general public in recent decades, according to food industry representatives. This fear is based, for the most part, on the idea that additives could represent a serious cancer risk. In the last three decades, the carcinogenecity of food, many experts have argued, has been perhaps recklessly associated with food additives, which include colorants.

Consequently, the use of flavoring agents, colorants, anti-caking agents, emulsifiers, thickeners, surfactants and antioxidants in food, has caused "naturalist" advocacy groups to make a lot of noise. One would hope, however, that if protests of that nature were to be successful in provoking changes in food products, that the position taken by the groups would be based on sound research and reliable information. Manfred Kroger, a food science researcher and associate professor at Pennsylvania State University in the 1970s, believed that there was an irrational and distorted perception of the risk of food additives. It is a question of risk-benefit analysis, and determining what constitutes a real threat. Dr Kroger assessed the population's fear of the food system in the following manner:

The fear of food additives is totally out of proportion. Much of this fear is fanned by people who can gain by it, and not out conviction to create a better world.[26]

Have our perceptions of food safety really become distorted to such a degree that we are now preoccupied with irrelevant issues? Or more importantly, with issues that are far more complex than the media would lead the public to believe?

For instance, of all the compounds found in foods, food additives should cause the least concern because they have undergone the most research and testing. The North American food supply, taken as a whole, has been described by Kroger as the safest and the most wholesome in the history of mankind.

Yet, there seems to be enough concern in the scientific community, to justify the creation of a new field of study called "food safety", which is really a blend of chemistry, microbiology and nutrition. In contemporary thinking, this form of science is called interdisciplinary and provides a sense of completeness or thoroughness. Dr Hall, Vice President of Science and Technology at McCormick & Company, refers to food hazards in terms of microbiological hazards, nutritional issues, contaminants from environmental pollutants, natural toxicants, pesticide residues and food additives.[29] He points out that chemicals added to food are seen with alarm by consumers, whereas they remain uncritical of those things seen as natural. In a 1977 interview he admits:

In part the pesticide residue and food additives risks are extremely low because a great deal of scientific and regulatory effort has gone into their evaluation, prevention and control. The microbiological hazards are large because they are affected by the way the 238 million people in the United States and Canada handle and choose foods, and few are experts.[29]

In the 1970s there was a perception that the natural world could, in fact, be controlled and kept in check by well tested chemicals, which were regarded as safe. Interestingly, the scientific opinion began to shift, as large population studies began making surprising links between heavily processed foods and disease by the turn of the new millennium. The World Cancer Fund 2007 Expert Committee[38] in addition to the American Institute for Cancer Research 2010 report[2] recommended a decrease in red meat consumption and a total avoidance of processed meats all together, after convincing studies began to surface. Following an exhaustive review of the literature, the expert committee concluded that eating in excess of 500g or 17oz-wt of red meat per week increased the risk of bowel cancer. This means that to remain healthy, a person should not consume more than 2.5oz-wt of cooked red meat per day, or three 5.67oz-wt servings of red meat per week. Processed meats, which include ham, sausage, hotdogs, and bacon, in addition popular sandwich meats like salami, corned beef and pepperoni, were found to be more strongly correlated with bowel cancer than fresh red meats. Dr Ute Nothlings and his team, from the University of Honolulu's Cancer Research Center, followed a cohort of 190,545 people over a 7 year period.[21] They concluded that regularly consuming processed meats increased the risk of pancreatic cancer by 68%. By comparison, those regularly ingesting pork and other red meats, experienced a 50% increase in risk. They could not find any link between poultry, fish, dairy, eggs and pancreatic cancer. If processed meats are indeed associated with greater cancer risks in the population, should the public trust that the food industry will correct the situation? Will they change the way processed meats are made?

Food manipulation was initially self-regulated by the food industry, with the understanding that maintaining a flawless track record from the standpoint of (a) safety, (b) quality and (c) cost, would ensure the survival of the industry.

> **For the most part, the food industry was entrusted to ensure that the products they produced and sold were safe for the consumer.**

The assumption that the food industry would take care of the welfare of the consumer was, however, never taken for granted by everyone, even though most Americans still believed, at the turn of the century, in the sacredness of Government and the integrity of American business.

Although early on there were clear indications that the Government's hands-off policy, intended not to impede any of the food industry's economic growth, would hopefully favor maximal growth in technology and advancements in food safety, president Lincoln in 1862, nevertheless created the U.S. Department of Agriculture (USDA). This was a clear indication of the federal government's interest in regulating the food supply. The idea at the time was that the USDA could be valuable in the protecting of the family farmer against pests that could ruin the crops. The Department of Agriculture did not take long before presenting the 1905 Pest Prohibition and 1912 Quarantine Acts, which eventually led to subsequent acts in the 50s that protected the farmer against 32,575 separate pests.

This government refrained from getting involved in the food industry, but was strictly focused on the protection of the farmer. For the government, these were policies that protected agricultural exports, and were perceived at the time as ensuring the continued economic growth of the nation. Up until the creation of the U.S. Department of Agriculture in 1862, the food industry was totally self-regulated. However, this independence from the government's watchful and critical eye was to be short lived.

Professor G.W. Wigner proposed federal legislation in 1880 that would ensure the prevention of food adulteration, as there were frequent examples of poor quality food being sold to the consumer. The act that reflected this proposal was never passed by Congress. However, Wigner's attempt provided the impetus necessary for several States to pass legislation regulating food, like the 1881 New York Food and Drug Law; the 1884 Food Sanitation Law of Illinois; the District of Columbia's 1891 Food and Drug Law.

The Federal Government decided to also step into the arena of food legislation not long after these state initiatives. One of the earliest Federal legislation, regulating the safety of the food supply, was the 1890 inspection of salted pork and bacon, a measure aimed at securing access of these products on to the international market. U.S. meat exports were threatened by trichinella, a parasite that causes gastroenteritis, and that eventually lodges in the muscle. On the side lines were individuals who felt that the government's involvement in the manufacturing of food products should extend beyond meat.

Brosin's Pure Food and Drug bills, which were sequentially presented between 1897 and 1902, exemplified the strength of this belief, and yet in the end, the bills went down to defeat. This was a clear indication of the Federal government's reluctance to control the industry, but also of the industry's powerful lobbying capacity.

However, the government mobilized some money to establish a very innocuous "pure food standard". It wasn't clear what this was supposed to accomplish, since there was no apparent Congressional empowerment attached to the creation of these standards.

Nevertheless, governmental involvement with the regulation of meats continued, with the successful passing of the 1906 Meat Inspection Act, which further enforced the first 1890 meat inspection requirement. This 1906 Act successfully sailed into Congressional approval along with President Theodore Roosevelt's Food and Drug Act.

Afterwards, the Meat Imported Act of 1930 and finally, the Poultry Products Act of 1957 followed. The Food and Drug Act was certainly one of the earliest forms of legislation that attempted to protect the consumers, in the District of Columbia and in the territories where Congress's authority was supreme, against misleading and potentially dangerous foods.

The legislation specifically banned chemical preservatives such as boric acid, salicylic acid and formaldehyde, products that were regularly used up until that time; it prohibited the interstate sale of fraudulent or unhealthy products; it forbade the practice of misbranded products or the production of adulterated food products. Adulteration was understood to mean:

the addition of poisons and deleterious materials, the extraction of valuable constituents, the concealment of inferiority, substitution of other articles, and the mixture of substances that adversely affect health.

> Legislation was apparently required to specifically ban poisons from manufactured food.

In considering the passing of the different laws, regulating the food supply, one can draw conclusions with respect to the need to table such legislative proposals. Was the food industry actually incapable of self-regulation? There must have been some concerns, because the landmark passing of the Food and Drug Act in 1906 ended up impelling the eventual creation of the 1927 Food, Drug and Insecticide Administration.

Within four years, it would be renamed The Food and Drug Administration, known today as the FDA. One of the most powerful forms of legislation that was presented to Congress was known as the 1938 Federal Food, Drug, and Cosmetic Act.

It kept much of the legislation enacted in 1906, but in addition, legally defined food; established food standards; and prohibited food adulteration, as well as the use of misleading labels.

The 1938 Act basically restricted the use of chemicals in the manufacturing of food, however some quantities of compounds could be argued as safe. Allowances were made either for chemicals that were judged as necessary in the manufacturing of a food, and defined as **"intentional additives"** or for those chemicals for which avoidance was not possible, and thus described as **"unintentional additives"**.[18]

The notion that there even existed chemicals that could not be avoided was troubling. What contaminants were they legislating into our food supply? They were essentially made up of a broad category of environmental pollutants that encompassed everything from pesticides, fungicides, rodenticides, and insecticides, to name a few.

Subsequently, the Miller Pesticide Amendment Act was passed in 1954, and created safe residue concentrations of pesticides. The decision that there could be such a thing as a safe pesticide residue stems from concepts that were tossed around irresponsibly for some time, and that were eventually published in the U.S. 1966 Year Book of Agriculture, entitled *Protecting our Food*.[32] The text compares the harmfulness of chemicals to that of electricity, a pen or money. The issue for these authors appeared to revolve around the quantity of chemical used. The 1954 amendment came about fourteen years after the introduction of synthetic pesticides, which included rodenticides; herbicides, in 1939; fungicides, in 1940; DDT, in 1942; denticides, in 1944; and organic phosphate insecticides, in 1947.

Still despite the 1954 amendment, it took several years before DDT was regarded as a serious carcinogen, regardless of the quantity used, and was unilaterally banned in the 60s.
Was this an embarrassment for the original chemists who claimed that chemicals were no more dangerous than a pen? It turns out, of course, that chemists are not physiologists, and did not understand that chlorinated hydro-carbons, like DDT, bio-accumulate in the fat reserves of the body, eventually leading to toxic concentrations even though the exposure may have been at regulated concentration levels.

This was serious business and caused many nutritionists and other health advocacy groups to raise concerns regarding the actual safety of the food supply. All these Amendments were the Government's attempts at trying to get a handle on something that was growing so rapidly, that no form of legislation could be practical enough, and no enforcement agency thorough enough, to ensure that the strict laws and regulations were being followed.

The FDA's monitoring activities were limited to samples of products taken randomly and not to thorough examinations of complete production outputs.

For instance, in 1965 the FDA collected only 19,000 samples from imported products, and 109,000 samples from domestic food products. Although these numbers of samples were promoted as very elevated, costing the tax payer $39 million for the fiscal year 1964-65, and clearly portraying a Government that is taking every initiative, and making every effort to assure a safe food supply, it became clear that with the supervision of 100,000 factories and workhouses as well as 700,000 other establishments, the total number of samples per establishment and per year, amounted to 0.14 samples.

> Due to the vastness of the food industry, the FDA could only sample and test a minute proportion of the food supply.

In other words, the FDA was capable of conducting $1/_7$ of a sample per company per year. Don't even assume that one company could possibly be manufacturing more than one product. The simplified fraction above assumes that every company produces only one product per year that needs to be monitored.

Clearly the government was not coping very well with this rather cumbersome responsibility. This was further magnified by the staff and budget increases, resulting in 1700 additional persons, and an additional $7 to $8 million between 1959 and 1965.

This represented a 121% increase in personnel and roughly a 22% increase in budget. Since that time, the number of manufactured products has increased, along with the number of companies, not to mention the rise in imported goods. And so it may appear unreasonable to expect the FDA to fully inspect and monitor the food industry. In contrast, the idea that companies should monitor the quality of their own food products became more popular. Internal corporate monitoring has been called all sorts of names; quality assurance, quality control, program evaluation and review technique (PERT), and critical path method (CPM).

These are techniques that ensure the thoroughness and quality of the work that is being done. If there is no quality, or it is not consistent, then the consumer will choose to buy elsewhere. In that sense, the market self-corrects in order to purge the companies that produced poor quality. Of course, in such a system, the company that doesn't monitor its own quality will fail. As consumers, we must see reality for what it is; the FDA is an arm of the Federal Government, which raps the knuckles of those that break food and drug laws. Its arm, however strong it may be, is not long enough to be far reaching, and therefore its power is exercised by the surprise factor and the randomness of its visits. Let's be clear, the quality of the North American food supply is not in the hands of Government, rather it is in the quality assurance programs and the integrity of North American, and International business communities.

Of course, it is reasonable to expect that if international products or compounds are legally banned by the Federal Health agencies in Canada and the US, that food products domestically produced, will not contain these compounds either. That means no residues coming from banned pesticides, or illegal food additives should be found on or in our food. Opening the borders to international trade was a good thing from many perspectives, except for food quality in many instances because the association between food and environment is excessively strong.

The dramatic impact that a highly contaminated environment has on the food, is to be understood in terms of the type and the quantity of residue left on the food. The repercussions of these residual compounds on the biological system are not fully understood, although it is clear that the bio-accumulation of some chlorinated chemicals in the body represents a tremendous physiological burden over time.

Hence, importing fruits and vegetables from a country like Chile, that has very little governmental policies regulating the use of pesticides, can be a practice that overwhelms the FDA's valiant efforts at controlling dangerous substances entering the American food supply.

If one was to think that the extent of preventative measures, aimed at protecting the public against "unavoidable chemicals" in food, is the complete

> **Plastics are highly absorbable to some chemicals and these can**
>
> **Importing foods increases the availability of seasonal foods, but also increases the risk of unknown contaminants and pesticide residues.**

avoidance of these chemicals in our food, then think again. The question is really, how much of these chemical residues are permissible? The tolerance limit for any residue is set by the Food & Drug Administration of the Public Health Service based on research evidence submitted by the manufacturer.

In fact, the Food Additive Amendment of 1958 stipulates that the safety of the additive must be shown, by the food company, before any authorization for sale is given. Equally alarming, was the commercial use of antibiotics to accelerate the growth of domestic animals in 1951. Such misuse of pharmaceuticals was justified on the grounds of economics; a faster turnover of cattle meant a greater profit. This practice did not contravene American law, although, most would agree that it should have. This is because there is a fine intricacy of American law that states that the main goal is to:

protect the public without discouraging free enterprise.

This fundamental philosophy of American law was responsible for the extraordinary growth of the food industry and of its distribution system, allowing a wide availability of products for public consumption.

This chapter is not about bashing the use of food additives, for it is clear that there is a necessary use of such compounds in food production.

Food additives became historically important elements in establishing a diverse, stable and safe national food inventory. These additives facilitated the access of the population to this inventory. Originally, there were only eight dyes used in food production in 1900. However, because there was no legislation regulating the quality of these dyes, it wasn't uncommon to use the same textile dyes both in clothing and in foods.

The Pure Food & Drug Act of 1906, restricted such abuses, and kept the total number of dyes to seven: orange-1, erythrosine, ponceau 3R, amaranth, indigotine, naphthol-yellow, and light green. But as the number of additives grew, and the color of the products became less natural-looking, public concern and awareness also intensified; suspicions that there were links between additives and disease began to worry some of the public. In 1960, as public awareness and concern about cancer risks grew, the Food Additive and the Color Additive Amendments were adopted to restrict the use of substances found to cause cancer in either man or animal.[20] This sounded good except for the fact that the Amendment did not cover any additives, previously classified by experts as *"generally regarded as safe"* (GRAS). The amendment did not pertain to *incidental* or *unintentional* additives; it omitted pesticides, which fall under another jurisdiction, as well as color additives and other substances that had previously obtained legal status.[18]

It was the 1960 Delaney clause of The Food Additive & Color Amendments that introduced a very rigid standard with respect to the presence of carcinogens in the food. The clause was interpreted as a "zero tolerance" standard for carcinogens, something the public applauded. It was essentially a piece of legislation that appeared to heighten the food standards for the sake of protecting the health of the American people. The clause introduced stringent standards that were criticized by scientists and the industry on operational grounds. In other words, it became difficult and impractical to abide by them. Before becoming too critical, it is important to understand the historical context of the law. It was written at a time when the causes of cancer were associated with cigarette smoking, radiation, soot, and chemical dyes, and detection concentrations were expressed in parts per million (ppm). Subsequent technological advancements, permitted the detection of carcinogenic compounds in concentrations equivalent to one part per billion or even per trillion. More sensitive measurements were picking up carcinogens in such minute amounts, that it was questionable whether there really was a risk of cancer. Were such detections needlessly alarming the public? Well the answer was more or less answered when the law gradually fell into disuse. Indeed, such infinitely small amounts, many concluded, had no real biological impact. They called the pesticide residues "unintentional food additives" and dropped the idealist goal of no residue limit. It became clear that a zero tolerance policy was not practical, for indeed, these residues could not be eliminated. The government established instead, tolerable and safe limits. So it was argued that the dangers of pesticides could be found least of all, on the fruits and vegetables grown in North America—organically grown least of all **(Figure 4.6)** — but more with imports coming from countries that have not banned certain

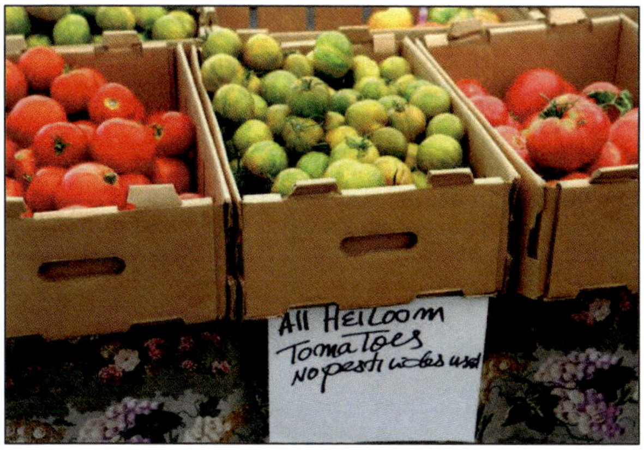

Figure 4.6: Pesticide Free Produce in Organically Grown Tomatoes © Don Bendickson.

pesticides. Consequently, as the U.S. consumer buys his fruits from the grocery store, he may be finding pes-ticide residues that our government cannot really protect him against.

The problem of food contamination must be considered also from the perspective of the migration of packaging contaminants into the food. At the University of Missouri's Department of Biochemistry, Dr T.D. Luckey conducted a series of experiment that nicely illustrated this problem of substance migration into the container.[18]

He mixed dry powdered grass with some Lindane (insecticide), which was then placed in a plastic container with baby crickets. After feeding on the grass, the crickets died as expected. The plastic container was then repeatedly washed out with water, then a dilute alkali, a dilute acid, a detergent and finally alcohol. The experiment was repeated after every cleaning, using fresh grass but no insecticide. The results were alarming; the crickets would die every time they were placed in the grass-filled container even though no chemical was added to the grass. It was specifically the insecticide that was initially placed on the grass that migrated into the plastic of the container thanks to the plastic's high absorbency.[18] It would appear that no amount of washing was enough to remove the Lindane from the plastic. More rapid migration of compounds from the plastic into the food would be expected when exposed to heat during microwave cooking.

DISCUSSION QUESTIONS

1. Discuss the potential dangers associated with the abundant use of plastics in food preparation and food storage on health.

2. Discuss the pros and cons of the use of additives in the food industry.

3. What is the significance of the US trend towards wanting a pure food supply in the late 1800s?

4. What was Louis Pasteur's role in the advancement of the food industry worldwide?

5. Discuss the differences between food intolerance and a food allergy.

References

1. Adams County Nebraska Historical Society. The Koo-Aid Story. Retrieved on October 10, 2013 from: http://www.adamshistory.org/index.php?option=com_content&task=view&id=32&Itemid=4

1b. American Extrusion International. Standard Direct Expansion. Retrieved July 19, 2013 from webpage: http://www.americanextrusion.com/direct_expansion.html

2. American Institute for Cancer Research (2010). Food, Physical Activity, weight, and Colon Cancer. Ritva Butrum et al. (eds). 17pp.

2b. Bahsin, K. Coke Vs Pepsi: The Story behind the Never-Ending Cola Wars. Business Insider; Retrieved from website July 27, 2013: http://www.businessinsider.com/coca-cola-vs-pepsi-timeline-2013-1?op=1

2c. Berridge KC, Robinson TE. What is the role of dopamine in reward: hedonic impact, reward learning, or incentive salience? Brain Res Brain Res Rev. 1998;28(3):309-69.

2d. Biello, D. (Feb 29, 2008). Plastic (Not) Fantastic: Food Containers leach a potentially Harmful Chemical. Scientific American. Retrieved on November 10, 2016 from: https://www.scientificamerican.com/article/plastic-not-fantastic-with-bisphenol-a/

3. Bobrow-Strain, A. White Bread: A Social History of the store-Bought Loaf. Boston: Beacon Press, 257pp

3b. Bobrow-Strain, A. (2007) Kills A Body Twelve Ways:Bread Fears and the Politics of what to Eat Gastronomica: The Journal of Food and Culture; 7(3): 45-52 retrieved August 8, 2013 from: http://comenius.susqu.edu/biol/312/killsabodytwelveways.pdf

3c. Brown, K,[†] DeCoffe, D,[†] Molcan, E, and. Gibson, DL. Diet-Induced Dysbiosis of the Intestinal Microbia and the Effects on Immunity and Disease. Nutrients; 4(8): 1095–1119. Retrieved from the US National Library of Medcine, National Institute of Health on July 10, 2013: http://www.ncbi.nlm.nih.gov/pmc/articles/PMC3448089/

3d. BUHLER Pasta & Extruded Products—Breakfast Cereals. Retrieved from website July 19, 2013: http://www.buhlergroup.com/global/downloads/Breakfast_Cereals.pdf

3e. CDC (2014). Overweight and Obesity. Adult Obesity Facts. Retrieved 06/19/2015 from: http://www.cdc.gov/obesity/data/adult.html

3f. *Coca-Cola Annual Report for 2012.* Retrieved July 8, 2013: http://www.coca-colacompany.com/annual-review/2012/pdf/form_10K_2012.pdf

4. Committee on Use of Dietary Reference Intakes in Nutrition Labeling. Institute of Medicine of the National Academies (2003). Dietary Reference Intakes: Guiding Principles for Nutrition Labeling and Fortification. Washington DC: The National Academies Press. 224pp.

4b. *Cookery As It Should Be: A New Manual of the Dining Room and Kitchen,* by A Practical Housekeeper and Pupil of Mrs. Goodfellow [Philadelphia:Willis P. Hazard] 1853 (p. 310)

5. Daniel CR, Cross AJ, Koebnick C, Sinha R. (2011). Trends in Meat Consumption in the US. Public Health Nutr. Apr;14(4):575-83

5b. Dominguez-Bello M.G., Costello E.K., Contreras M., Magris M., Hidalgo G., Fierer N., Knight R. Delivery mode shapes the acquisition and structure of the initial microbiota across multiple body habitats in newborns. Proc. Natl. Acad. Sci. USA. 2010;107:11971–11975

6. FDA and IFIC, Overview of Food Ingredients, Additives and Colors (2010). Retrieved on October 10, 2013 from: http://www.fda.gov/Food/IngredientsPackagingLabeling/FoodAdditivesIngredients/ucm094211.htm

6b. Frank D.N., St. Amand A.L., Feldman R.A., Boedeker E.C., Harpaz N., Pace N.R (2007). Molecular-Phylogenetic characterization of microbial community imbalances in human inflammatory bowel diseases. Proc. Natl. Acad. Sci. USA. 104:13780–13785

6c. *Gale Group Inc.* High Beam Business. Food Manufacturing Industry Reports. Cereal Breakfast Foods. Retrieved July 5 2013 from: *http://business.highbeam.com/industry-reports/food/cereal-breakfast-foods*

6d. *Global Industry Analysts Inc (2010).* Global Nutraceutical market to cross US$243 billion by 2015 according to a new report by Global Research Analysts Inc. Retrieved July 5, 2013 at: http://www.prweb.com/releases/nutraceuticals/dietary_supplements/prweb4563164.htm

6e. *Global Industry Analyst, Inc. (2012)* Nutraceutical: A Global Strategic Business Report. Retrieved October 30, 2015 from:
http://www.slideshare.net/GlobalIndustryAnalystsInc/nutraceuticals-a-global-strategic-business-report

7. Goldblight SA and Maynard JA. (1964).An anthology of food science: milestones in nutrition. Vol 2. Westport, Connecticut: The Avi Publishing Co, Inc

7b. Hayes, Jack **Biography of Dr. John S. Pemberton** Article by. Nation's Restaurant News. Part of Library of Congress Coca-Cola advertising history collection. URL: www.memory.loc.gov/ammem/ccmphtml/colainvnt.html

8. Himich Freeland-Graves, J. and Peckham, G.C. (1987) Foundations of food preparation. Fifth ed. New York: Macmillan Publ. Co.

8b. Hunt, P. A., et al. (2012). "Bisphenol A alters early oogenesis and follicle formation in the fetal ovary of the rhesus monkey." Proc Natl Acad Sci U S A **109**(43): 17525-17530

9. Jansen B.C.P. (1956). Early nutritional researches on beriberi leading to the discovery of vitamin B1. Nutrition Abstracts and Reviews, 26:1-14.

10. Jacobs EJ, et al.(2002) Vitamin C And Vitamin E Supplement Use And Bladder Cancer Mortality In A Large Cohort Of US Men And Women. Am J Epidemiol. 156: 1002-10.

11. Jarvis, W.T. (1983) Food faddism, cultism and quackery. Ann. Rev. Nutr. (3): 35-52

12. Johnston, B.F. (1951) Agricultural production and economic development in Japan. J.Pol.Econo. 49:498-513.

12b. Kaas Boyle, L. (2014). Plastic is Food Poisoning. Huffington Post. Retrieved November 10, 2016 from: http://www.huffingtonpost.com/lisa-kaas-boyle/plastic-is-food-poisoning_b_5219189.html

13. Kellogg, JH. (1877). Practical manual of Hygiene and Temperance. Battle Creek MI: Good Health Publishing Company, 242pp

14. Klein, B.P.(1992) Fruits and vegetables. In: Food, theory & application. 2nd ed. (Bowers, J. ed) New York: Macmillan Publishing Co. p: 688-777.

15. Klose, R.E. and Glicksman, M. Gums. (1968) In: CRC Handbook of food additives. (Furia T.E ed), Cleveland, Ohio: The Chemical Rubber Co. pp: 314-375.

16. Kreutzer-Hodson, T. (2007) Kool-Aid. Nebraska State Historical Society. Retrieved October 10, 2013 from: http://www.nebraskahistory.org/publish/publicat/timeline/kool-aid.htm

16b. Kuisel, Richard F., "Coca-Cola and the Cold War: The French Face Americanization, 1948-1953," in *French Historical Studies* Vol. 17, No. 1, (Duke University Press, 1991), 97-98.

16c. Lepine, JP. The Epidemiology of anxiety disorders: Prevalence and social costs. J. Clin. Psychiatry, 2002; 63 (suppl. 14): 4-8

17. Lorenz, A.J. (1954) The conquest of scurvy. Journal American Dietetic Association, 30:665-670.

18. Luckey, T.D. (1968). Introduction to food additives. In: CRC Handbook of food additives. (Furia T.E ed), Cleveland, Ohio: The Chemical Rubber Co. pp: 1-23.

19. Margotta, R. (1996) The Hamlyn History of Medicine. P. Lewis ed. Reed International books Ltd, London; 192 pp.

19b. Moss, M (2013) Salt, Sugar and Fat: How the Food Giants Hooked Us. New York: Random House Publishing

19c. National Institute of Mental Health. The Numbers Count: Mental Disorders in America. Retrieved on July 16, 2013 from: http://www.nimh.nih.gov/health/publications/the-numbers-count-mental-disorders-in-america/index.shtml

20. Noonan, J. (1968) Color additives in food. In: CRC Handbook of food additives. (Furia T.E ed), Cleveland, Ohio: The Chemical Rubber Co. p: 25-49.

21. Nothlings, U. et al. (2006) Meat and fat intake as risk factors for pancreatic cancer: the multiethnic cohort study. J Natl Cancer Inst. 7;98(11):796

21b. Pecina S, Smith, KS, and Berridge, KC Hedonic Hot Spots in the Brain NEUROSCIENTIST 2006; 12(6):500–511

21c. *PepsiCo Brands.* Retrieved July 8, 2013: http://www.pepsico.com/Brands.html

21d. PepsiCo Inc Annual Report for 2011. Retrieved July 8, 2013: http://www.pepsico.com/annual11/downloads/PEP_AR11_2011_Annual_Report.pdf

22. Peterson M.S. (1963) Factors contributing to the development of today's food industry. In: Food technology the world over. Vol 1. Peterson M.S & Tressler, D.K. eds. Westport Connecticut: The AVI publishing Co. p:45-68.

23. Peterson M.S. (1965). Establishing a modern food industry: The resources of the technical literature In: Food technology the world over. Vol 2. Peterson M.S & Tressler, D.K. eds. Westport Connecticut: The AVI publishing Co. p:3-37.

24. Pollan, M. (2008). In Defence of Food. New York: Penguin Books, p: 147

25. Potter, N. (1973) Food science. 2nd edition. Westport Connecticut:The AVI Publishing Company, inc.

26. Powell, L. (1977) Food was Never Safer, Penn State Expert says. Observer Reporter, Washington, PA, January 17. Retrieved October 12, 2013 from: http://news.google.com/newspapers?nid=2519&dat=19770117&id=u-VdAAAAIBAJ&sjid=E18NAAAAIBAJ&pg=933,2106524

26b. Pure Food and Drug Act 1906. Retrieved April 12, 2013from: http://www.ncbi.nlm.nih.gov/books/NBK22116 Retrieved on April 12

27. Randell, A. (1995). Codex Alimentarius: How It All Began. FAO Corporate Document Depository. Agriculture and Consumer Protection. Retrieved on October 7, 2013: http://www.fao.org/docrep/v7700t/v7700t09.htm

28. Rose. D. (1963). Food technology in Canada and the United States: Canada. In: Food technology the world over. Vol 1. 20. Peterson M.S. & Tressler, D.K. eds. Westport Connecticut: The AVI publishing Co. 1963:359-372.

29. Rossiter, A.(1977) Science Today: Safe at the Plate. Nashua Telegraph December 21.

29b. Ryan, T. The Making of I'd Like to Buy the World a Coke. Retrieved from Coca-Cola's website July 27, 2013: http://www.coca-colacompany.com/stories/coke-lore-hilltop-story

30. Schlereth, T.J. (1991) Victorian America: Transformations in everyday life. New York: Harper Collins.

31. Schoenthaler, S et al (1997). The Effect of Randomized Vitamin Mineral Supplementation on Violent and Non-violent Antisocial Behavior Among Incarcerated Juveniles. *Journal of Nutritional & Environmental Medicine 7*, 343-352

32. Schultz, H.W. (1966). Education for 500 careers. In: Protecting our food:The yearbook of agriculture. Washington D.C.:U.S. Government printing office: 236-246.

32b. Sebrell, W.H. Urgent problems of Nutrition for National Betterment. Am. J. Publ. Health; 1942; 32: 15-20. Retrieved online on August 14, 2013 from: http://www.ncbi.nlm.nih.gov/pmc/articles/PMC1527075/pdf/amjphnation00703-0023.pdf

33. Spears, M.C. (1991) Foodservice Organizations: A managerial and systems approach. 2nd Ed. New York: Macmillan Publishing Co.

34. Spiekermann, U. (2011) Redefining Food: The Standardization of Products and Production in Europe and the United States 1880-1914. History and Technology, 27(1): 11-36
34b. Schwartz, L.O. et al., (2008). Examining the nutritional quality of breakfast cereals marketed to children. JADA 108(4): 1866-1871
35. Taylor, S.L. (1985). Food allergies. Food Technology; February: 98-105.
35b. The Anxiety & Depression Association of America. Irritable Bowel Syndrome. Retrieved from website on July 16, 2013: http://www.adaa.org/understanding-anxiety/related-illnesses/irritable-bowel-syndrome-ibs
35c. **The Coca-Cola Company. History of Coca Cola Retrieved July 20, 2013**(URL: www.coca-cola.com)
36. The Cornucopia Institute Report (March 2013). Carrageenan: How A Natural Food Additive is Making Us Sick. Retrieved October 8, 2013 from: http://chicagotonight.wttw.com/sites/default/files/article/file-attachments/Carrageenan%20Report-March%202013.pdf
37. The Pure Food and Drug Act 1906 http://www.ncbi.nlm.nih.gov/books/NBK22116 Retrieved on April 12, retrieved April 12, 2013
38. Thompson, D. (2010) Why is American Food so Cheap. The Atlantic, January 11. Retrieved October 10, 2013 from: http://www.theatlantic.com/business/archive/2010/01/why-is-american-food-so-cheap/33259/
38b. U.S.D.A Budget Summary and Annual Performance Plan 2012. Retrieved from the USDA website August 3 2013: http://www.obpa.usda.gov/budsum/FY12budsum.pdf
38c. U.S.D.A. Profiling Food Consumption in America. In Agriculture Fact Book chapter-2. Retrieved from the USDA website on August 3 2013: http://www.usda.gov/factbook/chapter2.pdf
39. Vial R. (1989). Moeurs, sante et maladie en 1789. Paris: Londreys.
39b. Wight, H. The History and Processes of Milling. Hum. J. 2011: Jan 25. Retrieved July 9, 2013 from secondary source: http://www.resilience.org/stories/2011-01-25/history-and-processes-milling
39c. Wong et al.: Gut Microbiota Diet and Heart Disease. Journal of AOA C International 2012; 95(1): 24-30
40. World Cancer Research Fund (2007). Red and Processed Meats: Finding the Balance for Cancer Prevention. The 2007 Expert Report. Retrieved October 14, 2013 from: http://www.wcrf-uk.org/PDFs/processed_meat.pdf
41. Wyman, C. (2001) Jell-O: A Biography - The History and Mystery of America's Most Famous Dessert. New York: Harcourt Inc. Publishing

CHAPTER 5

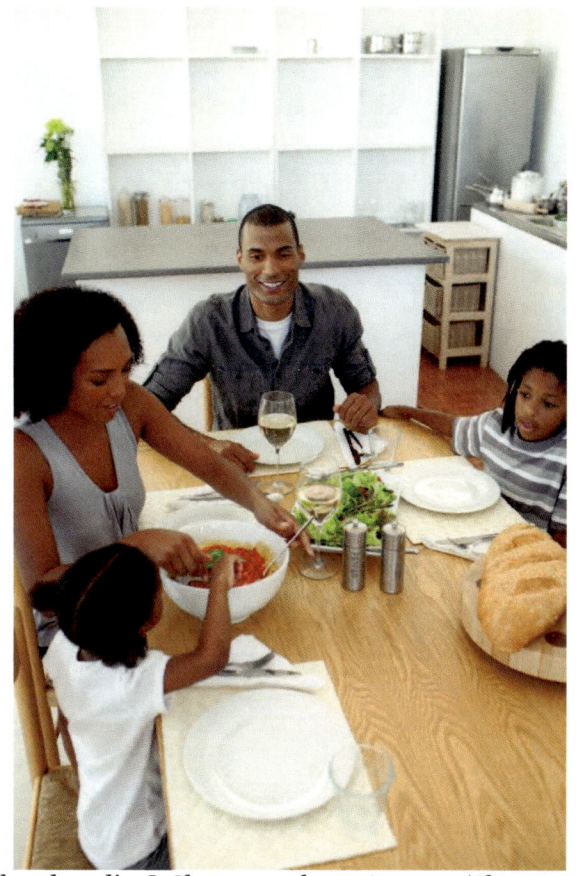

FAMILY AND CHILD NUTRITION

5.1 The Role of Nutrition in Pregnancy

5.1.1 Fertility and Birth Rates in the U.S. and Worldwide

The reproductive capabilities of a population, speak volumes about the health of a nation, for indeed, if a population were made up mostly of elderly people then that country's economic and industrial engines would come to a grinding halt. It is from the youth that new ideas are formed, and energy for change can be channeled. It is the youth that become the fuel that feed commerce in a country, because of the great material needs of a younger population.[67]

The reproductive capacity of a population then becomes the corner stone of economic progress for that nation. [89b] We may have reached, in the U.S., a point of such criticality—U.S. fertility rate is below the replacement value of 2.1—that it behooves us to stop and ponder the widespread devastation that awaits us in the coming decades, and centuries if we are unable to reverse our low birth rates, and improve our impoverished nutritional habits.

Stone [87b] writes in the January 27, 2020 issue of the National Review:

The change in the United States in recent years has been particularly rapid: Fertility rates have declined from about 2.12 children per woman in 2006 to just 1.72 today. The figure could head even lower in the near future, especially if another recession hits. In the long run, if fertility remains low, the result will be increasing economic stagnation, greater intergenerational economic and political tension, and, ultimately, strategic insecurity.

The problem is also now international with countries like France dropping from a fertility rate of 2.9 in 1960 to 1.9 in 2017. Saudi Arabia likewise saw a drop from 7.2 to 2.4 in the same time period. China and its one-child policy provoked a drop in fertility rates from its 1960s value of 5.8 to 1.7 in 2017. [89b]

Our diminished ability or willingness to reproduce, in addition to the unhealthy diets of our families, mothers and children, are now threatening the very health of our population. [55b]

What happens when a nation's birth rate consistently declines? What then if a people were to feed their unborn babies inadequate diets that prevent neurological systems from optimally developing and thriving? What happens to a nation such as the United States that aborts 20% of its pregnancies, and that sees 15% of its infants die yearly? What is going on?

Birth rates declined significantly in the U.S. between 1910 and 1930, going from 30.1 to 25.1 in 1915—the second year of World War-I—and downward to 18.9 per 1000 population during the economic crisis of 1929. Rates subsequently fell again to 18.0 during the economic relapse of 1931. This was the time that brought the roaring twenties to a close with the most severe economic collapse in U.S. history. [53]

Birth rates subsequently exploded between 1940 and 1958 in the aftermath of World War II with the birth of the baby boomer generation that populated streets, schools and parks for the next twenty five years. Neighborhoods teamed with those rowdy kids running everywhere; it was a time of economic recovery and hope.[30]

However, since 1962 and despite growing financial prosperity, birth rates have been steadily declining, reaching the lowest rate in 2009 with 13.8 births per 1000 people. It subsequently dropped to 12.7 in 2011.

Another marker of population growth is fertility rate. This measure reflects the number of births per woman assuming each woman lives through their full reproductive age. In 1971 fertility rates fell below the replacement rate of 2.1 children per woman, hitting its lowest point at 1.7 in 1976. As birth control was introduced in the 60s, birth rates and fertility rates dropped dramatically, and never really rebounded to the higher birth rates generally forecasted during economic growth.

Demographers have estimated that it takes approximately 3 generations or roughly 75 years, for a population fertility rate less than 2.1 to begin to cause a decline in the general population. Sociologists refer to this phenomenon as a "demographic winter".

> **Population with fertility rates of less than 2.1 will begin to decline after approximately 3 generations.**

Fertility rates remained under 2.1 between 1989 and 2000, at which point, according to U.S. statistics, rates returned to the replacement level for the first time in 30 years.[47] Specialists attributed the upswing in fertility rates to immigrant populations with religious beliefs that do not condone contraception. Subsequently, however, fertility rates turned downward to 2.08 again by 2008—below replacement rate—and further declined to 1.93 by 2010.[45, 46] The Pew Research Foundation[67] speculates that this new decline is the consequence of economic hardship, resulting from the crash of 2008. The U.S., like many other European nations, has surprisingly moved towards the rather serious demographic winter that was being defined through the 70s. In fact, according to the 2012 international birth rate statistics, the United States has dropped to 1.93, which is still above the rates reported in other industrialized nations for that year. For instance, Canada's rate is at 1.59, and most of Europe averages 1.5 with Greece and Italy having the lowest fertility rates in Western Europe at 1.38 and 1.39 respectively. Eastern Europe fertility rates are by far the most worrisome with mean rates in the vicinity of 1.25 births per woman, a rate that is clearly insufficient to ensure the renewal of the population. For these countries, a decline in population is expected to begin in the next fifty years. Until increases in costs of living give some indication of relenting, sociologists do not foresee birth rates climbing back to those levels documented in 1910, either internationally or domestically. The Pew Foundation claims the drop after 2008 was also greatly related to a 13% decline in birth rates among immigrant women in addition to a 5% drop in U.S.-born women.[67]

The American family has indeed changed and so, as a society many argue that we must adapt our definition of family, recognizing that it is in transition, changing as it were, from a previous standard of many children, to a new ideal of fewer to no children—a standard embraced by the Millennials. This is a trend that may actually reflect the selfish desires of a more narcissistic youth that emerged after 1982, writes Jean Twenge, [92] author of the 2006 best seller: "*Generation Me.*" Using surveys of 1.2 million youth going as far back as the 1920s, Twenge detected a growing trend towards individualism. She advances that this heightened concern about "Me" may actually be the darker consequence of parents pushing self-esteem, self-importance and high expectations about their children's accomplishments. The August 12, 2013 issue of TIME magazine likely captures the more nefarious side of this generation. The magazine featured a cover titled: "*The Child-Free Life: When having it all means not having children.*" Lauren Sandler[78] describes a childless generation that has caused national child birth statistics to plummet across all ethnic groups according to a 2010 Pew Research report. Currently, about 1 in 5 women end their reproductive years maternity-free. This is a shocking decline from the 1970s statistics that confirmed that 1 in 10 women were childless at menopause.[63] A closer look at U.S. data reveals that birth rates are compromised by a worrisome practice that has insidiously made its way into the regular lifestyles of most societies. Of the 6,408,000 U.S. pregnancies reported by the CDC in 2005, only 64.6% ended in live births, 18.85% ended in induced abortions, and 16.54% in fetal losses. [45, 46, 47]

There is something deeply troubling taking place here, that only becomes evident when we stratify the information. The percent of teenage pregnancies—among 15-17 year olds—that ended in abortion were very high, during the period 1980 to 1988, representing 42% of the pregnancies. More disturbing still, birth rates among teenagers in the United States, during that same time period, almost equaled abortion rates. It isn't clear what happened in 1989 that caused abortion rates to decline, leading toward an all-time low in 2005 of 25.6% of teenage pregnancies, but it is likely tied to a more widespread availability of contraception.

Abortion rates tend to be lowest in nations that make contraception more readily available. The decline in abortions translates into fewer future pregnancy complications and less emotional disturbances that lead to depression and anxiety. There are several concerns that emerge from the declining fertility rates of a population, however, a drop in pregnancy rate specifically among teenagers, is generally regarded as a good thing, as they tend to be high risk. Educational efforts directed at teen sexuality have caused pregnancy rates among 15-17 year old girls to shift from 70 per thousand women to 42, representing a 40% drop between 1980 and 2005. But still the prevalence of unplanned pregnancies remains a problem nationally and internationally, and is reflective of risky sexual behavior that feeds an intricate network of STIs. Stone, [87a] writes:

…every year [internationally] some 80 million women experience an unplanned pregnancy, 45 million of which end in an abortion; an estimated 500 million people acquire at least one of the four primary curable STIs (Neisseria gonorrhoeae, Chlamydia trachomatis, Trichomonas vaginalis, and syphilis); there are around 2 million new cases of HIV infection; and many millions are infected with the genital herpes virus, HSV-2.

This was a significant achievement in attempting to decrease infant deaths and stillborn rates in the U.S., and a valiant effort at trying to reshape and consolidate the American family. However, the importance of nutrition and healthy lifestyles in this newer family model cannot be overstated, especially at the prenatal level.

5.1.2 The Impact of Alcohol on Fetal Development

The reality is that pregnancy is one time in the life of a woman for which procrastination can be a serious game changer. Nowhere but during pregnancy, can the importance of both nutrition and lifestyle be seen as prime importance. Some and perhaps many procrastinate in embracing better eating habits, es-pecially when the likelihood of motherhood is con-templated. Some young women more or less say to themselves: *"I will soon be changing my diet once I clear my overcharged agenda…eventually"*.

Indeed, the health of the fetus, and of that child after birth, greatly depends on the mother's diet during pregnancy. The field of teratology—the study of the malformations and defects of the fetus—truly only gained importance following the seminal paper published by doctors Smith and Jones in 1973. The paper clearly described the visible facial and physical characteristics of Fetal Alcohol Syndrome (FAS). It was a discovery that clearly demonstrated that the uterus was not impervious to the external world. It's not that the social concern, for the effects of alcohol on children, only began to emerge after the identification of FAS, rather it is clearly docu-mented even in old testament writings. The biblical book of Judges chapter 13 verses 3-5, reveal very clearly that knowledge of the devastating effects of alcohol on the fetus were indeed well known more than 2000 years ago.

An angel of the Lord appeared to the woman and said to her, "Though you are barren and have had no children, yet you will conceive and bear a son. Now, then, be careful to take no wine or strong drink and to eat nothing unclean. As for the son you will conceive and bear, no razor shall touch his head for this boy is to be consecrated to God from the womb. It is he who will begin the deliverance of Israel from the power of the Philistines" (Judges 13:3-5).

There is also a mid-1700 lithograph by English artist Hogarth, titled: *Gin Lady, depicting an intoxicated woman dropping her child from her arms.* The artist's portrayal clearly condemns the practice of women drinking, and recognizes alcohol as part of an abusive environment for children. The earliest suspicion of a teratogenic impact of alcohol was documented in the medical literature around 1899. At that point, evidence was emerging that stillbirths and mortality, in infants born of alcoholic mothers, was twice that of the general population. Between 1900 and 1922, animal research confirmed that the placenta did not act as a barrier to alcohol, but was rather pervious to it, thus causing clear physical defects in the offspring of parents fed alcohol. Despite the mounting evidence being documented by the scientific community in the early 20th century, the eugenics movement, which was strong during the early 1900s, was responsible for delaying the propagation of this vital information.

The goal of the eugenics movement was rather nefarious as it envisioned itself as a promoter of practices aimed at improving the overall genetic composition of a population. And while alcohol, taken during pregnancy, was frowned upon and discouraged by eugenecists,—they believed that a stronger offspring was born when no alcohol was consumed— the eugenic movement had also expanded their philosophy to include a social Darwinism. It advocated the principle that a stronger and fitter social class would eventually emerge through a natural selection facilitated by alcohol.

Dr. Wasson, in his article published in the August 1913 Vermont Medical Monthly, describes the eugenic thinking that was emerging at that time:[96] *To use a term cacogenic—the study of Bad Heredity— coined by Doctor Southard, we might well call immorality, imbecility and epilepsy the cacogenic triplets derived from alcoholic parentage.*

The good doctor concludes in his article that most alcoholics are mentally defective or incorrigible, and thus should be sterilized, in order to prevent offspring from emerging from that subclass of defective genetics. However, by 1915 the scientific validity of eugenics began to be questioned. But it was its link to the Nazi movement in the 1940s that sealed its fate as a socially accepted precept. Eugenics quickly disappeared from the social radar for a time, having gone underground in order to redefine itself. It reemerged once again by the end of the 20th century as Planned Parenthood, with the popular surge in genetics, genomic and reproductive technologies. This time its eugenic practices fell below the public's radar, as it continued to facilitate abortions and contraception, primarily targeting the poor and those of the lower social classes.[43, 70, 71, 72]

Between the 30s and 50s there was very little scientific interest in the effects of alcohol during pregnancy. By this time the earlier work, published in the beginning of the 20th century, was long forgotten or the data regarded as inconclusive. In fact, many physicians of that time frequently recommended the intake of a little alcohol as a method to relax the mothers; they assured them that the alcohol would have no deleterious effects on the fetus.

Teratology, as a science, only truly emerged as a high profile field of study following two historical events: the first were the nuclear bombs in Hiroshima and Nagasaki in 1945. Interest in the effects of irradiation on the fetus became galvanized by the reported clusters of physical malformations that were emerging from the first generation of offspring after those bombs.

The second event was the thalidomide scandal that shook the western world in the 50s and 60s. Developed by the German pharmaceutical company Grünenthal in Stolberg near Aachem, the drug was sold in 46 countries, between 1957 and 1962, as an antiemetic and a cure for morning sickness. The latter frequently occurred during the first trimester of pregnancy.

> **Between 10,000 and 20,000 babies were born with serious physical deformities due to the maternal ingestion of the drug thalidomide.**

It is estimated that roughly 10,000 to 20,000 babies were born during that period with serious physical deformities caused by the thalidomide drug (**Figure 5.1**). The drug's teratogenic effects impacted the fetus during the period of greatest **hyperplasia** or cell development. This was a critical time during which the fine anatomical and neurological blueprints were being laid down. Although banned by the FDA in the United States, the drug did filter into the U.S. via other countries. Nevertheless, this FDA ban protected most of the U.S. population from the wave of debilitating birth defects that swept through other nations such as United Kingdom, Canada, and Australia.[101]

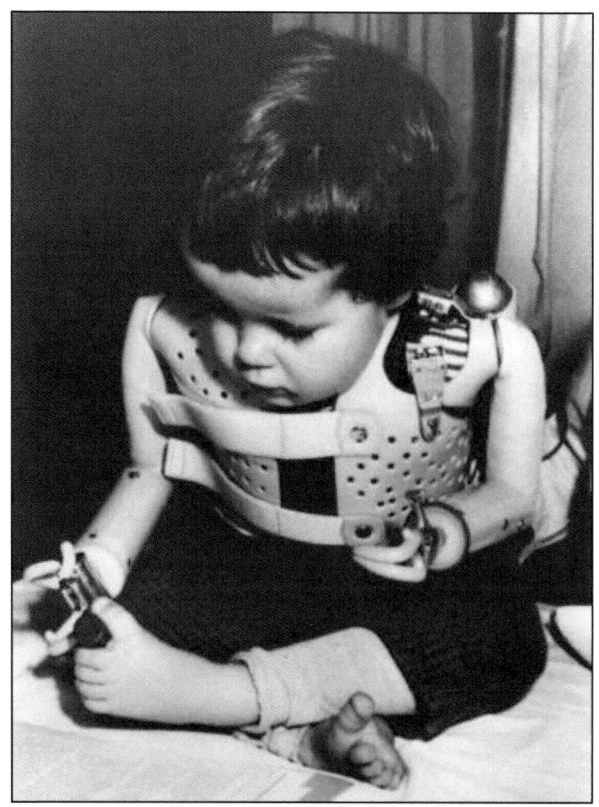

Figure 5.1: A three-year-old thalidomide toddler using power-driven artificial arms. Thalidomide was a drug prescribed during the late 1950s and early 1960s to pregnant women as a cure for morning sickness. The drug was inadequately tested and caused severe birth defects. By: Omikron-Omikron © Getty Images

In 1962, President John F Kennedy honored Frances Oldham Kelsey, the FDA pharmacologist who denied the Richardson-Merrell company's FDA application to distribute thalidomide in the U.S., insisting that further studies were needed.

> **Medical professionals remained skeptical about the teratogenic effects of alcohol on infants despite the growing research findings.**

Now despite the higher interest in teratogenic research, alcohol was not on the radar of the medical community until the late 1960s, when a Belgian researcher, Lemoine, published in 1968, a paper that described a set of common physical defects he observed in infants born from alcoholic mothers. His observations, however, for the most part, went unnoticed by the medical establishment. Finally,

Jones published findings in the early 70s, that appeared in the high profile medical journal, Lancet, that were similar to those of Lemoine. He reported craniofacial, limb and cardiovascular defects, developmental delays and growth retardation identified by height, weight and head circumference under the 5th percentile.

But it was in his second paper in 1973, that the term Fetal Alcohol Syndrome (FAS) was coined; at that point the scientific communities around the world began to take notice. Jones was able, in that second paper, to describe the microcephaly in addition to five easily identifiable facial traits associated with FAS: the thin upper lip, the epicanthic folds of the eyes, the indistinct philtrum under the nose, the short nose, and widely spaced eyes.

Afterwards, research papers abounded that documented the teratogenic effects of alcohol. Yet the medical establishment remained somewhat skeptical, since physicians commonly used alcohol to treat premature labor. Moreover, they felt that since alcohol use was so widespread, that if such a causal relationship between birth defects and alcohol was real, it would have been seen long before 1973. Most physicians felt that there were many more viable causes, behind these observed birth defects, that were much more likely than alcohol. For instance doctors believed that poor nutrition, lack of prenatal care, poly-drug abuse, such as nicotine, confounded the association with alcohol. It was felt that women who drank alcohol also smoked heavily. Also, doctors believed that traumatic insults to the fetus in utero, resulting from the mother falling, were more in tune with the kind of physical abnormalities that were seen at birth.[65]

Scientifically, physicians questioned the accuracy of FAS on the basis that there were no controls in the studies. Hence no serious momentum for change really occurred in medical practices, until well controlled animal studies were performed. Soon after, the research began to show abnormal facial and kidney development, heart defects and microcephaly that were consistent with the defects observed in human infants. They showed dose-dependent effects of alcohol on the abnormalities observed in the animal litters.[19] In addition, research demonstrated that alcohol effects were dependent on timing and genetic susceptibility.

> Fetal Alcohol Effects described a collection of subtle behavioral changes in infants exposed to maternal drinking of even half an ounce of alcohol per day. There now remains zero tolerance for alcohol during pregnancy because of the high risk to the infant.

Indeed, alcohol appeared to have its most devastating impact during the brain's growth spurt period involving synaptogenesis. Still the problem remained, that not every pregnant woman who abused alcohol had a baby with FAS, however, it became clear that FAS did not occur without alcohol.[75]

The decisive blow to the theory that alcohol was safe during pregnancy came from the emergence of behavioral teratology. This was a discipline that focused on brain development and behavior. Although the early autopsies conducted on fetuses born of alcoholic mothers, revealed widespread diffuse and non-specific brain damage, it was the neuroimaging techniques, such as Magnetic Resonance Imaging (MRIs) and computerized tomography (CT-scans) that provided irrefutable evidence. Created in the 1980s, the neuroimaging showed that defined and very specific regions of the brain were being affected by alcohol. There was a clear agenesis of the corpus collosum, lesions in the cerebellum, and a decreased size of the basal ganglia.[19, 21, 51] These aberrations to the brain translated, in many cases, into various degrees of behavioral abnormalities without the distinct physical anomalies normally expected in FAS. Consequently, while no physical features could be observed in the infant at birth, many parents, who had consumed alcohol in the early stages of pregnancy for instance, were falsely reassured that the alcohol had not impacted their baby. The truth of alcohol's real effect would show up later in the form of symptoms of attention deficit hyperactivity disorder (ADHD), impulsivity, delayed learning, poor memory and physical coordination, in addition to impaired executive functioning and social abilities in the pre-school and school years.[85] The main abnormalities, detected by behavioral teratology, were eventually coined Fetal Alcohol Effects (FAE) and fetal alcohol spectrum disorders (FASD).[13] These behavioral changes became apparent with as little as 0.5oz-wt of alcohol per day.[21]

From an epidemiological perspective, a problem was emerging: there was no way to document the prevalence of FAE since the symptoms were often mistaken for learning disabilities. The implications were serious, as the problem could not be monitored at a clinical level. There was, in fact, no way to know if the problem, from a societal perspective, was getting worse.

The surgeon general of the United States, Richard H. Carmona,[13] clearly stated in 2005, that there was a zero tolerance for alcohol during pregnancy. From his analysis, he concluded that the risk from alcohol intake, during pregnancy specifically, was so great that it outweighed any benefits that could be obtained from its consumption. It does not matter what way you look at it, the risk-to-benefit analysis does not favor alcohol intake during pregnancy under any circumstance.[13]

This intolerance to alcohol, during the gestational period, needs to be emulated when it comes to nutritional habits during pregnancy as well. If the foods consumed by expectant mothers are, for the most part, inadequate for optimal health, then should not the ingestion of junk food during pregnancy be loudly discouraged? Is it not time to advocate for zero tolerance here also?

5.1.3 Prenatal Nutrition

The notion that nutrition could influence pregnancy outcomes was novel, and stemmed from the studies conducted by Bertha Burke at Harvard in the 1940s. She provided the first evidence that robust birth weights of 7lbs 15oz in girls and 8lbs 8oz in males could be achieved with diets of good or excellent nutritional quality.[12]

The most convincing findings that nutritional quality during pregnancy was vital to the baby, emerged from the severe food rationing, imposed by the Germans on the Dutch during the winter of 1944-45. The food restrictions produced a significant number of low birth weight babies from women affected during the third trimester of pregnancy. Even before the numerous studies conducted during the 1940s, there was an underline understanding of the consequences of poor nutrition. Economic strife from the late 20s followed by a difficult economy in the 30s, created an environment where the poor suffered high degrees of food insecurity.

Subsequent studies after the 1940s, confirmed these earlier findings, and opened the door to the importance of prenatal nutrition. The idea that good quality nutrition could prevent poor pregnancy outcomes, such as low birth weights, was recognized more than 30 years ago in the U.S. By an act of congress, the Women, Infants and Children's (WIC) program was instituted in 1972, and administered by the United States Department of Agriculture (USDA).[22] Its goal was: *safeguarding the health of low-income women, infants, and children up to age 5 who are at nutritional risk*. The significance of this legislation was that it gave a strong message that poor nutrition affected the health of infants, and was preventable. The evidence was strong that the WIC program, for those lower income women who participated in it, did diminish the risk of delivering babies of low birth weight (LBW), very low birth weight (VLBW) and premature deliveries.

The poor dietary habits, and prevalence of overweight and obese pregnant women, currently seen worldwide, are also creating serious health concerns. Gestational diabetes, presently documented in Norway, is at a prevalence that is 5-times greater than fifteen years ago. The consequence has been a national surge in large babies, and a concomitant increase in the risks of fetal malformation, damage to mother and child at parturition, obesity, and type-2 diabetes in mother and the baby, leading up to adolescence.

In the United States, NIH data reveals that the prevalence of gestational diabetes represents between 2% and 10% of pregnant women. Of those mothers who do develop gestational diabetes, between 5-10% will progress to type-2 diabetes right after delivery, but surprisingly, within the following 10-20 years, roughly 35-60% will eventually develop diabetes mellitus.[60]

Using newer diagnostic techniques, physicians are now reporting a jump from 2-10% to 18% of pregnant women exhibiting symptoms of gestational di-

> **5-10% of mothers who develop gestational diabetes during pregnancy will remain diabetic after delivery.**

abetes. This translates into serious health issues, with long term implications for mothers for as many as 35-60% of those with gestational diabetes, will go on to develop type-2 diabetes over the following 10 to 20 years. There is much to be concerned about, as diabetes was, in 2007, the seventh leading cause of death in the U.S.[60] Diabetes is a devastating disease because of the degenerative path that it follows over time due to its many secondary diseases such as hypertension, heart disease and stroke, blindness, kidney and nervous system diseases, and amputations.[60]

Is this not a sign that demonstrates the way in which the American family is slowly collapsing? If the mother, who is the heart of the family, is now becoming ill at a greater frequency, then how will

> **Excessive weight is a problem often encountered by physicians managing pregnant patients and is a risk factor for developing pre-eclampsia and eclampsia. The highly processed foods and meat-based Westernized diet are actually responsible for a high prevalence of chronic diseases such as diabetes, obesity and cardiovascular disease.**

the babies, of the new generation, be affected? Will they not also be more susceptible to chronic disease?

Prenatal nutrition truly becomes a strategy that can begin to turn this crisis around. There are three fundamental reasons why pre-natal nutrition is so important:

First, the mother's diet feeds herself and her baby. But what she ingests as a young girl and adolescent, in preparation for future pregnancies, is also likely to establish a template for the health outcomes of her progeny and herself. There is strong evidence emerging that young women of reproductive ages (20-39 years) are now more frequently overweight and obese, and that this elevated pre-pregnancy weight is specifically associated, not only with increased medical and obstetrical risks, but also with multiple fetal complications.

It appears that obesity, prior to pregnancy, carries more serious health implications for baby and mother than the weight gain during pregnancy. There is a cold wind blowing in the horizon as the obesity crisis deepens and the quality of nutrition, among the young, continues to nosedive in the United States.

The National Health and Nutrition Examination Survey (NHANES)[62] documented, between 1999 and 2002 that 26% of women of reproductive age considered themselves overweight, and 29% claimed to be obese. In total then, 55% of adult women were potentially beginning their pregnancy already suffering from a weight management problem that could potentially impact the fetus directly.[62] This would have increased the risks of neural tube defects, spontaneous miscarriage, preterm delivery and neonatal respiratory distress. Moreover, when a woman is obese and depositing fat in the abdominal area, she is also producing more atherogenic lipoproteins in the blood, in addition to excess adipocytokines and free radicals. These compounds threaten the integrity of the vascular lining and other cells. During pregnancy it is unclear to what extent these nefarious byproducts of obesity make their way past the placenta, thus affecting the baby directly. We do know that medical practitioners are increasingly treating mothers who begin their pregnancies overweight or obese. They must manage these women by prescribing calorie-controlled diets aimed at limiting the total weight gain, in addition to the rate of weight gain over the duration of the pregnancy.

Weight management is a significant problem that is now routinely encountered by obstetricians and family physicians, and places pregnant women at high risk of **pre-eclampsia** and **eclampsia**.

Pre-eclampsia is a condition characterized by protein appearing in the urine, along with a noticeable rise in blood pressure and swelling; eclampsia, on the other hand, involves significant protein in the urine, a dangerously elevated blood pressure, seizures and kidney failure that put both mom and fetus at high risk of complications and death. It's very costly to treat obese pregnant mothers, who now represent a significant public health problem. Consequently, there are now very clear guidelines outlining the number of calories that need to be consumed at each trimester and the recommended rate of weight gain over the 40 weeks of a pregnancy (**Table 5.1**).

TABLE 5.1 Caloric and weight gain recommendations for obese, overweight, normal weight and underweight women during the three trimesters of pregnancy

Calories/weight gain	1ST TRIMESTER	2ND TRIMESTER	3RD TRIMESTER	Mean rate of weight gain in 2nd & 3rd trimester
Extra calories	0 KCAL	350 KCAL	450 KCAL	
Under Weight gain BMI<19.8	7-9lbs	10.5-15.5lbs	10.5-15.5lbs	1.0lbs/week
Normal Weight gain BMI: 19.8-26	5.5-7lbs	10-14lbs	10-14lbs	0.90lb/week
Overweight BMI: >26-29	4-5.5lbs	5.5-9.75lbs	5.5-9.75lbs	0.60lb/week
Obese BMI>29	0-4lbs	5.3-8.0lbs	5.3-8.0lbs	0.50lb/week

*Turner, E.R Nutrition during Pregnancy In: Modern Nutrition in Health & Disease 10th Ed. M. Shields et al. Editors Lippincott, Williams and Wilkins, Baltimore Pub, 2006: 771-783
**Institute of Medicine. Weight Gain during Pregnancy: Reexamining the Guidelines. Report Brief 2009. [35]

During the first trimester, there is essentially very little weight gain compared to the subsequent two trimesters. This is because hyperplastic growth of the fetus or in other words, **hyperplasia**, is mostly occurring in that early phase; it is characterized by the synthesis of new cells. Table-1 above indicates that in the first trimester no extra calories are required. It is during this very intense and crucial phase, that fine anatomical details are being defined with great precision along with a complex neurological network. The first trimester is therefore a period during which the risk for teratogenicity is greatest. So the biological system, in the first trimester, is not concerned so much with calories, as it is not particularly focused on growth, but rather on establishing the template/blueprint for future growth and development of the fetus.

Notice how the caloric requirements increase by 350 kcal in the second trimester (Table-1), concurrently with the shift from hyperplastic to hypertrophic growth. And while there is still some hyperplasia taking place during the second trimester, there is progressively more growth in the size of the cells, thereby explaining the more significant weight gain compared to the first trimester.

The third trimester necessitates, yet again, an increase in the number of calories per day by 450 kcal

> Contrary to popular belief, no additional calories are necessary for healthy fetal growth in the first trimester of pregnancy.

compared to pre-pregnancy needs; the fetal development is now primarily hypertrophic. Hence, the mother's caloric intake directly impacts the baby's weight at birth. In practice then, this means that insufficient calories consumed during this last trimester of a full term pregnancy, can translate into a low birth weight baby.[11]

Low birth weights can also occur because of premature deliveries. Low birth weight infants are defined as weighing less than 5.5 pounds, whereas preterm infants are those born at or before 37 weeks of gestation. About 8.2% of children born in the United States, according to CDC data from 2009, are underweight and roughly 12.5% are born too early or are premature. This percent is the highest in the western world.

The normal prevalence range for premature babies, in most of the European nations and in countries like Canada and Australia, varies between 7-9%. Hence, U.S. statistics of 12% give good reason to be concerned, since the prevalence of underweight babies in the United States has been increasing since the year 2000.

> Premature births in Canada and Australia occur in 7% - 9% of deliveries. In the US, the prevalence of premature infants is about 12% and has been increasing since 2000.

The rise in preemies in the U.S. has been linked to the surge in teen pregnancies, and to a greater number of women older than 35 having their first baby.

The recent drop in teenage pregnancy rate is considered a good outcome from a public health perspective for two reasons: first, teenage pregnancies invariably lead, in most cases, to economic strife; and second, there is generally poor health care for a teenage mom and her baby, and increased medical complications for the infant. This stems from the reality that many teenagers give birth to low birth weight babies who have higher risks of infant mortality and medical complications. Now that more teenagers are overweight and obese, the prospect of healthier pregnancies and babies looks rather grim. Indeed, the numbers of birth complications, infant mortalities and cases of teratogenicity are expected to climb. Scientists also know that there is a relatively strong mother-fetal relationship during pregnancy that can cause epigenetic changes in the fetus, depending on whether the mother is overeating or under-eating. This translates into undernourished mothers transmitting, to the underweight fetus, a greater tendency to synthesize fat more efficiently after birth, thus leading to obesity in adulthood. In the obese mother, it means pre-programming the fetus for obesity and insulin resistance early on in life.[7, 80]

More recently, evidence emerging from 13,000 subjects in the Nurses' Health Study, reveals that a diet elevated in animal fat and cholesterol, prior to pregnancy, leads to a 45% greater risk of gestational diabetes. More surprising still, are the new studies that demonstrate that the physical activity levels of young women before pregnancy, and early in the pregnancy, significantly decreases the risk of developing gestational diabetes.[91]

> Folate fortification of wheat and grain was highly successful and led to a decrease of about 1000 cases of NTD annually.

The higher quartile levels of exercise were linked to a much lower risk of developing gestational diabetes. The studies also reveal that the drop in risk was likely tied to a lowering of fat mass, to an increase in lean body mass or muscle tissue, and to improved insulin efficiency in controlling blood sugars.

Birth defects are not entirely associated with obesity and high fat intake. We do know that a young woman, of child bearing years, who does not consume enough folate in her diet prior to pregnancy, places her fetus at a higher risk of developing neural tube defects (NTDs) such as Spina-bifida. Public health programs, in the early 1990s, had previously promoted the importance of regularly consuming abundant fruits and vegetables, which are rich in folate. Because it became clear that not even public awareness was enough to sway future moms away from suboptimal eating habits, wheat and grain fortification programs were initiated in the United States in 1998, as it was generally regarded as a food group that almost everyone consumed.

The fortification program was driven by the knowledge that the folate status of young women needed to be adequate prior to pregnancy in order to significantly decrease the risk of neural tube defects in the fetuses. The fortification program was successful as the prevalence dropped from 4000 cases of NTDs in 1995-1996 to 3000 cases in 1999-2000.

5.2 The Importance of Infant Nutrition

5.2.1 Breast Milk—The Perfect Food

During American colonial times, it was common for all mothers to breastfeed their babies for 1.5 to 2 years. It wasn't until the mid to late 19th century that breastfeeding began to dwindle as mothers supplemented their milk with unpasturized cow's milk, usually before the child was 3 months old. And although the practice of initiating breastfeeding was very common—an estimated 100% of mothers began breastfeeding as the earliest form of nutrition for the newborn infant,—the practice of weaning the baby early from the breast was popular by 1910. The custom was commonly found among women of the mid to upper social classes who customarily entrusted their babies to servants, but also among working-class women who, for economic reasons, needed to leave their babies at home while they returned to the labor force. This was also a time when new expectations for marriage were being redefined as more centered on love rather than on economics and procreation. It was common to find articles in women's magazines, dated from the late 1800s, that described women's preferences to be the companions of their husbands rather than being caregivers of their children.

Late 19th century health statistics, out of the city of Baltimore, documented mortality rates among the infants of working-class mothers to be 59% greater than the average; by contrast the infant mortality rate was 5% lower than average among infants of stay-at-home mothers. The shocking difference in infant mortality rates was related, at the time, to continued breastfeeding practices among middle and upper-class women. Other studies during that period corroborated that infant mortality rates were consistently found to be greater among the working immigrant populations, living in crowed neighborhoods, who fed cow's milk to their babies.[77]

> In 1897, the Chicago Department of Health estimated that bottle-fed babies were dying at a rate of 15:1 compared to those who were breastfed.

In 1897, Chicago's mortality statistics clearly documented that 18% of babies died before their first birthday, and that 53% of these deaths were attributed to diarrhea. Chicago's Department of Health further estimated that fifteen bottle-fed babies were dying for every one breastfed child.[99]

In the early 1900s, physicians were unanimous in decrying the dangers of feeding cow's milk to infants. They contended that breast milk was indeed the optimal food, and that the practice of breastfeeding needed to be revived and more greatly promoted.

By 1910 poor health was generally associated, in the medical community, with artificially fed infants. Hence public health efforts, urging mothers to breastfeed as long as they could, were becoming more popular. Meanwhile, on the other end of the spectrum, health reformers, belonging to municipal governments, medical charities, private physicians and newspapers, led a crusade to clean up the milk supply.

These groups headed public health strategies, in big cities like Chicago that focused on the underprivileged immigrants, since infant death rates were at their highest in this group. They were also seen as the consequence of non-acculturation problems rather than poor nutrition. Public health nurses were sent into the poor neighborhoods, armed with a multifaceted educational program that included the promotion of breastfeeding, among other practices; the goal was mass education blitz.

By contrast, Dr. Julius Parker Sedgwick, who was chief of the Department of Pediatrics at the University of Minnesota, strongly advocated for breast milk as the single most vital component for infant health. He did not believe infant mortality, among immigrant populations, to be a non-acculturation issue, but rather the consequence of not breastfeeding. By 1912, his philosophy was beginning to spread into medical circles. Breast milk could be the cornerstone in the prevention of infant mortality.

It did not take long for Sedgwick's public health measures to translate into important declines in infant mortality. His approach inspired the creation of the Feeding Investigation Bureau of the Department of Pediatrics of the University of Minnesota in 1919. The Bureau was instrumental in ensuring that every new mother who gave birth would receive as many home visits, from a public health worker, as deemed necessary over the ensuing 9 months; the workers' only focus was to assist new mothers with initiating breastfeeding and dealing with lactation difficulties.[99]

> **Infant mortality rates began to drop in the 20s, largely related to the practice of breastfeeding.**

The program was so successful, that 96% of babies born in Minnesota were breastfed for 2 months, and a surprising 72% of infants breastfed for as long as 9 months during the early 1920s. But more importantly, the true evidence that breastfeeding was accomplishing its purpose, was the dramatic 20% drop in infant mortality rates as early as 1920.

The reformers, however, persisted in their crusade for clean milk, advocating for a more sanitized dairy industry. It was common for dairy farms in the early 1900s, to have filthy and decrepit walls, floors, and ceilings in the barns holding the cows. It was becoming untenable that the nation's milk was being supplied by such horrifically maintained establishments. Clean surrounds were becoming the norm expected by the public. This is not surprising as the population's awareness, of the bacterial contamination of food, had increased with Pasteur's research. Louis Pasteur's innovative work showed that increased food shelf stability and freshness could be attained through a high temperature treatment process later called pasteurization.

Hence, reformers pushed for pasteurized milk that would need to be collected from healthy cows, bottled and sealed under sanitary conditions, and finally shipped in refrigerated rail cars.

As cow's milk became safer to drink, the trend was for women to rely once again on cow's milk as a supplement to breast feeding, and for early weaning from the breast. Pasteurization was seen as successfully eliminating any difference between breast and cow's milk. In fact, by the 30s, the new generation of physicians, who had never known the devastating impact of adulterated cow's milk on infant deaths back in the late 19th and early 20th centuries, now promoted the safe cow's milk as superior to human milk. This shift in medical advice resulted in larger numbers of women choosing not to breastfeed at all. This trend to artificially feed rather than breastfeed babies persisted right up to 1971. That year, national statistics revealed that the practice of breastfeeding had declined to an all-time low, with only 24% of mothers initiating breastfeeding while still in hospital, according to the Ross Laboratories Mother's Survey, which began in 1954.

It wasn't, however, until the women's health reform movement, that took shape in the late 70s, that breastfeeding began to make a comeback. This feminist inspired movement took place within the backdrops of very prominent forms of social activism that cultivated a sort of hippie communalisms that nurtured newer forms of infant care. Although the hippie movement may have embraced breastfeeding, as a newer form of natural expression, it still had not caught on to the extent that most health officials wanted. In fact, the hippies only represented a relatively small fringe of American society; the infant formulas, introduced by pharmaceutical companies, in the late 60s and early 70s, and formulaically bolstered with vitamins, minerals and micro-minerals, were marketed as superior to breast milk. They were promoted as an effective way of liberating the woman from the cumbrous role of sole caregiver. The bottle effectively allowed the father to now participate in this previously exclusive female task of feeding the baby. This was a time of technological innovations that was capable of putting men on the moon. There was a sense that science knew better, and that we were in the midst of a scientific revolution that was going to change the way we lived for the better. The North American population quickly embraced these new formulas, which effectively liberated women from the confines of the home, and allowed them to emerge in the workplace in greater numbers.

Westernized women were being liberated from the subjugation to men, and empowered with career opportunities, the likes of which, they had never known before. Although the National Center for Health Statistics reported a decline in the initiation of breastfeeding by the early 70s, as early as the 80s the initiation of breastfeeding dramatically jumped to 61.9% but only to take a downward turn again between 1984 and 1989.

Finally, a promising turnaround took place in 1995, with the initiation of breastfeeding shooting back up to 60%. This sudden change in practice came in the wake of strong health promotion programs that sought to repopularize breastfeeding; new research was beginning to identify clear unmatched benefits associated with breast milk.

Since 1995, the practice of breastfeeding continued to spread nationally with 69.5% of U.S. mothers choosing to initiate breastfeeding (**Figure-5.2**); more recent data from 2002 indicated initiation rates exceeding 70%. The impact of this public health effort was certainly more widespread as evidenced by the greater numbers of black women, women with high school educations and women enrolled in WIC programs who were choosing to breastfeed.[99]

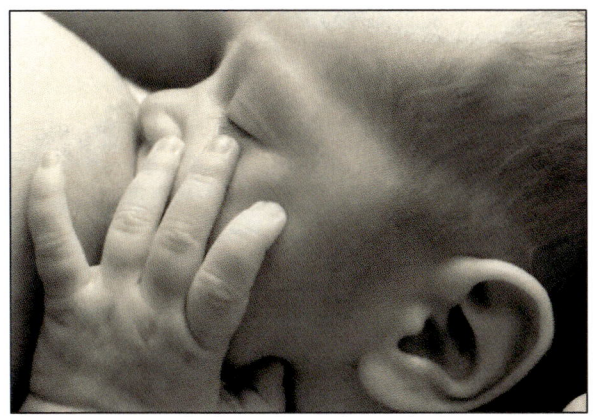

Figure 5.2: Breastfeeding Baby © Elena Yakusheva

In previous programs, historical data confirms that during the 1970s, predominantly white college-educated women tended to breastfeed their babies. And while these numbers are impressive, they do not reveal the rather sad reality that most North American women tend to supplement breastfeeding with formulas before six months.
In fact only 17% of American women follow the American Academy of Pediatrics (AAP) and the World Health Organization (WHO) recommendations to exclusively breastfeed for six months in order for the child to reap the maximal benefits.[59, 99]

Tragically, as many as 50% of mothers introduce formula before one week of age, by two months, 68% had introduced formula, and most worrisome, a total of 81% of women feed their babies formula by four months. This is detrimental from a public health perspective, since this early introduction of formula tends to shorten the overall total length of breastfeeding, which inclines to make infants particularly vulnerable to poor health.

Again, the AAP encourages women to breastfeed for at least one year, whereas the WHO takes a stronger stance and recommends at least 2 years while giving other foods; these demanding guidelines are supported historically by strong epidemiological evidence from the early 90s, that identified a much higher prevalence of respiratory, ear and gastrointestinal infections among infants who received little or no breast milk. Additionally, more recent studies have suggested that infant formulas, not only increase the risk of acute illnesses in babies, but may even set down the template for serious chronic diseases and conditions such as sudden infant death syndrome (SIDS), obesity, leukemia, breast cancer, asthma and diminished IQs. The implications of these findings are so serious that, viewed from a sociological lens, the practice of bottle feeding babies may actually be responsible for the devastation of entire populations.[99]

Consider for instance, that babies breastfed for less than 16 weeks, have a 5-fold greater propensity to develop SIDS compared to babies breastfed for more than 16 weeks.

The link between bottle feeding and obesity is also very concerning when compared to the clear benefits imparted to infants that are breastfed longer than one year.

Studies published in the British Medical Journal in 1999, and the Journal of the American Medical Association in 2001, reported that infants who were breastfed for less than 2 months had a 4 times greater likelihood of being obese, by elementary school, than babies breastfed more than 1 year.[99]

Lymphoid malignancies are also three times more likely to be diagnosed in infants, breastfed for 6 months or less, compared to those babies receiving breast milk for longer than 6 months. According to the Behavioral Risk Factor Surveillance System (BRFMS), the incidence of asthma has also been climbing worldwide since 1980, and was responsible for close to a half of a million hospitalizations and 4,500 deaths in 2000 alone. The spike in incidence raised concerns about some of the environmental changes that have taken place in recent decades, notably the effects of pollutants on health. Environmental contaminants, such as industrial waste, pesticides, herbicides, and fertilizers have insidiously made their way into lakes, ponds, wet lands and forests. Interestingly, the medical literature has tied some of the spike in childhood asthma to formula feeding. It is currently understood that there are only three primary factors that contribute to the development of asthma: First, gestational age less than 37 weeks; second, secondary smoke in the home; and third, the introduction of formula before the age of 4 months.

An important consideration does surface, however, when many of the studies are controlled for household smoke, low birth weights, and low maternity education—all conditions and situations that appear to magnify the risk of asthma in children. The recommendation for breastfeeding duration gets magnified to longer than 9 months in order to minimize the risk of developing asthma.

It was the findings of a Danish study that followed 3,253 men and women, which caught the attention of both the medical community and the popular media. Published in the May 2002 edition of the Journal of the American Medical Association, the scientists concluded that children, breastfed through 9 months, had more elevated IQ scores as teenagers and young adults, compared to those kids who received less or no breast milk.[99]

The literature also clarifies the benefits, imparted to mothers who commit to prolonged breastfeeding. Indeed, those mothers who breastfed for only 1 to 6 months had a 2-fold likelihood of experiencing pre or post-menopausal breast cancer compared to those mothers able to breastfeed for longer than 2 years.

The evidence was mounting as early as the mid-1990s that moms and babes benefited very clearly from breastfeeding. It also became apparent that the scientific community was no longer equivocal about infant formulas; it was the AAP's 1997 policy statement that identified breastfeeding as a most powerful and effective form of preventive medicine, that really became a game changer in the area of infant nutrition.

The AAP identified the clear health benefits of exclusive breastfeeding for 6 months, and highlighted

> Worldwide incidence of asthma has been increasing since 1980, and was responsible for almost half a million hospitalizations and 4500 deaths in 2000. Some research has linked the spike in childhood asthma to formula feeding.

the lower risks of chronic diseases in infants who are breastfed for as long as one year. Health and Human Services (HHS) weighed in three years later in 2000, urging health professionals to become strong advocates for prolonged breastfeeding, and dissuading the public from opting for formula feeding. Suddenly, public policy was being rigorously framed to define *optimal nutrition*, achieved through breastfeeding, as the new normal for infants; by contrast, infant formula was no longer going to be peddled as "normal nutrition". HHS further labeled the lack of exclusive and prolonged breastfeeding in American society as a clear "public health challenge" in their Blueprint for Action on Breastfeeding campaign. It was the first time, in over seventy years, that formulas were going to be vilified through the HHS's marketing campaign, which intended to explain the dangers associated with formula feedings. The goal of the campaign was to dramatically change breastfeeding practices in the U.S. and meet Healthy People 2010 goals (**Table-5.2**). The Healthy People 2020 goals are even loftier, as the push to incite more women to breast feed escalates.

TABLE 5.2 Healthy People 2010 & 2020 Breastfeeding Goals

HEALTHY PEOPLE		LENGTH OF BREASTFEEDING
2010	2020	
75%	81.9%	of mothers will initiate breast feeding in the post-partum phase
50%	60.6%	of mothers will still be breastfeeding at 6 months
25%	35.1%	of mothers will breastfeed at 12 months
40%	46.2%	of mothers will exclusively breast feed for 3 months
17%	25.5%	of mothers will exclusively breastfeed at 6 months

Breastfeeding Report Card—United States 2010—Center for Disease Control and Prevention[59] Retrieved May 12 2012: http://www.cdc.gov/breastfeeding/data/reportcard/reportcard2010.htm

Internationally, the U.S. was really only trying to bridge the incredible gap separating breastfeeding practices between the United States and the rest of the world, where up to 79% of infants are breastfed for 12 months. This contrasts greatly with the 17-20% of U.S. mothers who are breastfeeding for that length of time.

Despite the courageous government policy changes that were implemented in 1997 and 2000, and even the planned Ad Council's publicity campaign[2] geared towards highlighting the importance of breastfeeding, there has been a considerable waning in the American breastfeeding initiative.

In fact, it would not be an exaggeration to say that these efforts have been a complete failure, given that, as of 2008 only 8% to 24% of women received encouragement and guidance to breastfeed from their family physicians.

What exactly went wrong? A little investigation into the Ad Council's campaign, which was scheduled to launch in December 2003, revealed that the ads were stalled because of the formula industry's opposition to the release of what they called scientifically inaccurate and misleading ads.[2]

The formula industry hired a hard-hitting Washington lobbyist by the name of Clayton Yeutter, once secretary of Agriculture for the elder President Bush, and a past Republican Party chairman. But most surprising, the AAP also opposed the ads, referring to them as too idealistic, and geared towards giving many American women a guilt trip for not breastfeeding long enough. The watered down Ad Council's ads were finally released in June of 2004, but with the deletion of any references implying higher risk of leukemia and diabetes in babies who were not breastfed. In the end, the lobbyists were too strong in protecting the pharmaceutical industry's interests.

5.2.2 The Prevalence of Pediatric Obesity in American Society

CDC statistics from 2009, estimated that 17% of children and adolescents, ages 2 to 19, were obese and that, when stratified into specific genderless age groups, the most shocking increases in the prevalence of obesity, between 1963 and 2008, occurred in the age groups 6-11 and 12-19 years of age according to the NHANES cross-sectional studies.

Pediatric obesity was barely on the radar of most pediatricians in 1963. At that time NHANES only detected rates of between 4.2%-4.6% in the two age categories 6-11 and 12-19 respectively (**Figure 5.3**). What unfolded between 1963 and 2008, reveals troublesome changes specifically in the lifestyles of American children and adolescents. During that 45 year span, the prevalence of obesity rose

366% in the 6 to 11 year olds and 293% in the 12 to 19 year old children and adolescents.

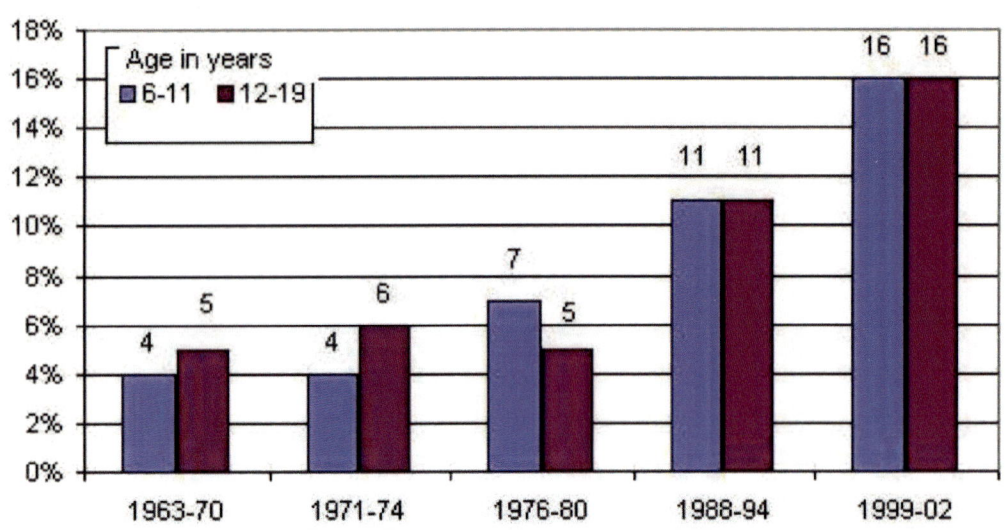

Figure 5.3: Prevalence of Overweight children and adolescents in the US population Source: CDC/NIHS, NHANES[33]

Pediatric obesity in the U.S. has now become a national crisis; 35-36% of children in the U.S. were either overweight or obese in 2003-2004, according to NIH data, whereas it was only 13-15% in France in 2006-2007.

> Costs for managing pediatric obesity from 1970 to 2000 increased from $35 million annually to $227 million.

The cost to manage pediatric obesity alone, between the 1970s and 2000, was linked to a staggering increase to the financial burden. It grew from $35 million a year to $227 million representing a 549% increase.[7a] This alarming jump in the cost to manage obese children and adolescents, acted as a sort of harbinger for the approaching storm clouds that were about to impact our health care financial system.

Medical practitioners and epidemiologists, with many years of experience treating and tracking diabetes, are alarmed by the trends they are now seeing. Epidemiologists are concerned specifically about the 9.5% obesity prevalence recorded among infants and toddlers under the age of 5, and are alarmed by the degree of obese and overweight children among the lower socioeconomic classes and disadvantaged ethnic groups.

According to the National Survey of Children's Health, published in 2007, it is the non-Hispanic blacks, the Hispanics and the Hawaiian/Pacific Islanders ages 10 to 17 years of age, who are particularly suffering from higher rates of obesity. In fact, between 41 to 44% of these ethnic groups are either overweight or obese.[17] Fast food intake and soft drink consumption, especially among the young, have been driving the weight gain (**Figure 5.4**).[61,88]

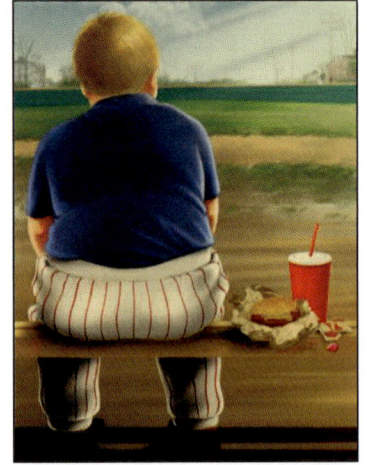

Figure 5.4: Illustration of a Fat Kid Eating Fast Food © The Turtle Factory

The threat of obesity has become so serious, that it is imperative that parents regulate the eating habits of their infants, right at the beginning. The American Heart Association (AHA) has formulated several recommendations that are consistent with their belief that cardiovascular risk begins early in life (**Table 5.3**).

TABLE 5.3 AHA dietary recommendations for infants living in the U.S.[4]

1. Breast-feeding is ideal nutrition and sufficient to support optimal growth and development for about the first 4–6 months after birth. Try to maintain breast-feeding for 12 months. Transition to other sources of nutrients should begin at about 4–6 months of age to ensure sufficient micronutrients in the diet.

2. Delay introducing 100 percent juice until at least 6 months of age and limit to no more than 4–6fl-oz/day. Juice should only be fed from a cup.

3. Do not over-feed infants and young children. They can usually self-regulate the amount of calories they need each day. Children shouldn't be forced to finish meals if they aren't hungry as they often vary caloric intake from meal to meal.

4. Introduce healthy foods and keep offering them if they're initially refused. Don't introduce foods without overall nutritional value simply to provide calories.

5.2.3 Obesity a symptom of a much greater social malaise

Weight loss diets have been the main therapeutic modality for weight management problems as far back as Hippocrates, and still today it is the single most utilized weight management strategy. [32d, 7b] Yet, studies have found that caloric restrictive diets, despite causing rapid and significant weight loss over the short term, are not efficacious in sustaining weight loss over the long term [29b, 35c, 44] Other initiatives have failed to show substantial results in combating rising obesity rates such as the 2010 Let's Move campaign and the Supplemental Nutrition Assistant Program (SNAP). [14b, 17c, 35b, 99b] The CDC has shown no significant decrease in obesity rates between the year 2011 and 2014, alternatively obesity has increased significantly in households supported by government programs during that time span. [14b, 25c, 17b] Food policies implemented such as taxation on high caloric and low nutrient-based foods and subsidies on wholesome food have yielded similar low success results.[25b, 61b] In fact, despite all of these public health initiatives, it has been estimated that by 2030 as many as 51% of the US population may be obese. [24b] Consequently, a more comprehensive understanding of the root cause of obesity is needed for the development of a more effective treatment strategy. Indeed, a new paradigm that involves the true social demographic reality behind the rising prominence of obesity needs to be considered.

The literature appears to point to the breakup of the American family as the single most influential vector that is driving this serious epidemic. The best image that can justly reflect this paradigm, is the castle used as a symbol of the home or family. Once the walls of the castle are breached--with the disappearance of the father--it is then that the castle residents become vulnerable to more nefarious outside influences and attacks.

Consequently, a set of changes or disruptions take place which lead to family dysfunction.

Meal-Time Disruptions—The beginning of dysfunctional family dynamics, primarily caused by busy schedules, could be seen, as early as the 1960s through to 2008, with the high frequency at which meals were eaten away from home. [83b] In fact, by 2008 approximately 42% of dollars dedicated to food, in the US, was spent on food eaten away from home compared to 25% in the 1970s. [51c] Despite a rising frequency of eating out through the latter part of the 20th century, it appears that the trend stabilized by the first decade of the new Millennium with two thirds of daily calories still consumed at home. [83b] However, meal time focus has currently shifted away from home cooked nutrient-rich meals to convenience pre-prepared and ready-to-eat meals. The trend towards frequent snacking of nutrient-poor but calorically-dense processed food products eaten on the go is also on the rise [83b] and contributing to less than 20% of Americans meeting Dietary Guidelines for Healthy Eating. [37b] This has invariably led to adolescents consuming nutritionally suboptimal meals and missing family meals more frequently. [81b] It has also resulted in more children eating in isolation. [88b]

A decrease of family meals is linked to eating habits such as suboptimal nutrient consumption, meal skipping, eating out and picky eating preferences. Increased family meal times with a focus on conversation have shown increased key nutrient consumption such as calcium, fiber, B12, A and E in adolescents. [11b, 23b] By contrast, increased soda consumption has been tied to decreased family meal times. Family relationships may not be the tightest when members do not get along with each other; they may find it hard to sit around a dinner table together comfortably. It has been shown that using a television to distract from the negative relationships can help increase fruit and vegetable consumption in these families, and can be way to help them re-establish a positive relationship with one another. [23b] In contrast, television viewing and snacking behaviors in adults has a positive correlation to metabolic syndrome. [90b] In fact, aggressive television advertisement campaigns has been shown to increase snack food consumption in children. [32c]

Poverty & Single-Parent Families—It has been proposed that obesity is more of a symptom emerging from a greater social malaise. Indeed, the breakdown of the family has been proposed as the cornerstone behind much of the obesity crisis, but also, it appears to fuel depression, anxiety, the rise in risky sexual behaviors, promiscuity, sexually transmitted infections, [32b] childhood adverse events, and substance abuse. [51b, 35d, 87a, 2b] The social disruptions are widespread, affecting many different segments of societal activity. It is interesting that one of the most immediate consequences of the family breakdown is poverty, from which arises distress. The research households can raise well-adjusted children, [82b] but supports the high likelihood of experiencing poverty, neighborhood stress, and poor emotional support. [34b] Moreover, when compared to intact families, children from single-parent families tend to have more adjustment difficulties, higher incidences of substance abuse, academic difficulties and social deficits. [2b]

5.4 Assessing Pediatric Obesity Using Graphs

Growth charts developed by the Center for Disease Control and Prevention (CDC) are used to monitor the growth of children between the birth and 24 months (**Figures 5.5 and 5.6** and between 2 and 20 years of age (**Figures 5.7 and 5.8**).

The idea is to plot the infant's weight relative to his age over a 24 month period (figures 32 and 33) or between 2 and 20 years of age (Figures 34 and 35). The child should theoretically remain on the same percentile curve that was established by 3 months. If plotted on the 25th percentile, it means that 25% of the children, for that gender and age group, weigh less than him. Also, if plotted on the 75th percentile, for a specific age, it would suggest that 75% of the children that age weigh less than him. Whatever curve they are initially placed on, they should maintain the same percentile until adulthood. Deviation downward or upward by 2 per-centile lines or more is considered clinically significant, and would suggest either a failure to thrive, if there is a downward deviation or **excessive food consumption**, if the deviation is upward. In either case, a significant deviation requires some kind of intervention in order to rectify the distorted growth pattern.

Using the growth charts in figures 32 and 33, it is possible to plot the height as well as the weight relative to the age of either a boy or girl infant. Monitoring the height is especially important since the proper growth in stature reflects both adequate nutrition and energy.

A **stunted growth**, that is to say a height that remains under the 5th percentile for age, can reveal worrisome issues that may be preventing normal expected growth.[40] Conditions likely to influence the stature would be insufficient calories, protein, and deficiencies in vitamin A, vitamin K, calcium, zinc and copper.[40]

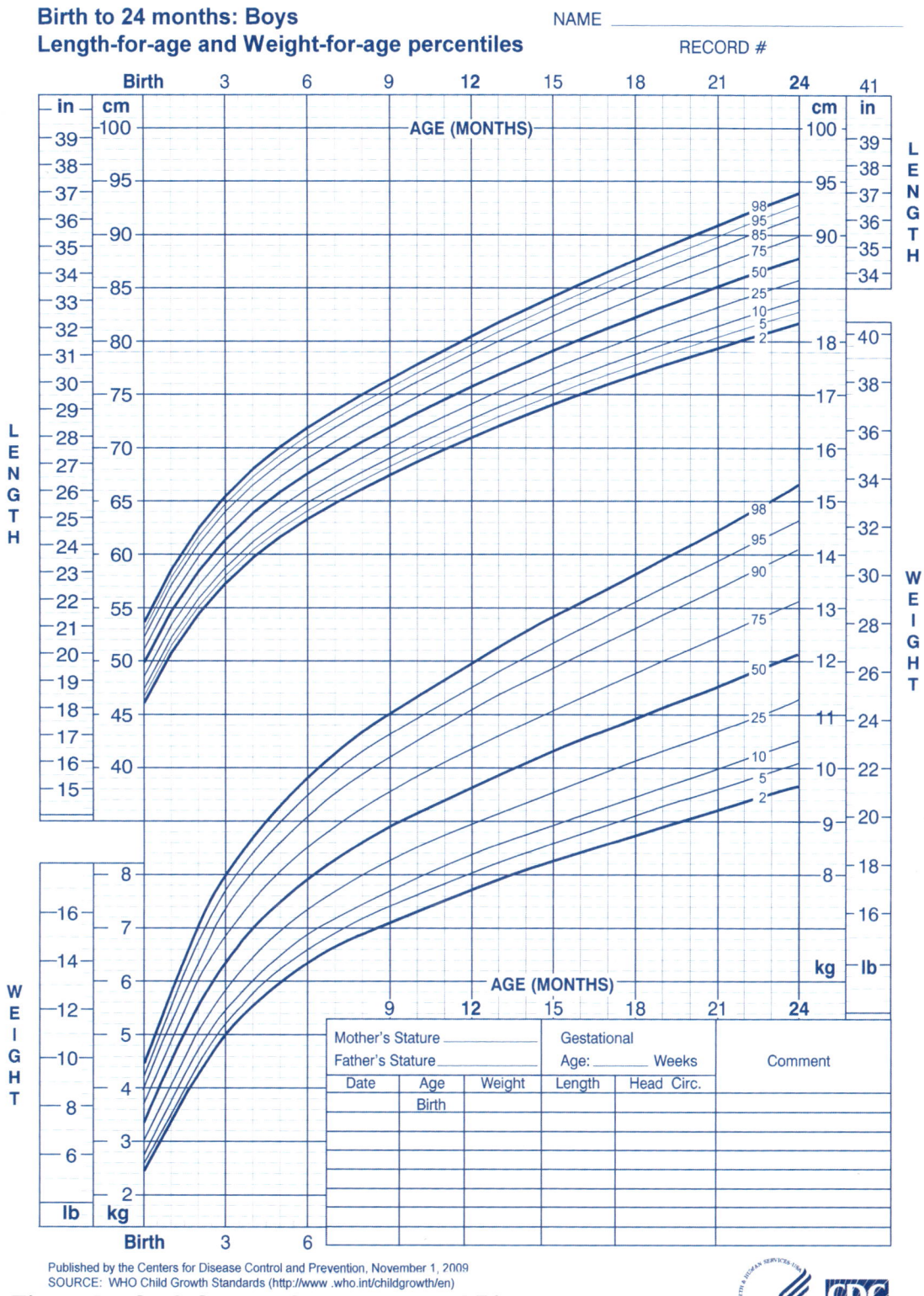

Figure 5.5 CDC Growth Chart Boys aged Birth – 24 Months

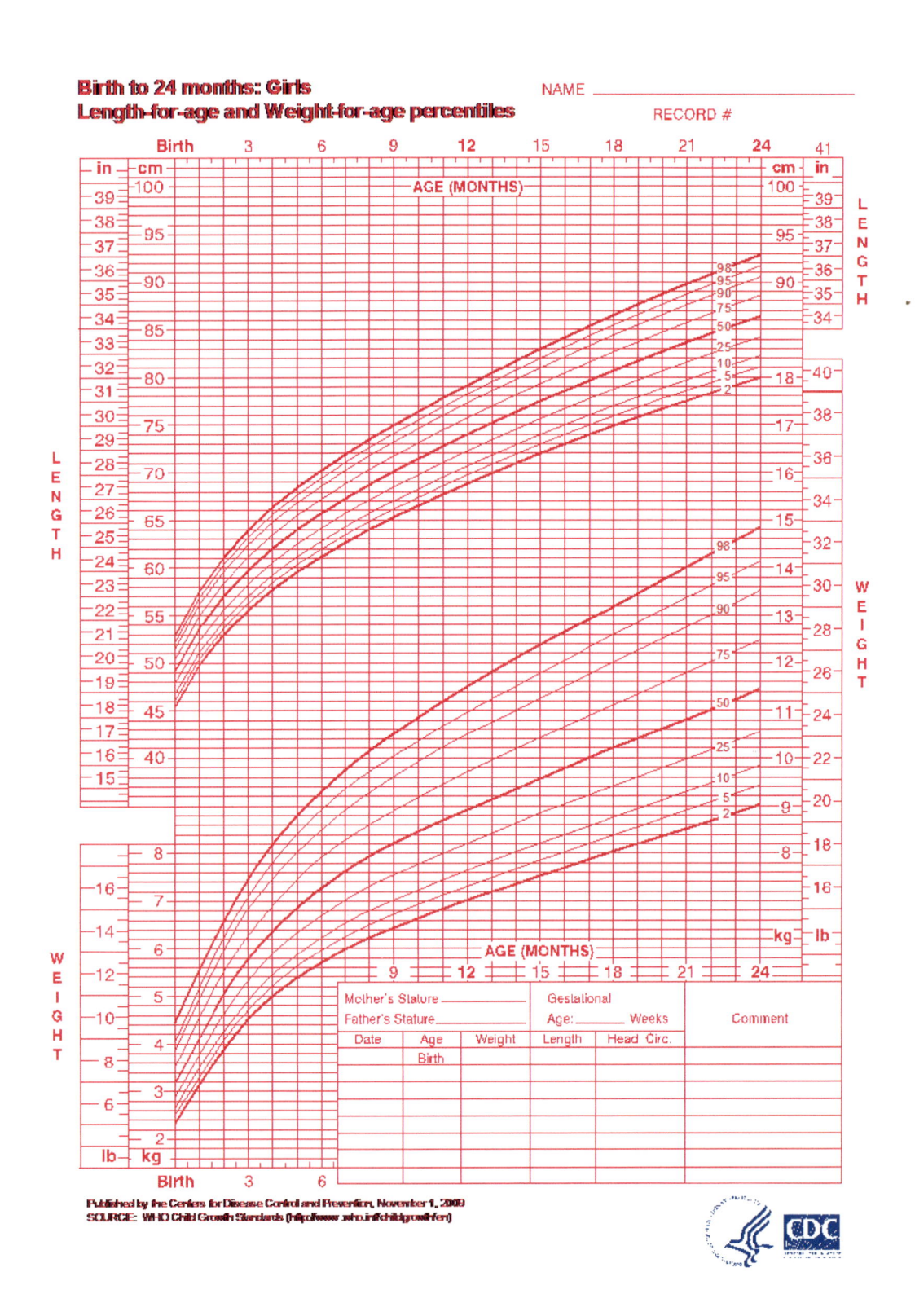

Figure 5.6 CDC Growth Chart Girls aged Birth – 24 Months

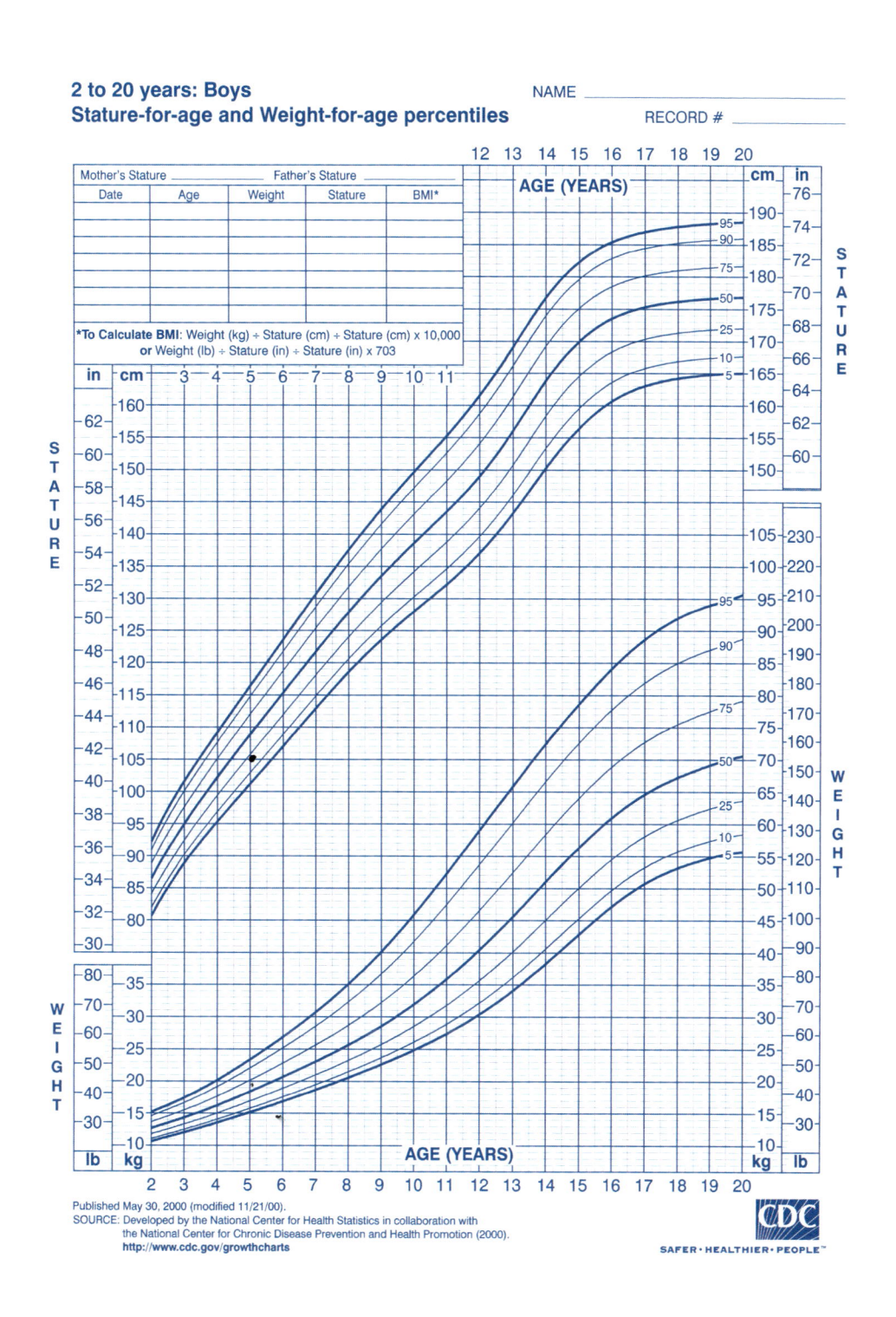

Figure 5.7 CDC Growth Chart Boys aged 2-20 Years

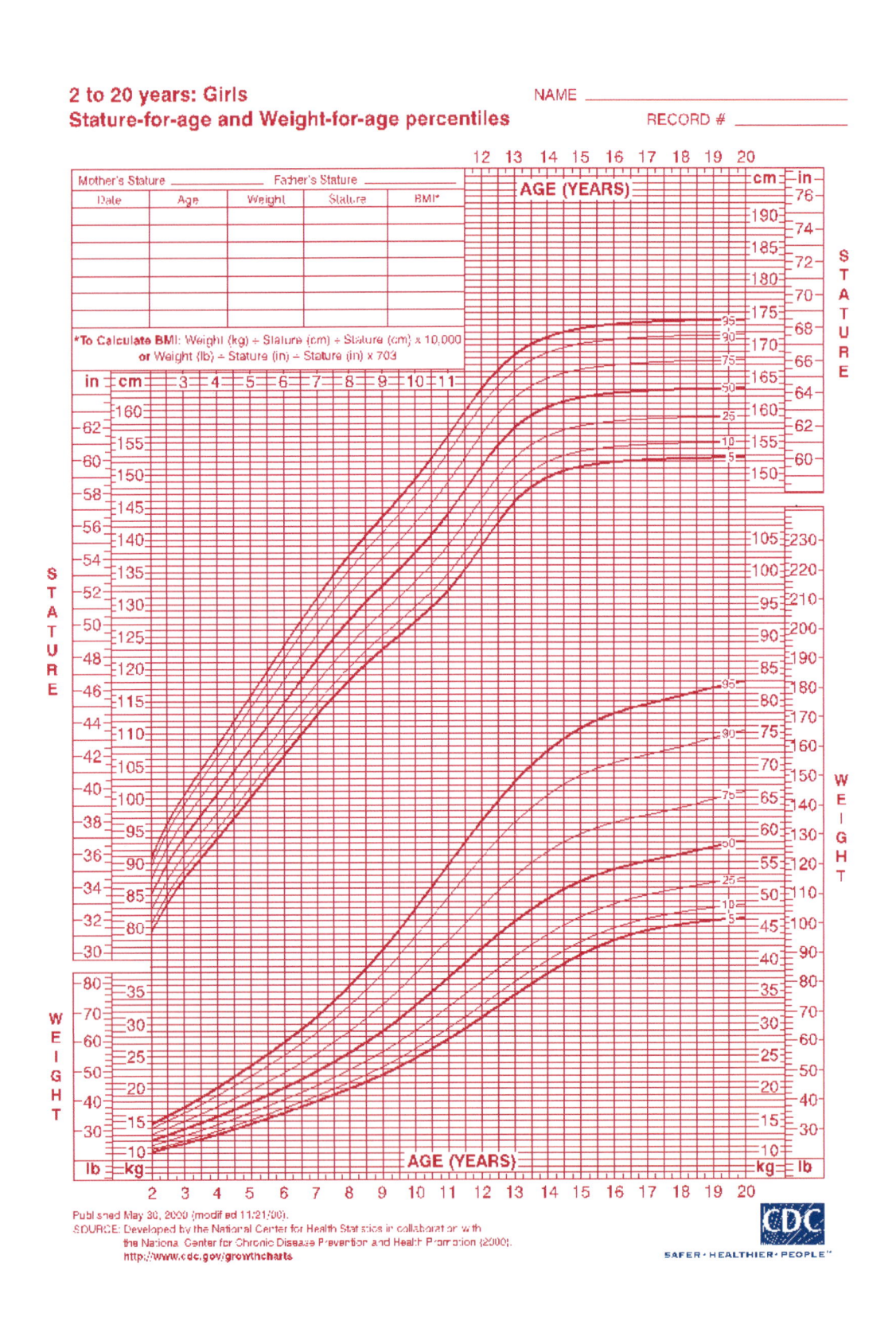

Figure 5.8 CDC Growth Chart Girls aged 2-20 Years

Using the specific weight-for-height percentile curve (**Figures 5.9 & 5.10**) or the BMI percentile-for-age curve (**Figures 5.11 & 5.12**), clinicians are able to more accurately assess the weight of a child, given that it is plotted against its own height. A *"normal stature"*, would be assigned, using either the height-for-age or the BMI-for-age percentile curves, if the height is greater than the 10th percentile and less than the 85th percentile. The most accurate and reliable of the two graphs, is the BMI-for-age; this is the one clinicians are encouraged to use when assessing pediatric patients.[25]

Also, the weight-for-age charts reveal how the children's weights compare with the weights of other children for the same gender and age. It can provide some evidence of emaciation and malnutrition if the weight-for-age percentile is < 5th percentile or it can provide somewhat of an idea of risk of an excessive weight problem if the weight is > 85th percentile.[17b]

It is important to remember, however, that the weight-for-age charts are the most unreliable, as there are too many false positives for obesity and malnutrition. False positive findings conclude there is a problem such as obesity or malnutrition when in fact, there is none.

The height of children and adolescents can also be monitored using the height-for-age percentile growth curve (**Figures 5.7 and 5.8**). It considers the height relative to the age of boys and girls between the ages of 2 and 20.

And while the curves can provide a reasonable estimation of height status between the ages of 2 and 12, the accuracy of these charts are significantly reduced between the ages of 12 and 16 because of the unpredictable growth spurts that affect girls and boys in those age ranges, thus leading to errors in percentile estimates.[27]

For instance, a young girl 13 years of age, who has a sudden growth spurt, could show up on the 75th percentile for height, when in fact she really is at the 50th percentile; this over exaggeration tends to get readjusted to the correct percentile a few years after the spurt. The same example could apply to boys as well, although their growth spurts tend to take place around 15 or 16 years of age.

In contrast with the weight-for-age percentile chart (Figures 6.7 and 6.8), the weight-for-height is actually far more accurate in its weight assessment. In fact, weight relative to height (Figures 6.9 and 6.10) can better predict a greater likelihood of obesity or malnutrition compared to the weight-for-age curve (Figures 6.7 and 6.8). This is because of the greater danger of inaccurately overestimating a child's weight if plotted on the weight-for-age curve; a child could be tall for his age, leading to an erroneous assessment of being overweight when in fact his weight could be perfectly average for his taller height. Hence, growth charts such as the weight-for-height (Figures 6.9 and 6.10) or the BMI-for-age table (**Table 5.4**) or the BMI-for-age percentile curve (Figures 6.11 and 6.12) are more widely used for their accuracy in assessing weights.[25]

In order to minimize the possibility of erroneously drawing false conclusions about body weights in young children, based on percentiles, health care providers consider a weight to be normal if it is situated anywhere greater than the 5th percentile and less than the 85th percentile using the gender and age-specific BMI growth table (**see Table 5.4**) and charts (**Figures 5.11 and 5.12**) or the weight-for-stature percentile curves (**Figures 5.9 and 5.10**).

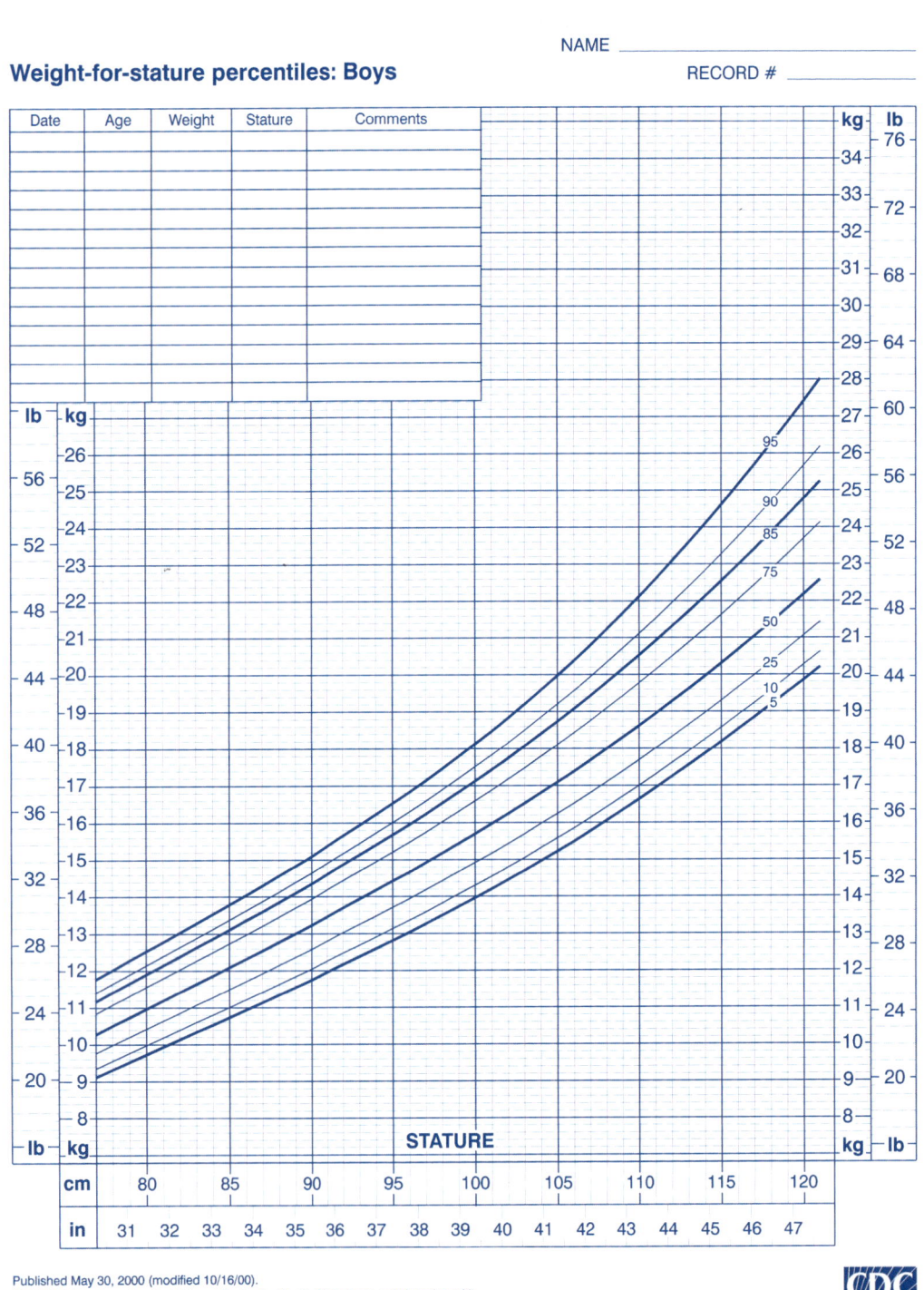

Figure 5.9 CDC Weight for Stature Percentiles: Boys

Figure 5.10 CDC Weight for Stature Percentiles: Girls

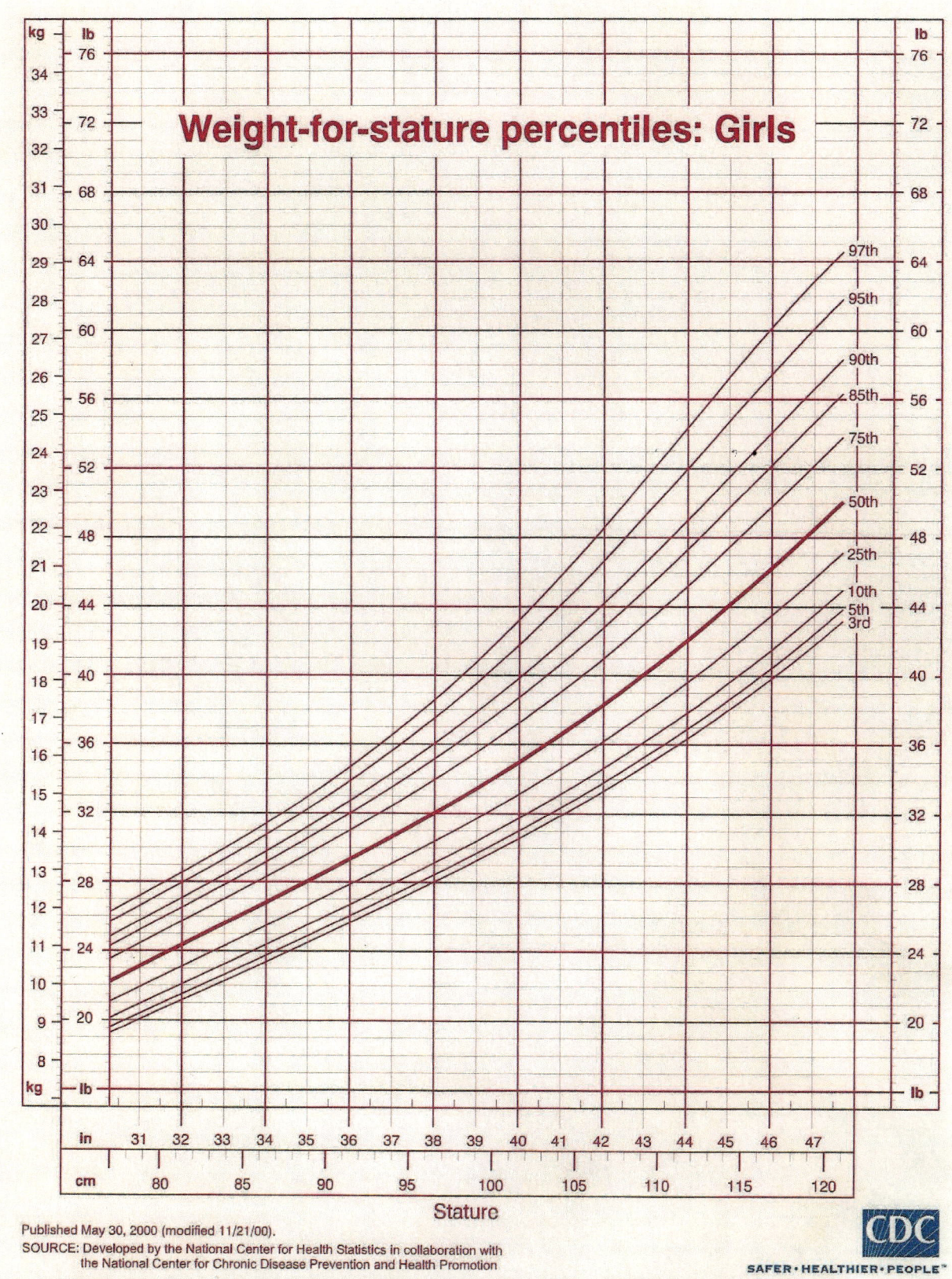

TABLE 5.4 CDC Percentile BMI Growth Table for Boys and Girls from 1 to 5

Nutritional Assessment
Obesity is when BMI> 95th percentile

BMI for children 1-5 years old

Gender	Age	5th	50th	85th	95th
Males	1	14.6	17.2	19.4	19.9
	2	14.4	16.5	18.2	19.0
	3	14.0	16.0	17.4	18.4
	4	13.8	15.8	16.95	18.1
	5	13.7	15.5	16.8	18.0
Females	1	14.7	16.6	19	19.3
	2	14.3	16.0	18	18.7
	3	13.9	15.6	17.2	18.3
	4	13.6	15.4	16.8	18.2
	5	13.5	15.3	16.8	18.3

Reference: Motil et al Sensitive measures of nutritional status in children in hospital and in the field. Int.J. Cancer 1998 suppl 11: 2-9

Source: Center for Disease Control and Prevention. Healthy Weigh-It's not a Diet, it's a Lifestyle! About BMI for Children and Teens. Motil et al Int. J Cancer 1998 suppl. 11:2-9

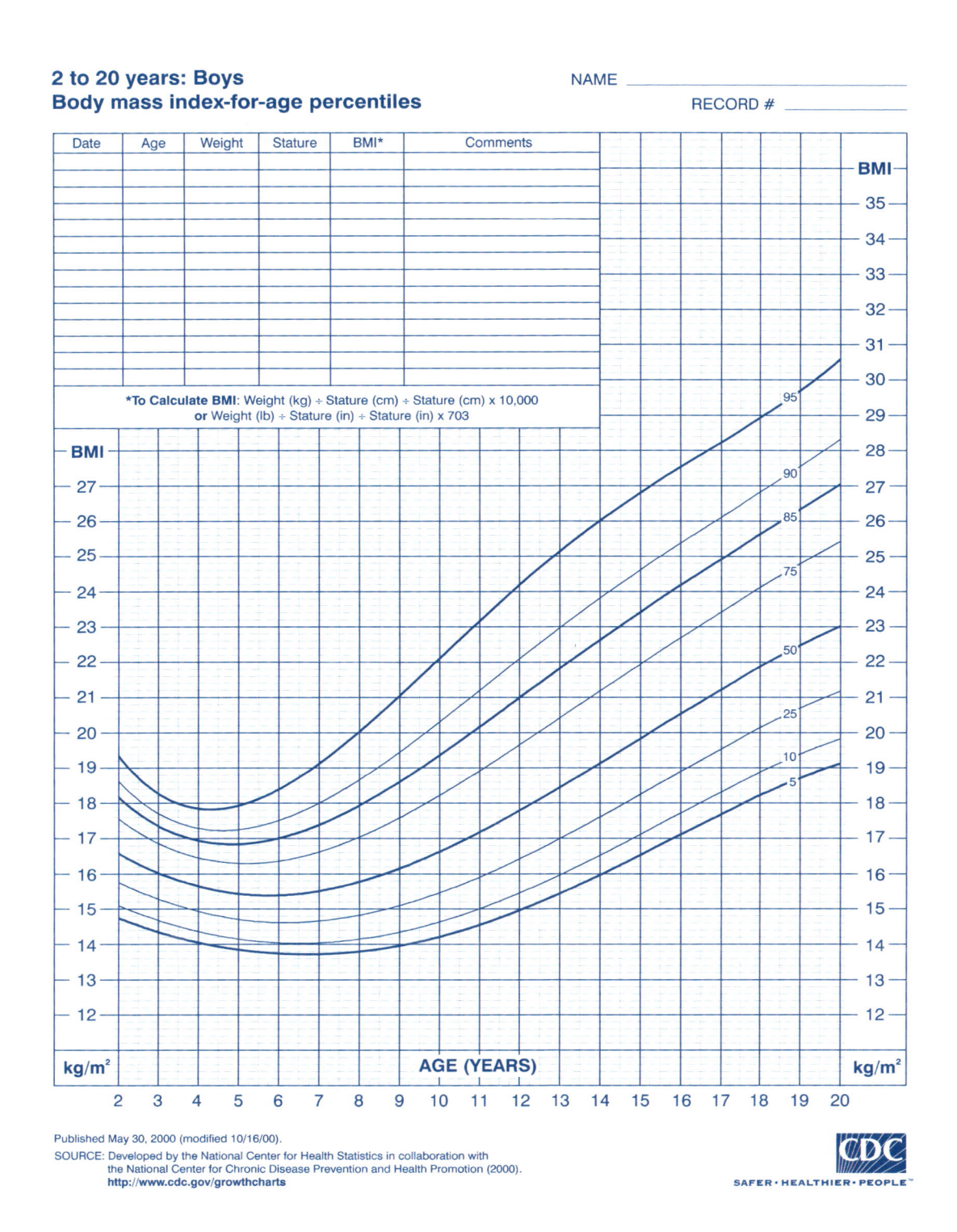

Figure 5.11: CDC BMI Percentiles: Boys ages 2 -20

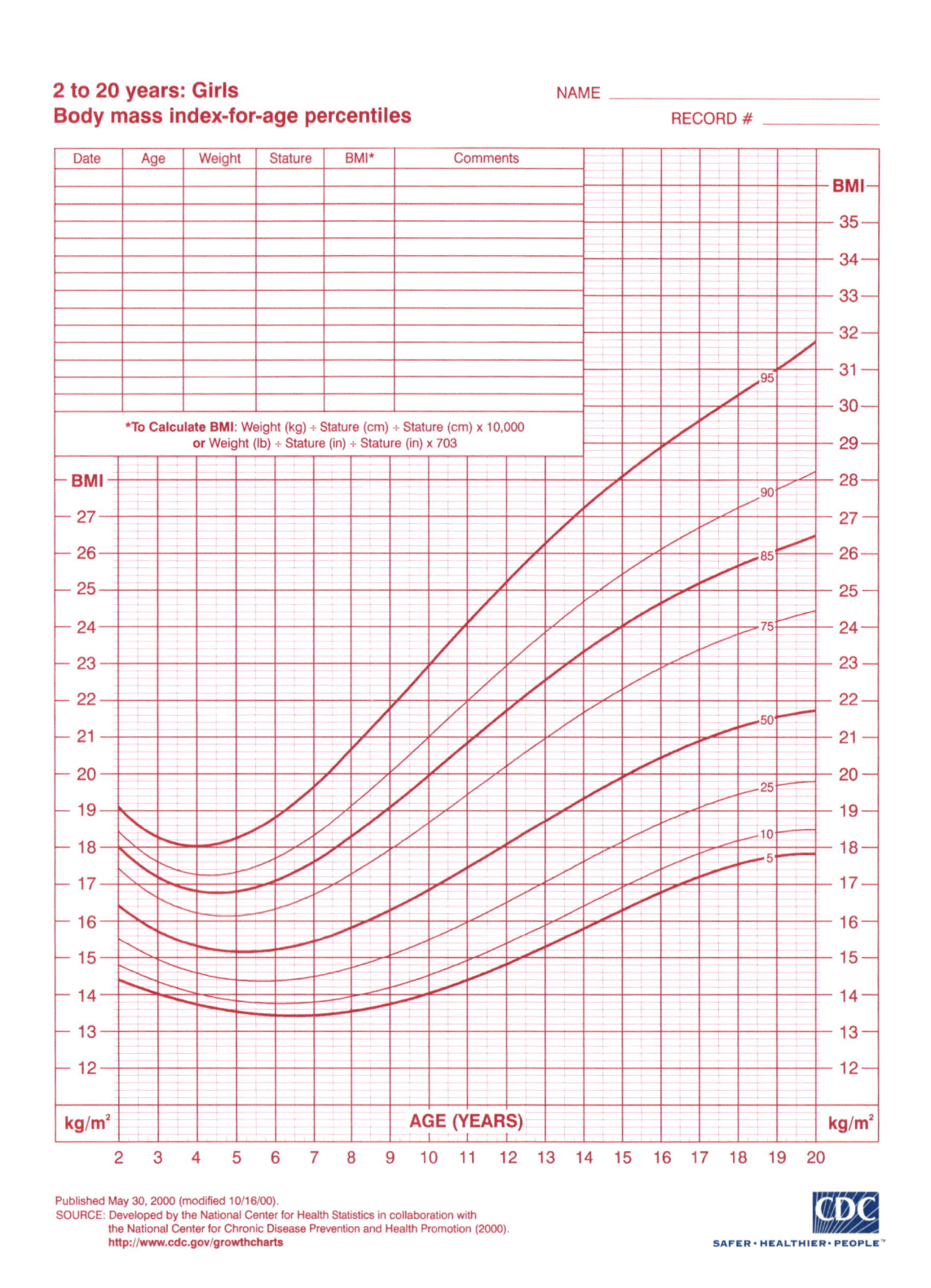

Figure 5.12: CDC BMI Percentiles: Girls ages 2 - 20

The weight-for-age charts (figures 5.7 & 5.8), while providing some indices of weight status, should still be cautiously utilized because of inaccuracies. The consensus is that a child can be at an elevated risk of overweight if he is equal to or greater than the 85th, but less than the 95th percentile. Obese is considered if he equals or exceeds the 95th percentile on the weight-for-height or the BMI-for-age growth curves and chart. The two boys depicted in **figure 5.13** illustrate how they are assessed differently even though they have identical BMIs. Indeed, the 10-year old boy is considered obese with a BMI=23, whereas a BMI=23 for a 15 year-old boy translates into a healthy weight.

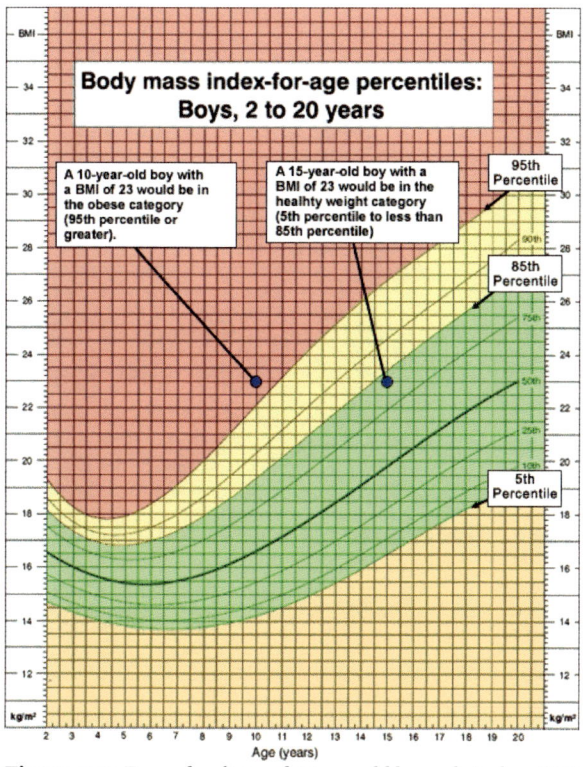

Figure 5.13 Example of 10 and 15 year old boys plotted on BMI for Age Percentile Graph. Source: Center for Disease Control and Prevention. Healthy Weigh-It's not a Diet, It's a Lifestyle! About BMI for Children and Teens.[15]

The jump in the pediatric obesity rates compared to the 5% prevalence in 1960s, suggests a large scale problem, which became more apparent around 1980.

The prevalence of obesity among children and adolescents, however, does vary according to ethnicity and geographic location. When the U.S. 2009 obesity map is examined more closely, 20.9% of American Indian and Alaskan Native children, for instance, were identified as the most obese in the nation.

> About 83% of obese children will become obese adults, carrying with them an array of comorbidities.

The implications are serious because 83% of obese children will eventually become obese adults, afflicted with an array of comorbidities; moreover, up to 25% of obese children suffer from an altered glucose metabolism that can seriously compromise their health.

The growth charts that plot weight-for-height or BMI-for-age can be used to plot a child's weight relative to the expected weight. When the percent is less than 60% of expected weight, then acute or severe malnutrition can be concluded; a percent between 110-119% indicates the patient is overweight; patients would be considered obese if the percent of expected weight varied between 120-140%; morbid obesity would be concluded, if the percent exceeded 140% (**Table 5.5**).

The red dots in **Figure 5.14** demonstrate that the patient's weight relative to expected weight crossed over 2 percentile lines: a notable and significant change requiring some kind of intervention. The clinician is comparing the actual weight to the expected weight at the 50th percentile, as there is no access to medical records in order to know the previous percentile curve. In such instances, the physician defers to a mean 50th percentile as the expected weight. If the patient's historical percentile curve is known, then it is used rather than the 50th percentile. The percent value is determined by dividing the actual weight of 43 Kg by the expected weight of 33 Kg and then multiplying that value by 100. The calculation is shown below:
(43 Kg / 33 Kg) x 100 = 130%
Using Table-4 below, this percent signifies that the patient is at high risk of being obese.

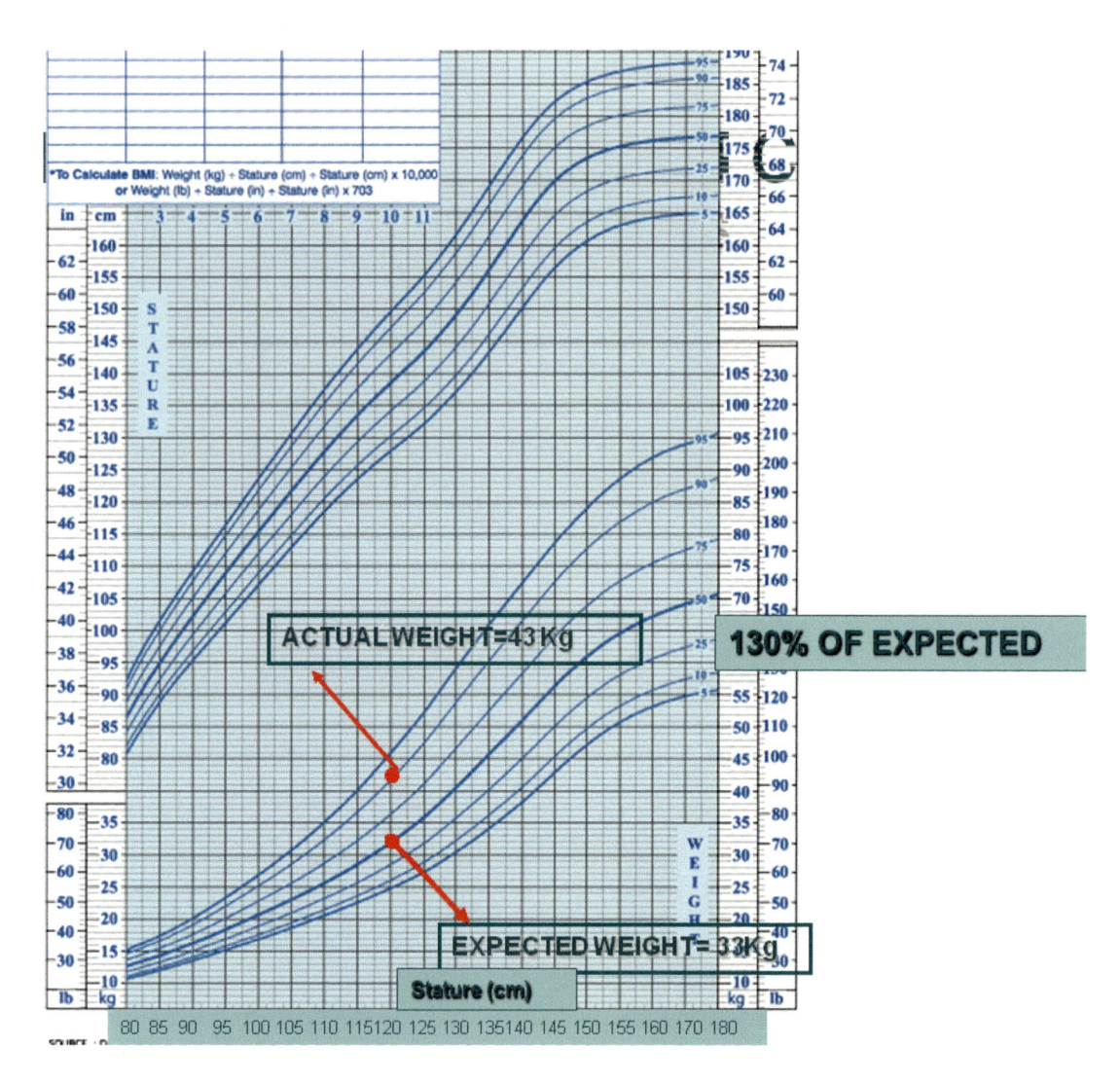

Figure 5.14 Child Body Weight Plotted as Obese Relative to Height in centimeters (cm).

TABLE 5.5 Assessing Weight and Nutritional Status using the Actual Weight Relative to the Expected Weight in addition to the BMI-for-Age Percentile Graph.

% of Usual Weight-for-Ht.	Assessment	Percentile BMI for Age	Assessment
<70%	Severe Malnutrition	<5th Percentile:	Underweight
70-89%	Mild to Moderate Malnutrition	✗	✗
90-110%	Adequate Nutrition	5th - 85th percentile	Health Weight
111-119%	Overweight	≥85th but <95th percentile	Overweight
120-160%	Obese	≥95th Percentile	Obese
>160%	Morbid Obesity	✗	✗

Source-1: Waterlow, JC (1972) Classification and definition of protein-calorie-malnutrition. British Med. J. 3: 566-569
Source-2: Center for Disease Control and Prevention. Healthy Weight, It's not a Diet it's a lifestyle. Retrieved October 18, 2013: http://www.cdc.gov/healthyweight/assessing/bmi/childrens_bmi/about_childrens_bmi.html
Source-3: National Institutes of Health; National Heart Lung and Blood Institute. How are overweight and obesity diagnosed? Retrieved October 21, 2013: http://www.nhlbi.nih.gov/health/health-topics/topics/obe/diagnosis.html
Source-4: Obesity Definition. www.TheFreedictionary.com Retrieved October 21, 2013 from: http://medical-dictionary.thefreedictionary.com/Morbidly+obese
Source-5: Lee, RD and Nieman, DC. (1996) Nutritional Assessment Boston: Mosby 2nd edition p: 454
Source-6: Y Graph Source: http://wellsinceyouasked.com/how-much-should-i-weigh-for-my-age-and-height/http://ygraph.com/chart/591
Source-7: CDC. It's Not a Diet, it's a lifestyle. About BMI for children and Teens. Retrieved on December 6, 2013 from: http://www.heart.org/HEARTORG/GettingHealthy/Nutrition-Center/Dietary-Recommendations-for-Healthy-Children_UCM_303886_Article.jsp
Source-8: CDC: Safer-Healthier People. Overview of CDC Growth Charts: Retrieved December 9, 2013 from: http://www.cdc.gov/nccdphp/dnpa/growthcharts/training/modules/module2/text/module2print.pdf

5.5 The Persistent Growth of Pediatric Obesity

he problem of obesity has become so significant that there are presently growing numbers of adolescents who are becoming morbidly obese (BMI ≥40) and super-obese (BMI≥50). These levels of fatness are likely to threaten the quality of life of these young teenagers. Indeed, more recent studies indicate that they become prone to depression, orthopedic problems such as tibia vara, slipped capital femoral epiphysis, and medical conditions like steatohepatitis, polycystic-ovarian syndrome, pseudotumor cerebri, and biliary disease. Add in the risks of diabetes, fatty acid liver disease, liver fibrosis, obstructive sleep apnea and cardiac hypertrophy, and these kids are looking at a poor quality life, diminished performances in school and work later in their adult years. [55] It is truly the equivalent of a death sentence, and so the medical community is now recommending bariatric surgery for those morbidly obese kids. This is a controversial strategy at best, as many professionals consider this kind of radical approach as futile, since the young patients do not commit to new and healthy lifestyles. The three of the most popular bariatric surgeries performed in the U.S. are: Roux-en-Y gastric bypass (**Figure-5.15**), sleeve gastrectomy and the adjustable gastric band.[9] The FDA has not yet approved the adjustable band in patients younger than 18 years of age.[66]

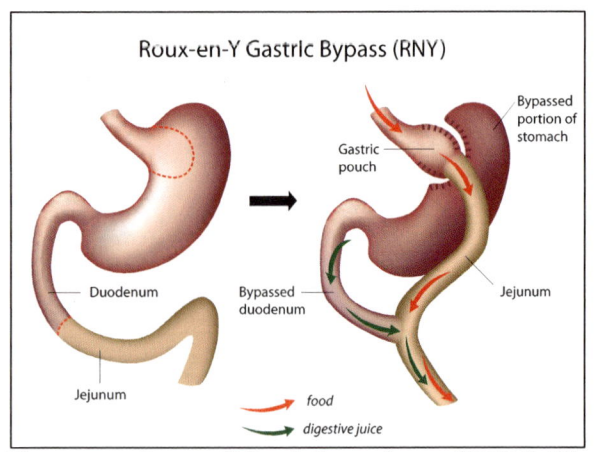

Figure 5.15: Roux-en-Y Gastric Bypass Surgery (RNY) © Alila Medical Media

Nancy Copperman, a registered dietitian from the division of adolescent medicine at Schneider Children's Hospital in New Hyde Park New York, explains that many of the young patients desire very much to lose the pounds in a way that does not involve lifestyle changes. They want an instant fix because they perceive that modifying a lifestyle would simply be too difficult.[66] It is not uncommon for frontline healthcare providers to encounter, either in urgent care or in family practice, a 16-year-old, 5 foot 2 inch teenage girl, weighing over 350 pounds, who presents with an array of medical complications, all originating from the obesity.

> Many physicians and nurse practitioners often do not prescribe diet restrictions for obese patients, nor refer to a dietitian because of a lack of time for counseling.

The physician rarely speaks to the patient about the obesity; there are so many more pressing medical issues to tend to. In many instances, physicians and nurse practitioners do not prescribe diet restrictions nor do they tend to refer patients to dietitians, in part because of time constraints—there is simply not enough time in a 30 minute time slot to discuss diet—but mostly the physician's perception of patient non-compliance is at the center of the problem.[66]

In the end, patients tend to not successfully lose weight and keep it off. Consequently, these morbidly obese young patients are very much left on their own to find the right diet, and they don't generally make wise choices. All too often they select crash diets, a practice that raises concerns since many of these teenagers will tend to overly restrict foods, possibly even starving themselves, therefore causing a further aggravation of the weight problem.[44]

Indeed, research by Stice[87] and Fields[24] suggest that extreme dieting may actually lead to continued weight gain. The problem becomes so overwhelming, that these morbidly obese teenagers, not seeing substantive weight loss over short time-spans, get discouraged and abandon their diet pursuits. Gastric bypass becomes then, a viable alternative that can promise concrete weight loss results that translate into improved blood sugars and blood pressure. In recent years, gastric bypass surgeries have significantly less complications, compared to the 1970s and 80s, and have therefore become a viable alternative.[9] In order to be eligible for surgery, patients must first undergo sophisticated screening that assesses whether previous dietary/lifestyle modifications of some kind had been attempted. The surgical team wants evidence that the candidate tried losing weight for at least six months. Second, the BMI must be 40 or more; third, patients must have reached their adult height, and finally, the candidates must be suffering from health-related problems such as type-2 diabetes or heart disease.[66]

Currently the National Institutes of Health guidelines for bariatric surgery, established in 1991, fail to include guidelines for adolescent surgeries. With the growing prominence of obesity among adolescents, there is interest in using bariatric surgery in order to manage many of the secondary diseases and conditions associated with obesity.

Controversial as a weight-loss strategy, bariatric surgeries, conducted on morbidly obese adolescents, are not a quick fix solution, but rather an extreme strategy to kick start the weight loss process. The problem is that the long-term implications of this kind of surgery, in developmentally immature adolescents, are not known.

> Bariatric surgery for obese adolescents is an invasive treatment option reserved for extreme cases of obesity.

So far however, the few studies conducted on the overall success rates in adolescents, have shown that they are indeed similar to those observed in adults. A five to ten year follow-up study of teenage bariatric surgical patients, ages 12 to 18, concluded that the procedure could be performed safely in adolescents, and that a mean 63% loss of excess body weight was observed in patients.[66] In addition, these patients experienced better socialization and self-image, and an improvement or resolution of their diabetes and high blood pressure.

Most troubling, however, 17% of teenage bariatric patients regained most of the lost weight by 5 or 10 years after the surgery. The primary reason for the weight regain was attributed to frequent snacking of high-fat foods.[66]

5.6 Causes of Pediatric Obesity

But what exactly is going on that our medical community is now considering such drastic and dramatic approaches to curbing the growth of obesity in children? Although bariatric surgery does reduce comorbidities, no one is really asking the question: how did these kids become so shockingly obese in the first place?

Dr. George Bray, a Boyd professor at Louisiana State University, and a professor of Medicine at the Pennington Biomedical Research Center in Baton Rouge, Louisiana, proposes that these paradigms of weight loss and weight gain revolve around energy balance and not changes in the human genome. This becomes obvious since the dramatic growth of obesity in the U.S. has only been going on since the 1980s—a time line regarded as insufficient to cause genomic changes. Bray will admit, however, that energy balance does not explain the whole story. For instance, it does not clarify the gender and eth-nic differences in body fat deposits, nor does it speak on the regulation of food intake, two signifi-cant determinants of obesity. Studies investigating the impact of heritability on obesity,—excluding identical twins studies— have concluded that the heritability factor varies between 10-50% according to Bray.[10]

As we look at the obesity crisis among the American pediatric population, it becomes clear that American children and adolescents live in an environment conducive to low physical activity, with boundless food availability and large portion sizes. The consequence is an inevitable excessive consumption of calories and little energy expenditure. A review of the literature, by Shutz and Jéquier in the 1990s, described a strong consensus that there was a relationship between low physical activity and body fat accumulation in the pediatric population.[83] There is simply no doubt that low activity levels, in children and adolescents, are fueling the crisis.

The million dollar question pertains to what our children are eating and why? Bray and Popkin argue that environmental agents, such as the food industry, are playing a key role in this epidemic.[8] Indeed, food companies have successfully marketed three significant changes to the food supply, and greatly affected our patterns of food consumption since the 1970s.

First, food companies began packaging larger portions and marketing frequent snacking as part of the "***shareholder value movement***" that was initiated, on Wall Street, in the early 1980s. It was a strategy to greatly enhance the short term earnings of shareholders.[61] They introduced highly processed, but tasty snack foods, using aggressive marketing tactics to increase food sales, and consequently changed the snacking habits of Americans. The food industry had effectively dumped such a significant amount of extra calories into the U.S food market that, between 1980 and 2000, the American public had access to an additional 700 kcal/person/day compared to the late 1970s. The U.S. consumer, by the beginning of the new millennium, was snacking in hair salons, bookstores, laundry mats, health clubs, schools and service stations; the total available calories had significantly jumped from 3200 kcals/person/day to 3900 kcals within a 20 year period.[61] Second, around the mid-1970s the food industry began to slowly use high fructose corn syrup (HFCS) in foods and especially sodas, and to promote the high consumption of sweetened beverages, which are the leading cause of obesity worldwide.[73] Dr. Barry Popkin, an epidemiologist at the University of North Carolina, Chapel Hill, interviewed by the English paper, The Guardian, in September 2013, claims that smoothies and juices are, much like soft drinks, contributing a sizable sugar load to the consumer, and raising his risks of heart disease and diabetes. He adds: *"It's kind of the next step in the evolution of the battle. And it's a really big part of it because in every country they've been replacing soft drinks with fruit juice and smoothies as the new healthy beverage. So you will find that Coke and Pepsi have bought dozens [of fruit juice companies] around the globe."*[8]

Finally, the third notable change was the explosion of fast food restaurants around the U.S.; the fast-food industry went into growth-overdrive, all through the 1970s and 80s, registering sales of $110 billion by 2001.[79] Fast food restaurants began to pop up everywhere—McDonald's alone was opening 2000 new restaurants per year[79]—affecting a fairly rapid change in the overall population's dietary habits, and became the most significant acculturative change of the 20th century.[79,88] In just two decades, the U.S. incorporated fast food, that was high in sugar, fat, calories and sodium, into a new cultural reality that drew people to eat food outside the home more frequently. In fact, between the 1970s and 2007, the percent of household food expenditure spent eating out, rose from 34 to 47.9%, a dramatic jump from 1950's estimate of 22%. This growth translated into $537 billion per year in restaurant sales according to the National Restaurant Association.[88] The popular practice of eating out invariably equated to much higher calorie and saturated fat intakes, often reaching between 1100 to 2350 kcals per meal.[88] It should then come as no surprise that studies are now clearly showing that the frequency of eating out positively correlates with weight gain and ultimately obesity.[88]

Popkin's research has shown that snacking frequency in the U.S. has played a big part of the obesity crisis. He advances that the average American child and adult have shifted from eating three times a day in the 1960's and 70's, to essentially 3 daily main meals in addition to two and half to three snacks daily. He claims that around 30 percent of Americans eat between 7 and 10 times a day, causing substantive increases in caloric intake, and an explosion in weight problems in kids.[8, 73]

> **Up to 80% of overweight adolescents currently exhibit one cardiovascular disease risk factor.**

Being overweight for children is a serious matter, as 80% of overweight adolescents currently exhibit one cardiovascular disease risk factor, and that as many as 20% already have two risk factors. The magnitude of the problem is substantive enough, that there is now a medical ethical obligation to screen children, so as to intervene in a timely manner to diminish their risk of heart disease and other medical complications. Internationally, the prevalence of obesity is growing as well. Countries like Mexico, where historically the proportion of overweight and obese has been low, have in recent times seen significant weight gain in their population, especially the women and children. The 1999 Mexican National Nutrition Survey has documented a surprising surge, going from a 33% prevalence of overweight or obese in 1988, to a shocking 59% by 1998. Paradoxically, at the same time, as many as 42% of children were suffering from undernutrition, and it is in the southern rural areas of Mexico that the poor nutrition was most notable.[49]

It is conceivable that, once cardiac risk factors begin to surface early on, such as hypertension, diabetes, hyperlipidemia and hyperinsulinemia, the newer generations will begin to show signs of poor health at younger ages. The problem with chronic diseases is that they are debilitating and cause a diminished quality of life.

Type-2 diabetes is an important disease that progresses from obesity, and that is degenerative in nature; indeed there appears to be a heightened risk of retinopathy and nephropathy in adolescents with type-2 diabetes.[31] In 2002 the cost to manage diabetes came with an alarming price tag of $131 billion in 2002. While it is understood that 90 to 95 percent of all diabetes mellitus patients are type-2, it is important to note that the prevalence of type-2 diabetes is still rare in the less than 10 year old children (0.4 per 100,000 cases). The most numerous cases in the youth, nevertheless, have been observed in the 10-19 year olds (8.5 cases per 100,000).

Type-2 diabetes, a disease that was historically documented in adults over the age of 40, was recognized as a growing problem in U.S. children and adolescents during the 1990s. A study by Pinhas-Hamiel[69] in 1996 found that the incidence of type-2 diabetes, among newly diagnosed diabetic children, jumped from 2-4% in 1982 to 16% by 1994, which, when stratified, represented 33% of the 10-19 year-olds. Since then, the prevalence has steadily increased, with a reported 21% jump in overall prevalence between 2001 and 2009 according to statistics released June 9, 2012 by the American Diabetes

Association. By 2005, close to 45% of newly diagnosed diabetic patients were classified as type-2.[68] The statistics were frightening enough at the national level, but dramatic increases in the incidence could be noted in region-specific medical centers; a 10-fold prevalence hike, in a New York Health Center, between 1990 and 2000, for instance, was discussed by Haine and colleagues.[31] The growth is not expected to relent. Epidemiologists foresee an estimated increase from the 13.9 million diabetics documented in the US in 1995 to an astounding 21.9 million by 2025. This 57% increase is likely to overwhelm the medical financial system.

The prevalence of type-2 diabetes becomes more accentuated if cases are stratified by ethnicity. Indeed, prevalence increases, of between 8 and 45%, have been reported in the population, depending on the ethnic heritage. The American Pima Indians, for instance, are particularly vulnerable with the prevalence of type-2 diabetes reaching 40%, which is 16-fold greater than non-Pima Mexicans.[80] In addition, Pima girls, ages 10-14, are very susceptible to the disease.[49] Between the decades 1967-76 and 1987-1996, the prevalence of diabetes in these young girls jumped 300%.

Also, the Asian Pacific Islanders, Hispanics and the Non-Hispanic blacks, ages 10-19 and residing in the U.S. between 2002-2005, are also specifically at risk, as close to 50% or more of the newly diagnosed diabetics in these groups tend to suffer from type-2 diabetes.

In the UK, the number of children, 18 years and less, diagnosed with type-2 diabetes increased 54% between 1996 and 2003, and first time hospital admissions with obesity jumped 70% during that same time period.[6] Wen the incidence was investigated between 2004 and 2007, rates were 2.5 fold greater compared to the previous study period. The story is most notable in the United Kingdom because researchers also found that the incidence of type-2 diabetes was 3.5 times greater among Asians and 11 times larger in black than in white children.[31]

The time is short, and so we must act in haste to reverse this epidemic. It does appear that government support for community health interventions is needed, if we are, as a society, going to get the upper hand.[88] In the end, the prevention rather than the treatment of this disease seems to be a more affordable and beneficial alternative.[7b]

5.6.1 Large Portion Sizes

Strategies aimed at triggering the hyper growth of the U.S. food industry in the 1980s, represented a true challenge for corporate executives. The problem was that the U.S. market was already saturated with food in the 1960s and 70s, with no visible path for growth. The food industry, nevertheless, began to aggressively market the idea of snacking on tasty foods that were developed by the sophisticated sensory evaluation labs. Suddenly, Americans began snacking on delicious and very addictive foods in bookstores, hair salons, schools, sports facility and mall. The idea of constantly eating became such an important part of the culture that an additional 600-800 kcal per person flooded the market by the year 2000. On average, this translated into kids actually consumed an additional 200 kcal/day, and adults a mean 300 kcal more per day compared to the 1970s. A closer examination of the foods, contributing the most significant calories, forcibly singled out soft drinks and other sweetened beverages as the driving force behind this pediatric obesity crisis worldwide.[7, 61, 73]

Consider that the size of soda containers has gone from the humble 6fl-oz serving bottle, typically seen in the 1950s, to the 32fl-oz serving of the 1990s and 2000, representing upwards of 400 kcal per serving. The problem with consuming larger volumes of soda is that liquids do not trigger the brain's satiety mechanisms the same way that solid foods do, thus facilitating larger calorie intakes by the end of the day.

American restaurants used increased portion sizes as a successful marketing tool—as early as the 1980s—that drew customers into eating and drinking more calories by promoting a false sense of value; visibly the customer got more food at a low cost, and free refills certainly compounded the illusion. The big portion campaign was so successful that the CDC 2006 report concluded that American caloric consumption rose 10% between 1989 and 1998, concomitantly with the growth of portion sizes.[28] This comes as no surprise as research clearly demonstrates that when served larger portions, the customer consumes greater calories. Obese kids appear particularly vulnerable to the negative impact of large portions, possibly because of their inability to identify normal size portions. Having been raised in the 1960s when 6-8fl-oz soda containers were the norm, a customer would be overwhelmed if presented with a 64fl-oz serving of soft drink. Having never seen a 6fl-oz soda bottle, American youth perceive the 64fl-oz soda as normal, and tend to consume it without too much mental anguish.

5.6.2 Sugar & High Fructose Corn Syrup

It probably isn't surprising that there is strong research now linking the consumption of soft drinks to greater risks of obesity and type-2 diabetes. Interestingly, the research sponsored by the soda companies finds no association between sweetened beverages and obesity.[61] What is the rational person to understand from such controversial and contrasting findings?

Scientists and health professionals claim that there is no controversy. In fact, as far back as 1942, the American Medical Association (AMA) already knew that the sugar content of sodas would invariably represent health problems for the American youth.[7a] Today, pediatricians and dietitians are accustomed to seeing obese children and adolescents who consume up to a 1000 kcal/day of soft drinks.[61]

> Ever increasing portion sizes appealed to consumer's sense of value at the detriment of their overall health.

Yet, despite an AMA position paper on the subject of soda, nobody really listened.

Dr. Barry Popkin, a leading epidemiologist in the field of international obesity, points towards sodas as the most influential dietary factor in this epidemic along with frequent snacking.[73] It would therefore be reasonable to push for a curtailing of soda consumption among our children. Consider that sweetened beverages now contain, on average, 10% high fructose corn syrup (HFCS), and that the prominent use of HFCS in sodas is now being regarded as an important source of the obesity and diabetes crisis.[8] In the 1900s, fructose coming essentially from fruits represented only 15g/day or 4% of total calories. Before World War II, fructose consumption had jumped to 24g/day and then to 37g/day by 1977. However, with the introduction of HFCS into sodas by 1994, fructose consumption sharply rose to 55g/day. Currently, when stratified by age, it is estimated that adolescents consume 73g/day.[7b, 42]

The consumption of fructose has in fact increased 5-fold since the early 1900s and doubled since the 1980s. If one considers high fruit juice intake in addition to sodas, the total fructose consumption per capita can be adjusted upwards to 194 g/ day or a total of 156Lbs per year.[42] The initial interest in fructose was fueled by the understanding that intakes of fructose did not increase blood glucose levels. So it seemed like the ideal sweetener for diabetics. However, elevated fructose consumption can drive denovo hepatic lipogenesis or in other words, new synthesis of fat from fructose. In a sense, the overabundance of fructose, consumed through soft drinks, can metabolically overwhelm the mitochondrial TCA cycle, resulting in the abundant synthesis of fat in the liver, leading to steatosis (fatty liver) and inflammation. In fact, when carbohydrate intakes exceed the energy expenditure of the body, hepatic fat synthesis increases 10-fold.[1] Most importantly, both fructose and ethanol metabolically produce reactive oxygen species (ROS) which increase the risk of hepatocellular damage (liver damage).

In response to this overabundance of sugar being consumed by the U.S., the American Heart Association recommends cutting sugar consumption by more than 50%. Health practitioners and dietitians need to revise current sugar intake standards as it is clear that things are getting out of hand. Harnack and colleagues[32] reported in 1999, that 12% of pre-

> Anyone consuming three 32 fl-oz sodas per day is consuming the equivalent of almost a full pound of sugar daily.

schoolers regularly drank a mean 9fluid ounces of soft drink every day. They also noted that as many as 33% of school-aged kids drank 9fl-oz or more per day, and 25% of adolescent ingested as much as 26fl-oz per day. These amounts of soft drink intake are worrisome because they are sufficient to also displace other foods and nutrients such as milk, juices, vitamins A, calcium, riboflavin, phosphorous, folate and vitamin C. Of special concern was the lower calcium to phosphorous ratio, which may cause increased bone resorption (breakdown). Researchers suggest that teenage girls, who consume soft drinks regularly, are especially at risk of suboptimal bone density in later years. Harnack writes:[32] *Epidemiological studies suggest that variations in calcium intake, early in life, may account for a 5 to 10% difference in peak adult bone mass. This difference may subsequently account for a 50% greater risk of hip fractures later in life.* The problem becomes even more concerning because of the abundant use of high fructose corn syrup in soft drinks. High fructose corn syrup doesn't act like other sweeteners. There is now evidence emerging that chronic intake of large amounts of fructose may actually prevent dopamine clearance from the brain. This generates a continued stimulation of the brain to produce additional dopamine, which in turn causes the body to desire more calories despite regenerated energy stores[5, 42, 52]

Simply stated, sweetened beverages need to be removed from school lunches and from the competitive foods sold outside the cafeterias. Very plainly, the kids are consuming too much of it. In fact, thirty-two percent of adolescent girls and 52 percent of adolescent boys are drinking in excess of 24fl-oz per day of soda. It's not hard to figure out the body burden that this load of sugar represents on children. One 10fl-oz soda contains about 10 teaspoons of sugars, totaling 40g of sugar per drink. Many teenagers are now consuming supersize portions that easily reach 32fl-oz on average. The larger portion is 3.2 times more than the standard 10fl-oz drink, used in the early 1990s, and delivers a power punch equal to 128 g (32 teaspoons) of sugar per drink. Imagine consuming three of these drinks per day—a habit easily achieved and maintained by many American teenagers, and possibly one of the reasons their health is deteriorating quickly. Consuming three 32fl-oz sodas per day would amount to ingesting a little over ¾ of a pound of sugar per day or 309 pounds of sugar per year. The impact on the pancreas alone would be alarming, as it would have to hyper-secrete insulin in response to the rapid rush of glucose entering the blood system through the gastrointestinal tract.

The evidence that our children are over consuming soda is troubling, and yet, Coke and Pepsi are still being dispensed from pop machines located at high schools and elementary schools throughout the U.S.

This average amount of excessive calories, consumed regularly by sweetened beverages, is estimated at 200 kcal/day,[61] which translates into 40lbs of sugar/year, and a possible additional 21lbs of weight gain after a year, should the beverage calories be in excess of a person's normal daily calorie needs. Because soft drinks displace other foods and drinks out of the diet[32] it is not uncommon to observe intakes of milk, fruits and vegetables plummet. The end result is an impoverished diet filled, paradoxically, with empty calories. And so, American children and adolescents are becoming obese and malnourished at the same time.

5.6.3 The Introduction of Highly Processed Foods

The food processing industry began, at a large scale, in the mid-19th century as canned food was manufactured for a population that was migrating in great numbers to the cities for work. Families were exiting the rural settings and converging towards the denser urban centers, causing a significant change in lifestyle. It was a time of great ingenuity, and mechanization was driving an industrial revolution in England during the mid-19th century. However, this revolution transitioned over to the United States near the end of the 19th century, and so, much like a vortex, it drew significant talent from Europe, fueling as it were, a second wave of brilliant industrial and technological progress that remains to this day unmatched.

Sterilization of canned foods was one of those advances that help make the food supply safe. Because of the heat treatment used in canning, there was, however, a noticeable loss of flavor in foods. Consequently, spices and flavoring agents began to make their way into many staples to heighten acceptability. England's perfume houses also began to produce a variety of food flavoring compounds that were included in many of those early processed foods. The success of the food processing industry depended greatly on imparting appealing flavors and aromas back into the foods. The second industrial revolution that was unfolding, in the latter half of the 19th Century, attracted the development of a flavoring industry which began to add man-made flavoring agents to baked goods, candies and sodas.

It was understood, early on, by food manufacturers, that food acceptability was greatly dependent on taste and flavor. It was around the 1950s, when processed food sales began to really take off—freezing and dehydration was used throughout the industry—that artificial and natural flavors were added to greater number of foods.

Scientific inventions, like gas chromatographs and mass spectrometers, permitted a much finer recognition and manipulation of food components than ever before. The technology, by the 1950s and 60s, permitted a detection of parts per billion and per trillion of compounds in foods, thus raising the bar of sophistication in food manufacturing. The food industry developed thousands of new products, and the consumer was never happier.

The industry grew from producing 2-3 thousand new foods per year to tens of thousands of novel foods yearly, grossing $1.4 billion in annual sales with most of these foods requiring flavoring agents.

The transformation of the American food supply was so complete by the year 2000, that 90% of the American food dollars were dedicated to purchasing processed foods. International Flavors and Fragrances (IFF), the largest flavoring company in the world, saw its annual revenues grow fifteen-fold since its creation in 1958.

The industry produced artificial flavoring products that imparted very marketable tastes to foods that have now become favorites of the American diet: potato chips, corn chips, breads, crackers, breakfast cereals, ice creams, cookies and pet food.

The technical wizardry involved in flavor development was spellbinding as it truly opened the door to the possibility of producing an altered food supply that tasted absolutely great. Point in fact, methyl anthranilate was used by General-Foods to manufacture grape Kool-Aid; and the strawberry milk shakes produced by Burger King® contained no strawberries. The list of ingredients (**Table-5.6**) utilized in the production of Burger King®'s strawberry milkshake is so extensive that it puts into question the wisdom of feeding these kinds of nutritionally impoverished and chemically-rich foods to children. Since the 1990s Burger King did improve its strawberry shake ingredient list, in the wake of the public alarm that grew from the release of the best seller Fast Food Nation.[79]

TABLE 5.6 Ingredient list of Burger-King®'s Strawberry Milkshake

Amyl acetate, amyl butyrate, amyl valerate, anethol, anisyl formate, benzyl isobutyrate, Butyric acid, cinnamyl isbutyrate, cinnamyl, Valerate, cognac essential oil, diacetyl, dipropyl, ketone, ethyl acetate, ethyl amylketone, ethyl butyrate, ethyl cinnamate, ethyl heptanoate, ethyl heptylate, ethyl lactate, ethyl methylphenylglycidate, ethyl nitrate, ethyl propionate, ethyl valerate, heliotropin, hydroxyphenyl-2-butanone, alpha-ionone, isbutyl anthranilate, isobutyl butyrate, lemon essential oil, maltol, 4-methylacetophenone, methyl anthranilate, methyl benzoate, methyl cinnamate, methyl heptane carbonate, methyl naphthyl ketone, methyl salicylate, mint essential oil, neroli essential oil, nerolin, neryl isobutyrate, orris butter, phenthyl alcohol, rose, rum ether, gamma-undecalactone, vanillin and solvent

Source: Fast Food Nation by Eric Schlosser, Harper Perennial Publishing, New York, 2002[79]

The secret behind the taste sensation that made McDonald's French fries so incredibly unique and flavorful had nothing to do with the type of potato selected, but more with the oil used for frying. Prior to the 1990s, McDonald's used an oil mixture consisting of 7% cottonseed oil and 93% beef tallow. The taste that Americans and the world fell in love with came from the unique taste of meat found in the beef fat. The bad press associated with their choice of a very saturated fat for their fries, forced McDonald's to change their formula to a pure vegetable oil in the 1990s supplemented with a highly secretive meat flavoring agent.

The flavor industry is tightlipped about the identity of their clients, and about the formulas of their various flavoring agents. Interestingly, flavoring companies are not mandated by any kind of FDA regulation to reveal the ingredients of their flavoring agents, which causes some concern about the possibility of meat components being potentially present in flavoring agents. There was a real risk, for instance, of contaminating the purity of meat-free vegetarian food.

In recent years, it is specifically the field of biotechnology that has prompted tremendous advances in flavors. It is the science of organoleptics, specifically, that creates high taste sensation with the goal of repeat customer purchases. The flavor industry no longer uses natural flavors that are extracted from food but rather, rely on fermentation, enzyme reactions, fungal and tissue cultures, to produce newer types of flavors that the FDA now classifies as natural. This is rather surprising, given that they are produced through biological and enzyme-facilitated reactions.[79]

So now the industry can produce dairy flavors that are indistinguishable from the real thing. Grocery shelves now feature butter flavor, fresh creamy butter flavor, cheesy butter and milky butter flavors.

Very realistic meat flavors are now available through heat treatments of sugars and individual amino acids. This has become a multibillion dollar industry, essentially created to produce authentic-tasting synthetic foods that have lost most of their natural ingredients through processes of dehydration, freezing, freeze-drying and canning. The children, now exposed to these foods, with highly developed flavors, become accustomed and trained to seek high taste sensations in these foods that are nothing but a defilement of the food supply; for indeed these enzymatically-derived flavors impart taste that deceive the costumer into believing they are eating something they are not. Rest assured that the cheese-flavored crackers, picked up from the grocery store, do not contain cheese.

5.6.4 Predominance of the Fast-Food Industry

Fast food has profoundly altered the eating habits of the young, and there is really no evidence that their lifestyles or taste preferences permit them to escape from these foods that have become part of the fabric of our culture.

In the 1970s, farm activist, Jim Hightower, warned of the "McDonaldization" of American society. In his book, Eat Your Heart Out, Hightower feared that the unprecedented growth of the fast food industry would result in only a few corporations controlling significant volumes of our food supply. He also felt that the standardization, espoused by McDonald's, would establish a new successful busi-ness model, grounded on standardized products and procedures that would reshape so many other sectors of the economy, and decimate small busi-nesses.

Much of what Hightower talked about did come to pass: McDonalds grew from about one thousand restaurants in 1968 to an astounding thirty thousand restaurants worldwide; McDonald's is the largest beef, pork and potato purchaser in the U.S., and is the second largest procurer of chicken in the country.

The success of the fast food industry was based on a model that ensured fast service, cheap delicious foods, and clean restaurants. There was also a need for cheap access to food, as the trend of women entering the work force, was becoming mainstream.

Indeed, U.S. statistics in 1975 identified that one third of women with children worked outside the home; by the late 1990s that proportion had risen to two thirds, and then to three quarters of mothers leaving home to go to work by 2003.[79]

With fewer mothers at home to prepare meals, the American family began to progressively migrate from the dining room to the fast-food outlets or drive-thrus. It simply made less sense to make home-cooked meals after a full day at work, especially when both parents earned incomes, and the children still had many after-school events, often times scheduled around supper time.

The time crunch was becoming a reality with brutal

> **Fast food was so popular that Americans were spending more money of fast food than on higher education.**

consequences: In the 1970's three quarters of the dollars spent on food in the U.S. was dedicated to meals prepared at home; within a generation, up to

50 percent of those dollars were spent in restaurants which often included fast food outlets. The financial growth of the fast food industry was impressive, going from $6 billion a year in sales in the early 1970s, to $110 billion by 2001. It is not surprising that the fast-food industry is now a controlling force of American agriculture.

Eric Schlosser in his best seller, *Fast Food Nation*,[79] claims that McDonald's acculturated the United States so thoroughly, that the golden arch is now more recognized than the Christian cross. It is so commonplace, that on any given day, 25% of Americans will purchase food at a fast food restaurant, representing 75 million customers per day. Stratifying fast food by age reveals that close to 33% of children and adolescents now purchase fast food on a daily basis.

Very quickly, U.S. children went from consuming 6.5% of their calories from fast food in the 1970s to ingesting 19.2% of calories by the mid-1990s. This is because fast-food has infiltrated every segment of society: high schools and elementary schools, universities, zoos, airports, amusement parks, big box stores, gas stations, and hospital cafeterias just for starters.

Americans spent more money on fast food, according to Eric Schlosser, than on higher education. The problem is that fast food is delinquent in many micronutrients, most notably fiber and phytochemicals, many vitamins and minerals, and is very high in fat, sodium, and sugar. This means that fast food is calorically-dense but has poor micronutrient density. The Big-Mac® contains, for instance, 590 kcal, 35g of fat and a whopping 1090 mg of sodium or 45% of the daily maximum cut-off of 2400 mg. However, the Big-Mac® only contains 3g of fiber, which is about 8.6% of a healthy daily recommended intake of 35g. Unless fruits and vegetables are consumed in abundance along with whole grains afterwards, there is little chance a person could meet recommended fiber intakes by the end of the day.

Taking a broader look at a full meal at McDonald's provides a more comprehensive understanding of the caloric wallop that is contained in a single meal. The assumption here is that a kid could easily consume a Big-Mac®, medium French Fries along with a hot caramel Sundae, containing a total of 2310 kcal, and representing the complete daily caloric needs of many adult Americans. The problem is that such a caloric intake clearly surpasses the energy needs of a typical non-physically active American kid.

The meal package also contains 56g of fat—again meeting the total daily fat requirement of a typical adult; the sodium content of that meal totals 1470 mg, representing 61.25% of the daily maximal allowance. This example of a fast-food meal simply demonstrates how easy it is to consume phenomenal calories in one sitting, and this is what our children are regularly doing.

You may argue that not all kids consume a caramel Sundae, but they certainly can drink either a 32fl-oz or 64fl-oz soda containing 373 kcal and 747 kcal respectively, and shocking sugar loads of 104g and 208 g respectively. It does send the message home more dramatically when these grams get converted into a more conventional and visually more familiar measure like the teaspoon. These quantities of sugar can be converted into 27 and 52 teaspoons of sugar by dividing the gram amounts by 4, as there are 4g of sugar found in a leveled teaspoon.

Consider as well, that a medium Blizzard® from Dairy Queen contains 1020 kcal, and a shocking 40g of fat. There has been, however, a kind of shift, in the fast-food paradigm over the last decade, as the idea of making fast-foods healthier became a more popular way of thinking among fast-food executive, especially in the wake of Morgan Spurlock's "*Supersize Me*," that hit the movie screens in 2004. But even before then, the American Heart Association was pushing for improvements in fat content. Indeed, while one sector of the industry positioned itself to appear as though its menu offered healthier options, the other sector offered foods that made the term "abomination," appear mild by comparison.

Hardee's® 2/3lb Monster Thickburger® is considered by some as a heart attack meal, packing 1320 kcal and a total fat load of 95g; it is considered by others as a healthy choice as it was a meal that met Doctor Atkins' diet prescription for a low carbohydrate meal. Most people simply did not eat the hamburger bun but only the meat and the fat. It's almost as if the marketing strategy was not to appear healthy, but rather to appeal to the "living dangerously" inclination of men; the Monster Thickburger® is an invitation to men to be real men who are seeking some risk and a high taste appeal and sensation.

This is a truly a paradox if we believe that every individual only wants to eat what is good and healthy. It is this perversion of the senses or more specifically of the pleasure center of the brain that has, since the 1960s, slowly caused a deviance in the eating habits of Americans. The concern about the dietary practices of American youth is serious because atherosclerotic development begins in youth, and comes to completion with the formation of arterial plaques some 20 to 30 years later. Consequently, prevention strategies strongly support intervening early in the life of children in order to effectively decrease cardiovascular risk factors later in life. The American Heart Association (AHA) revised its dietary guidelines for youth in 2005 (**Table-5.7**), in light of the growing obesity crisis among children and adolescents.

TABLE 5.7 Dietary Guidelines for American Youth Older than 2 Years of Age and Applicable to Families

===
1. **Balance dietary calories with physical activity to maintain normal growth**
2. **60 Minutes of moderate to vigorous play or physical activity daily**
3. **Eat vegetables and fruits daily, limit juice intake**
4. **Use vegetable oils and soft margarines low in saturated fat and trans fatty acids instead of butter or most other animal fats in the diet**
5. **Eat whole grain breads and cereals rather than refined grain products**
6. **Reduce the intake of sugar-sweetened beverages and foods**
7. **Use nonfat (skim) or low-fat milk and dairy products daily**
8. **Eat more fish, especially oily fish, broiled or baked**
9. **Reduce salt intake, including salt from processed foods**
===

Source: Gidding, SS et al. Dietary Recommendations for Children and Adolescents A Guide for Practitioners Consensus Statement from the American Heart Association, Circulation 2005; 112:2061-2075

5.7 Recommended Treatments for Pediatric Obesity

There are five main strategies that could be followed in order to assist children and adolescents in reshaping their eating habits and lifestyles in compliance with AHA guidelines,[3] (**Table 5.7**) with the intent of lowering their BMIs or realigning the percentile mark to under the 85th percentile on the weight-for-height or the BMI for age curves.

First Dietary Change: Regularly Consume Breakfast. Breakfast is considered the most influential meal of the day. Research certainly supports the notion that breakfast eaters have, in general, improved nutrition profiles compared to those individuals who purposely skip breakfast (**Figure 5.16**). The USDA's National Food Consumption Survey (1977-1996) noted a significant decline, among children of working mothers, in the frequency of consuming breakfast. This has also been confirmed in findings from the Bogalusa Heart Study (1973-1994).[33]

Also, cereal consumers tend to eat overall more milk and more calcium compared to non-cereal consumers. For children, the AHA recommends 2% milk right up to the age of 1 in order to favor continued brain development, as fat plays such a critical role in the expansion of neurological networks after birth.

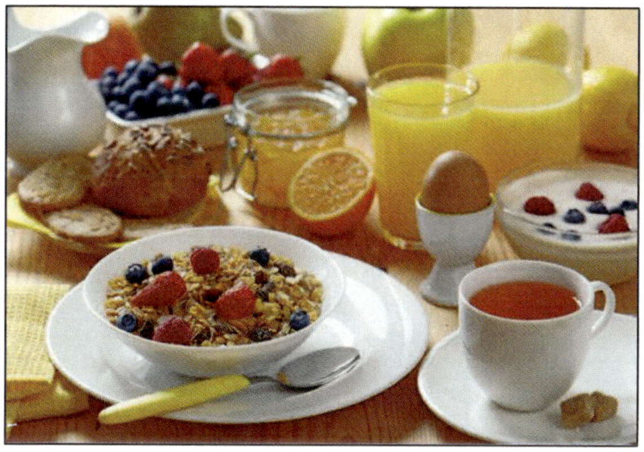

Figure 5.16: Healthy Breakfast with Fresh Fruit and High Fiber Cereal © MaraZe

Other countries like Canada encourage 2% milk right up to age 3 which is understood to be the time at which brain and neurological growth ceases.

Nevertheless, there are increasing numbers of children and adolescents who make it to school without having eaten a breakfast. Doctor Song, a research scientist in the department of Food Science and Nutrition at Michigan State University, reports that 20.5 % of 9 to 13 year-olds and 36.1% of 14 to 18 year olds frequently skip breakfast.[84]

A typical breakfast cereal, suitable for children and adolescents in today's fast-paced society, should include either a ready-to-eat breakfast cereal low in sugar or at least high in fiber. This means that it should include a minimum of 20% of the Daily Value (DV) for fiber or 5g of dietary fiber per serving or more.

Our diets are so refined that most children and teenagers would not find it possible to meet the minimum daily requirement of 25g of fiber/day. That goal is next to impossible to meet without the assistance of ready-to-eat high fiber cereals. The following ready-to-eat breakfast cereals contain excellent sources of fiber, and should be consumed regularly by children, adolescents and adults (**Table 5.8**).

It is remarkable that the nutrient content claims, featured on the breakfast cereal boxes, sometimes either falsely exaggerate how much of the nutrients are actually in the cereal or describe the nutrients as more wonderfully unique than they actually are. For instance, a study published by Schwartz and colleagues[81] in 2008, reported that on average, the breakfast cereals, claiming to be whole grain, only contained 1.4g of fiber per 1oz-wt serving, an amount considered to be a borderline poor source of fiber as it is just over the 5%DV cut-off. Cereals with the content claim: "low in fat," signify that they are 40% lower in fat compared to the mean of other cereals, however, the average fat per 1oz-wt serving for all breakfast cereals are under 3g per serving, and therefore are already legally low in fat.

So in the end, the advertised claim of being low in fat, actually applies to almost all ready-to-eat breakfast cereals. Schwartz and colleagues also reported that children's breakfast cereals contained on average 8% more energy, 15% more sodium and 52% more sugar compared to adult cereals. These findings reveal the misleading nature of mass marketing campaigns, promoted by the food industry. In the end, the food has to taste good if these companies are going to sell any. The Alliance for a Healthier Generation, which brings together professionals of the food industry and health professionals, has established healthy guidelines for competitive foods in schools. These guidelines suggest that foods in schools should contain 35% or less of calories from fat, 10% or less of calories from saturated fat, 35% or less of their weight from sugars, and should not exceed 230 mg of sodium per serving.

The breakfast cereal research, conducted by Schwartz, found that only 35% of children's cereals were in full compliance with these guidelines, a stunning outcome that seriously puts into question the intentions of breakfast cereal companies, especially since up to 56% of adult cereals did respect health content guidelines.[81]

In addition to a breakfast cereal, children and adolescents need to consume at least 1 to 2 servings of fresh fruit. Juices are generally discouraged throughout the day but certainly one 4fl-oz serving of a fruit juice is acceptable at breakfast; it is simply wrong to think that juices can serve as hydration throughout the day.

TABLE 5.8 Breakfast cereals that are excellent sources of fiber (20% or more of DV)

Breakfast Cereal	Serving	Kilocalories	Fiber (g)	Sodium (mg)
Fiber One Original	½ cup	60 Kcal	14g	105 mg
All Bran Buds ®	½ cup	70 Kcal	13g	200 mg
Kashi® GoLean	1 cup	140 Kcal	10g	85 mg
Grape-nut® Original	½ cup	200 Kcal	7g	290 mg
Raisin Bran	1 cup	190 Kcal	7g	320 mg

Shredded Wheat® Original	2 biscuits	160 Kcal	6g	0 mg
Cracklin" Oat Bran	¾ cup	200 Kcal	6g	150 mg
Chex® Multi-bran	¾ cup	160 Kcal	6g	270 mg
Mini-Wheats ®	5 biscuits	180 Kcal	5g	5 mg
Flax Plus ® Multi-bran	¾ cup	110 Kcal	5g	135 mg
Great Grains® Raisin, Dates & Pecan	¾ cup	200 Kcal	5g	160 mg
Bran Flakes	¾ cup	90 Kcal	5g	210 mg
Total® Raisin Bran	1 cup	160 Kcal	5g	230 mg
Crunchy Oatmeal Squares	1 cup	210 Kcal	5g	250 mg
Chex® Wheat	¾ cup	160 kcal	5g	300 mg

Source: Stephenson, J & Bader, D. Health Cheques TM Carbohydrate, Fat & Calorie Guide 4th Edition Appletree Press Inc Mankato MN 2012 pp139[86]

Juice is erroneously seen as a suitable method of hydration because it is naturally extracted from the orange, and a good source of nutrition. Excessive juice intake can be a problem because of the elevated sugar content found in each 8floz serving. Whether it's in soda or pure orange juice, sucrose, if consumed in abundance, can overtax the biological system.

Rather, fruit juice needs to be considered, much like milk, as a food. Consider that one ½ cup of orange juice contains a suitable 15g of sugar, but when a liter of juice is consumed over an entire day there is a potential to ingest 120g of sugar or 30 teaspoons of sucrose. This quantity of juice represents a considerable amount of added calories, and doesn't quite quench the thirst completely. Also, the fiber content and sense of satiety experienced with fruit intake are far better than with juice.

Second Dietary .Change: Consume Greater Varieties of Fruits and Vegetables.

Choices of fruits and vegetable are very narrow among American youth. Kid's taste buds are competing with food products with high taste sensation that overshadow the delicious, but more subtle-tasting fruits. It becomes a true dietary nightmare when the youth are unable to diversify their vegetable intakes as indicated in **Figure 5.18**. It is indeed, in this graph, that we see the true tragedy of the North American diet: 56% of the vegetables consumed by our young are potatoes with 46% prepared in the form of fried potatoes. The potato has dominated the food industry in the United States over the last 30-40 years to such an extent that it caused a tremendous growth in the frozen food industry. This is another example of the powerful influence the fast-food industry wields in the U.S.—it forcefully orchestrates and controls agriculture beyond what would appear to be reasonable.

The fact that only 8% of the youth include dark green and other colored vegetables (Figure 46) in their diet is a testament to the insidious way in which French fries have taken over menus in restaurants, school cafeterias and homes. The School Lunch Program in the U.S. affects some 32 million children per year, and so it make sense that First Lady, Michelle Obama, would champion the cause of increasing the nutrition quality of school lunches in the U.S. as part of her fight against childhood obesity. But the fight is not easy. An amendment to the Federal School Lunch Program, presented before the Minnesota House in January 2012, intended first, to declassify pizza from being recognized as a vegetable, according to School Lunch Program standards; second, to no longer define French fries as a vegetable, and third, to limit the number of times potatoes and French fries could be offered per week on a school menu.

From the outset, it seems like a strange amendment, but in truth it reveals the rather ludicrous nature of our laws, for indeed, in 2003, while President George W. Bush was in power, the USDA recognized French fries as a vegetable. The French Fries industry lobbied the USDA for at least 10 years to revise the Perishable Agricultural Commodities Act (PACA) in order to recognize frozen French fries as a perishable product. From there, the Frozen Potato Product Institute appealed to the USDA in 2000 to alter its definition of fresh produce, in order to now include fries. This was a stretch of the imagination at best, but for an industry thirsty for more growth, it was a brilliant move.[48] In 2003 the courts ruled that French fries were indeed a vegetable using the "batter-coating rule" which contends that simply rolling a potato slice in batter and then frying it was the equivalent to waxing a cucumber. This 2003 ruling shaped the way we have been feeding our children for close to a decade now.

The idea behind the 2012 Minnesota amendment was that legislators needed to recognize that pediatric obesity was getting out of hand, and that Americans needed to start feeding their children more vegetables and fruits as part of a healthy diet. But like so many attempts at fighting the food and beverage industries, this one failed as well. Wilson and Roberts write in Reuters in 2012: *In contrast, the Center for Science in the Public Interest, widely regarded as the lead lobbying force for healthier food, spent about $70,000 lobbying last year -- roughly what those opposing the stricter*[nutrition] *guidelines spent every 13 hours, the Reuters analysis showed.*[98]

Since Obama took office in 2009, the food and beverage industry has spent $175 million in lobbying efforts to fight taxes and marketing restrictions that have been levied at them, as public demands for healthier food are increasingly heard. There is not one battle they have not won, the Reuters' investigation claims.

Yet, nutritional scientists attest that specifically dark-colored vegetables are needed for good health, since they are richer in phytochemical content, and it is phytochemicals like flavonoids, phenolic acids, phytoestrogens and organic sulfur compounds, that offer various levels of protection against cancer and heart disease. And so it baffles the mind that the Minnesota House rejected the amendment, ruling in favor of continuing to recognize pizza and French fries as vegetables.[98] Corey Henry, the spokesperson for the American Frozen Food Institute, referred to the ruling as a victory, but for whom? Amidst the childhood obesity epidemic, a 2007 USDA report, documents very clearly that French fries and pizza are the two most commonly consumed foods in U.S. schools. So it was, in fact, a monetary victory for the Frozen Food Industry, but a grand defeat for those fighting against childhood obesity. Margo Wootan, nutrition policy director at the Center for Science in the Public Interest, clearly understands that the ruling is not good for children but sarcastically claims *"but it's good for companies that make pizza and French fries."*

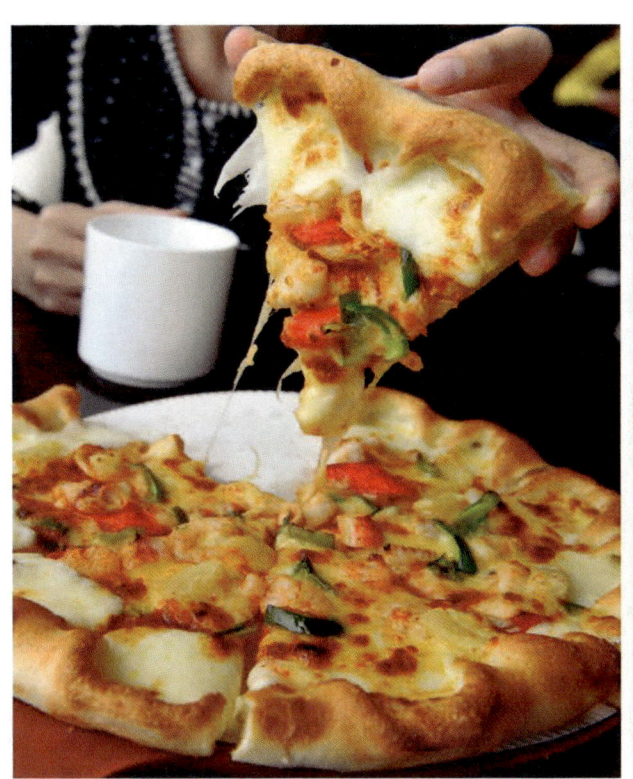

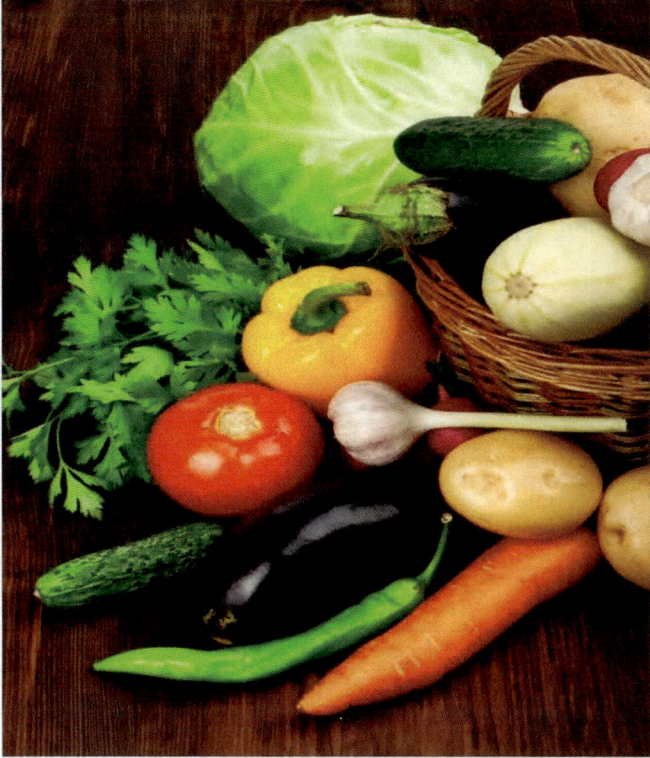

Figure 5.17: Fresh Vegetables displayed around a wooden basket © Sergiy Telesh. Combined with hand taking single slice of Italian pizza © hxdbzxy Which of these are legally vegetables?

This kind of failed amendment truly reflects the perverted nature of our political system certainly, but is a likely reflection of a loss of a social moral compass that reaches deep within the social construct right down to the family. It is here that the true failure has occurred for indeed, parents feed their children pizza and French fries regularly, and so then, why is it not correct to continue feeding the children what they are already receiving at home? This is the ultimate argument for why the obesity epidemic is not about to end any time soon; we have forgotten how to feed our children, and so the definition of vegetables can be redefined using relativistic notions that corrupt the purest of intents, that of feeding the children. In the end, **Figure-5.17** is a true conceptual test that many would likely fail.

It does not matter how you look at it, we are failing as society to properly nourish our children, and consequently, we are about to pay the price through significant spikes in chronic diseases in the next 10-30 years, unless we able to turn this mess around. Two food groups need to be promoted to a far greater degree than ever before: fruits and vegetables. It is the blueberries, raspberries, blackberries, the pineapples, peaches, apricots, and apples that need to replace those nasty desserts that we have been feeding our kids; these fruits contain profoundly protective phytochemicals. Flavonoids, for instance, tend to be elevated in berries, black and green tea, purple grapes and juice, citrus fruits, olives, soybean and whole-wheat. Similarly vegetables such as garlic, leeks, onions and cruciferous vegetables (broccoli, cabbage, and cauliflower) are all elevated in organo-sulfur compounds consisting of indols and isothiocyanate; these are the phytochemicals that protect against a wide variety of cancers.

There is in fact only a very narrow window during which taste preferences can be developed and formed in infants and toddlers; afterwards, the occasions to expose young children to good healthy nutrition practices become rarer, because highly processed foods, with abundant flavoring and coloring agents, dominate the marketplace.

These foods look attractive to children and have delightful flavors, consequently making a varied fruit and vegetable intake near impossible. NHANES 2000 concluded that as many as 79% of the youth do not meet minimum recommendations for healthy fruit and vegetable intakes.[56] The AHA identify fruits and vegetables as essential dietary components that needs to be included in the diet of the young if a reversal of obesity, diabetes and heart disease is to occur in this country.

"Serve a variety of fruits and vegetables daily, while limiting juice intake. Each meal should contain at least 1 fruit or vegetable. Children's recommended fruit intake ranges from 1 cup/day, between ages 1 and 3, to 2 cups for a 14–18-year-old boy. Recommended vegetable intake ranges from ¾ cup a day at age one to 3 cups for a 14–18-year-old boy". (Source: Dietary Recommendations for Healthy Children—American Heart Association AHA):[4]

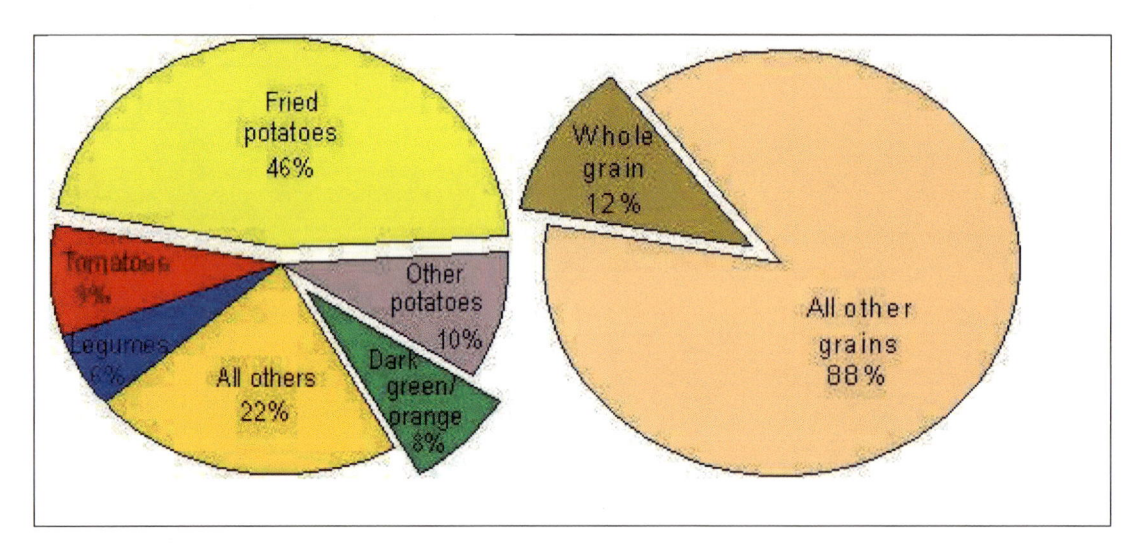

Figure 5.18: Intake of vegetable and whole grain consumption among children 2-19 years of age

Source: National Health and Nutrition Examination. Survey 1999-2000, NCHS, CDC[31]

Third Dietary Change: Increase the Intake of Whole Grain Products The NHANES 1999-2000 survey also reveals that only 12% of American youth regularly consumed whole grains (**Figure 5.18**). Poor whole-grain consumption by the young is troubling and is really the reflection of taste preferences that were cultivated and formed at very young ages **(Figure 5.19)**.

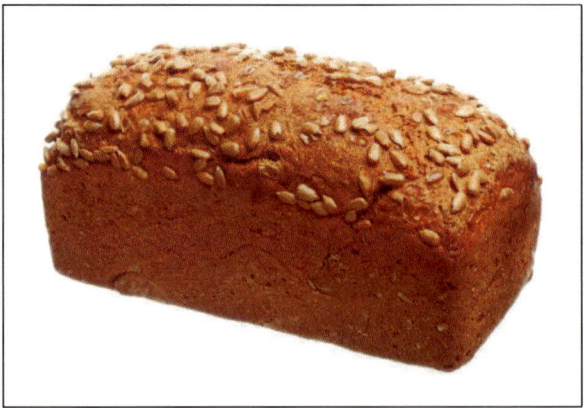

Figure 5.19: Whole Wheat Traditional Bread © L Saloni

Again, the AHA has clear directives for parents:

Serve whole-grain/high-fiber breads and cereals rather than refined grain products.

Look for "whole grain" as the first ingredient on the food label and make at least half your grain servings whole grain. Recommended grain intake ranges from 2oz-wt/day for a one-year-old to 7oz-wt/day for a 14–18-year-old boy.[4]

Whole grain products are important for the simple reason that they provide greater satiety and contribute significant amounts of fiber, which is essential for the health of the gastrointestinal tract. Furthermore, they tend to be nutritionally more complete, especially if they are not heavily processed.

Fourth Dietary Change: Decrease the Amount of Total Fat and Consume Healthier Oils.

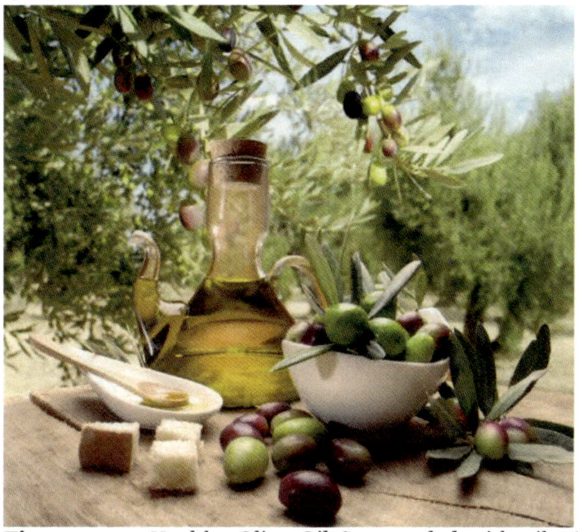

Figure 5.20 Healthy Olive Oil Surrounded with oils © JIL Photo

Fats and oils are considered essential for normal growth and development. The emphasis should be on ensuring that healthy oils are ingested by children. Olive oil (**Figure 5.20**) is considered one of the best oils for human consumption; it tends to decrease the risks of both cardiovascular disease and some cancers. Also, fat often becomes the vehicle through which fat soluble vitamins are absorbed and large quantities of calories are ingested. Because there are 9 kcal for every gram of fat, children can consume frightful levels of calories in one sitting, especially when exposed to fast foods, snack foods and desserts, on a frequent basis.

Given that snack, and fast foods are easily accessible to most children, it cannot come as a surprise that fat intake can rise so dramatically within a day. Consider that a large French fries from Burger King® contains 540 Kcal and 27 g of fat which is the equivalent of almost 5 1/2 teaspoons of oil.

These are hidden calories that become potentially dangerous for a child, over the long time, as fat gradually creeps on to the body. Putting total daily caloric requirements into perspective can help understand to what degree certain foods become significant calorie contributors.

The AHA strongly encourages parents not to overload their children with excessive calories, a practice that is all too common within the North American context. For instance, an infant right up to 1 year of age requires 40-50 kcal/lb of baby weight. Using the body weight-for-age percentile growth curves, a 6 month infant situated at the 50th percentile would weigh approximately 16 pounds; the typical caloric need for this infant would vary between 640 to 800 kcals per day.

Once children progress to the ages of 1 to 8 years of age, caloric needs vary between 1000 and 1742kcal per day according to Dietary Reference Intakes (DRIs) and activity levels. Children ages 9 to 13 years of age tend to jump up to between 1600 to 1800 kcal per day if leading sedentary lifestyles, but up to 2200 kcal if physically active. On the other hand, caloric requirements for active 14 and 18-year-old girls can be as high as 2200 kcal per day whereas for active boys in that age range, calorie requirements can reach 2600 kcals per day.[4]

In recent years, there has been a clear reduction in energy expenditure as many children have become more complaisant and sedentary.

The CDC estimates that on average, American children ages 8 to 18 spend 7.5 hours/day of idle time in front of either a computer, television or some kind of electronic device, such as a video game or cell phone, causing the total energy expenditure to drop 600 to 800 kcal per day.[15]

For boys ages 15 to 18, this more inactive lifestyle leads to a 1000 kcal reduction in energy expenditure per day. And so when a teenage girl ingests the complete contents of an 11.5oz-wt bag of potato chips, she is actually taking in the equivalent of 1920 kcal in fat alone or 43 teaspoons of butter equivalent.

The total caloric load of this one snack likely meets or exceeds the total daily energy needs for most sedentary female teenagers.

The problem is not just limited to total quantities of fat consumed, but also to the quality of the fat. The highly processed foods that have been consumed over the last 30 years were laden with trans-fatty acids. Researchers uncovered in the 1990s, that these fats, generally tied to hard margarines and shortenings, carried twice the risk factors for heart disease compared to lard and other saturated fats. Since the early part of the twentieth century, there was a shift in the quality of our fat intake, as we transitioned from saturated to trans-fatty acids, and shifted from omega-3 to omega-6 fatty acids concomitantly with a specialized corn and soy bean-dominant agriculture. The change was dramatic enough that by the end of the 1990s, we were consuming abundant polyunsaturated fats and oils, high in omega-6 fatty acids (**Figure 5.21**).

Dietary Fat Content Comparisons

Oil	Saturated Fat	Alpha-Linolenic Acid	Linoleic Acid	Mono-unsaturated Fat
Canola oil	7	11		61
Flaxseed oil	10	48		26
Safflower oil	10	Trace		14
Sunflower oil	12	1		16
Corn oil	13	1		29
Olive oil	15	1		75
Soybean oil	15	8		23
Peanut oil	19	Trace		48
Cottonseed oil	27	Trace		19
Lard	43	1		47
Beef tallow	48	1		49
Palm oil	51	Trace		39
Butterfat	68	1		28
Coconut oil	91			7

CanolaInfo 306.387.6610 www.canolainfo.org canolainfo@canolainfo.org

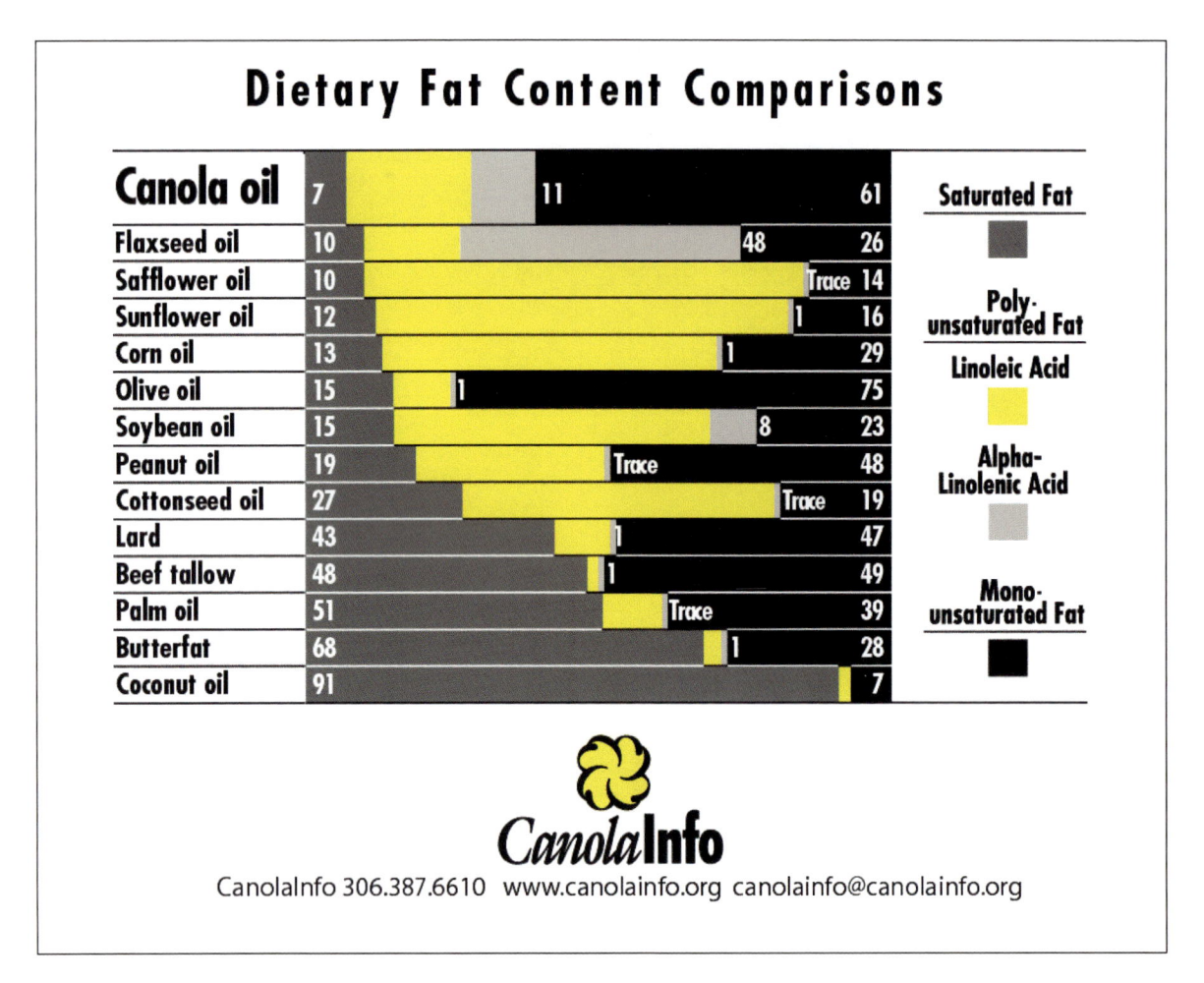

Figure 5.21 Dietary Fat Content Comparisons of Different Types of Oils. Source: wwwCanolainfo.org

The goal in feeding children and adolescents is to introduce into the diet oils rich in monounsaturated fats, as evidence now points to their protective role against heart disease and some cancers.

Families need to use more olive oil, peanut oil and canola oil, as these are the most significant contributors of monounsaturated fats in the North American diet.

At the same time, we need to limit the use of those oils and fats that are elevated in saturated fat such as coconut oil, butter, palm oil and beef tallow. There is some research now surfacing that suggests that the medium chain triglycerides (MCT) that make up coconut oil and butter are likely good for our health, despite being high in saturated fat.

It also appears helpful, to the diet and health of our young, to encourage the ingestion of those oils that contribute significant amounts of the omega-3 fatty acid, alpha linolenic acid. A review of **Figure 6.21** reveals that there are three vegetable oils that contain sizable proportions of omega-3 fats (grey bar): soybean oil, canola oil and flaxseed oil.

The goal here is to offset the large proportion of omega-6 fats that have slowly crept into the diet, by ingesting a greater amount of omega-3 fats.

There are two problems that emerge from this over-abundance of omega-6 oils: first, the metabolism of these fats, generate an elongated fatty acid by the name of **arachidonic acid**. This 20 carbon fatty acid causes the production of eicosanoids, among which is an inflammatory compound called thromboxane-2. It is responsible for the inflammatory damage seen in heart disease; second, the abundance of omega-6 fats in the diet, causes a slow-down of the omega-3 fatty acid pathway that produces anti-inflammatory eicosanoids, such as EPA and DHA, which are protective against heart disease.

To shield our children against the higher long term risks of heart disease, the goal is to focus at introducing the olive, peanut and flaxseed oils into the diet for starters; the omega-3 contained in vegetable oils can in theory generate EPA and DHA fatty acids, which carry important benefits.

If that omega-3 pathway is shutdown or slowed because of excessive omega-6 fats, then the next step should be the introduction of fatty fish containing the omega-3 fats, EPA and DHA. These provide such high levels of protection against heart disease but also improved neurological development in young children.

The fish that contain the highest levels of DHA and EPA are mackerel, salmon, bluefish, sable fish, herring, lake trout, sardines and tuna.

There is no doubt that much needs to be done to turn the eating habits of our young around, and we need to move promptly for there is much at stake. All of these bad food habits, documented in this chapter, have been tied to a compromised performance of our children at school. Is there any question that academics are suffering in this country, possibly because of a tired and undisciplined youth? Are we troubled yet that our children are underachieving, compared to other nations? There are 9 steps proposed by the CDC to reinvigorate our children's health and they revolve around exercise and healthy eating (**Figure 5.22**):[16]

1. Begin evaluating in a consistent manner the eating habits and physical activity levels of our youth
2. Develop school environments that serve only healthy foods and that foster physical activity in children
3. Ensure that our schools have quality meal programs, and that only healthy and appealing foods are offered outside of the school meal program
4. Implement a comprehensive quality physical activity program for the kids at school
5. Ensure that our schools have health education that provides nutrition knowledge, skills and experiences that help develop lifelong healthy eating habits
6. Provide students with health, mental health and social services that assist students with developing healthy eating, physical activity and prevention of chronic disease
7. Families and communities need to set up partnerships to encourage healthy eating and physical activity in cities and towns and neighborhoods
8. Implement school employee wellness programs to encourage staff to take positive and significant steps at improving food habits and exercise
9. Implement professional development opportunities that foster physical education, health and nutrition education, in addition to mental health support to staff who work with the kids.

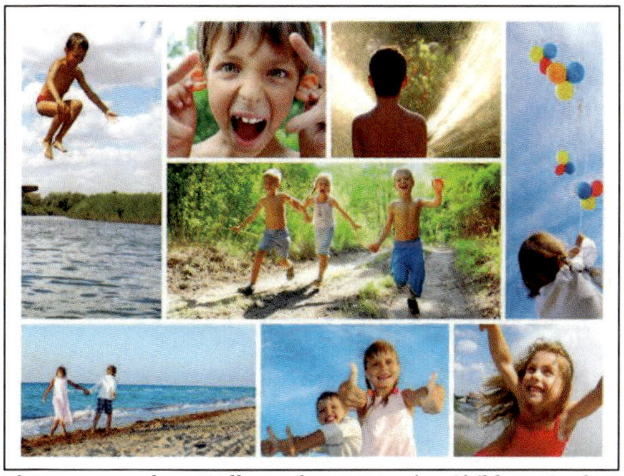

Figure 5.22 Photo Collage of Happy Active Children © Cherry Merry

Fifth, A Lifestyle change: Introduce Physical Activity in the Lives of Children Physical activity levels have declined so dramatically, among the youth since the 1950s that, in combination with a diet that is evermore calorically-dense, there is no doubt as to why obesity prevalence is increasing so dramatically among the young.[17]

Our young have gone from active to inactive lifestyles, because of the overpowering impact of the electronic entertainment age. As such, the total mean daily expenditure, in teenage girls ages 15-18, is now between 1700 and 2000 kcal per day. This is down from 2300 to 2800 kcal/day, when they were more active.

For boys 15 to 18, who are now sedentary or with low activity levels, total energy needs vary between 2100 to 2800 kcal/day instead of the more significant expenditures of 3100 to 3800 kcal, typically seen in active and very active boys. This daily drop in caloric expenditure, when compounded by the mean 200 kcal/day increase in food intake over the last 5-7 years in children, creates a nightmare scenario that has ignited an obesity crisis in our children.

The only solution that appears to offer some kind of hope is not found in dieting; to prescribe restrictive diets for these children and young adolescents with weight problems, is the equivalent to sentencing them to a lifelong struggle with weight from which they may never be able to escape.[44] Rather, the solution most likely to be successful on the long run, is to limit their access to poor quality foods and increase their physical activity, but by how much?

The 2010 Healthy Eating Guidelines for Americans are now aligned with the 2008 Federal Physical Guidelines for Americans, issued by the Department of Health & Human Services. They encourage children and adolescents to engage in 420 minutes per week of activity, performed at moderate and vigorous intensities for significant health benefits.[94]

Ideally 3 days per week need to be dedicated to strength building exercises, and another 3 days should focus on vigorous aerobic activities. This works out to be a dedicated 60 minutes per day of moderate to vigorous intensity exercise balanced between aerobic and anaerobic muscle strengthening workouts.

The caloric expenditure associated with this level of physical activity is surprisingly elevated. The physical cost to the children and adolescents would be substantive, and would tax their bodies to a high degree since American children and adolescents have lost most of the physical endurance seen in times past.

The guidelines are very much needed at this time, but the question is: Can parents successfully unglue their kids from the entertainment centers and cell phones long enough to get them into higher degrees of physical fitness?

The exercise proposed in **Table-5.9** below, is intended to assess the weight of a typical 15 year old teenage girl whose height=5'4" and whose weight=154lbs, and to prescribe a weekly routine of physical activity that involves 180 minutes/week of moderately intense to vigorous aerobic activity, another 180 minutes/week of strength building exercises of vigorous intensity and an additional 60 minutes of moderate leisurely activity for a total of 420 minutes. Then, calculate the total energy expenditure, using the table of physical activity below. Next, add that caloric value to the teenager's total sedentary energy requirement of 1775 kcals per day. The addition of both sets of calories provides the teenager's total daily caloric expenditure.

For the strength-building exercises, it is important to note that from a time management perspective, the 1 hour in the gym does not generally translate into 60 minutes of strength exercise but rather into 20 minutes of hard weight lifting and 40 minutes of resting and stretching. Hence, in using the table below, the 180 minutes/week of strength building at moderate to vigorous levels—using the circuit training—would only translate into 33% exercise time or 59 minutes. This teenager would only burn, from the circuit weight training, an extra 763 kcals per week.

In addition, she would have to do another 180 minutes of moderate to intense aerobic activity per week. If she chose vigorous aerobic dancing, she would burn an additional 1718 kcal per week. An extra 60 minutes of leisurely exercise could be walking at a brisk pace. For that one day, she would expend an extra 388 kcal.

Next, the idea is to add up all of the weekly caloric expenditures and divide by 7 in order to establish that person's extra daily energy needs. In this case, the young woman would be expending a total additional weekly expenditure of 2869 kcal. Next, divide this amount by 7 and then add the average daily expenditure to her daily expenditure at a sedentary level. So then divide 2869 kcals by 7= 409.86 kcals, which is roughly 410 extra kcals per day. Her total daily energy expenditure would then equal 1775 kcal (resting energy +sedentary activity) plus 410 kcal or 2185 kcal/day. This is a moderate increase that would help maintain her weight stable as long as her food choices are not calorically-dense processed snack foods. By following the Federal Physical Guidelines for American, this young lady went from expending 1775 kcal/day, when following a sedentary lifestyle, to burning 2185 kcal/day. Assuming she consumes no extra calories after exercising, she would lose 0.82lbs/week from only exercise or 3.56lbs/month because of the daily 410 kcals deficit (she would lose 1lbs for every 3500 kcal deficit)[73] At the end of the year, her disciplined workouts would generate 42.72lbs of weight loss at the end of the year. Her patience would likely pay off, over the long term, as there is a high likelihood of more permanent weight loss for two reasons: first, she did not calorically restrict her diet, and second, the weight loss, experienced from only exercise, was slow. Now using table-8 again, establish additional caloric expenditures, from a weekly 420 minute exercise routine, you are going to assign to yourself.

TABLE 5.9 Calories expended per pound per minute of exercise

Activity Subject's weight (lbs):_____	Expenditure/lb/min	Exercise time (minutes/week)	Total Kcal/wk
Bicycling at 25 mi/hr	0.139 kcal/lb/min		
Bicycling at 13 mi/hr	0.045 kcal/lb/min		
Running 10 miles/hr	0.114 kcal/lb/min		
Running 5 miles/hr	0.061 kcal/lb/min		
Cross count skiing (8ml/hr)	0.104 kcal/lb/min		
Vigorous Soccer	0.097 kcal/lb/min		
Vigorous basketball	0.097 kcal/lb/min		
Recreational basketball	0.05 kcal/lb/min		
Vigorous Aerobic Dancing	0.062 kcal/lb/min		
Walking at a brisk pace	0.042kcal/lb/min		
Swimming (crawl—45yards/min)	0.058 kcal/lb/min		
Roller skating (9 mi/hr)	0.043 kcal/lb/min		
Circuit weight training	0.084 kcal/lb/min		

Caloric expenditure values were taken from Pearson's MyDietAnalysis software.

DISCUSSION QUESTIONS

1. Using the Medline search engine, locate a peer-reviewed journal article that supports an association between low breastfeeding rates, and a high incidence of leukemia, diabetes, respiratory illness, or obesity. Discuss the main conclusions of the paper.

2. Discuss, in a one page document, how the blundered Ad Council's campaign, promoting breastfeeding, could have been successful with an alternative ad. Describe the contents of an alternate ad that could have reinvigorated the breastfeeding initiative.

3. Based on what you have learned, about fats and oils in this chapter, discuss how you

would change your fat and oil selections and explain why.

4. Consider the blundered Minnesota amendment to change the definition of a vegetable, according to the USDA, and write a one-page letter to the current state senator, urging him/her to retable another amendment based on your view of the importance of nutrition in battling the growing prevalence of child and adolescent obesity in this country.

5. Discuss why did the North American mother embrace infant formulas so thoroughly in the late 1960s, 70s and 1980s?

6. Using table-8 in the textbook, how many weekly calories would be expended, if a 176lb adolescent boy bicycled at 25 mph for 3 hours on Saturdays, then ran at 5 mph for 1 hour 3 times/week, and then played vigorous basketball for 1 hour/week. Show your calculations?

7. Discuss the changes that took place in the quality of fat consumed between the end of the 19th century and 2002?

References

1. Aarsland, A et al (1996) Contributions of de novo synthesis of fatty acids to total VLDL-triglyceride secretion during prolonged hyperglycemia hyperinsulinemia in normal man. J. Clin. Invest; 98:2008-2017
2. ABC News (2012) Exclusive report: Breast Feeding Ads Stalled and Watered down: Retrieved May 12, 2012: http://abcnews.go.com/2020/story?id=124271&page=1
2b. Amato PR, Keith B. (1991) Consequences of parental divorce for children's well-being: A meta-analysis. Psychological Bulletin;110:26–46.
3. American Heart Association (AHA) (2013). AHA's Diet and Lifestyle Recommendations. Retrieved December 6th 2013 from: http://www.heart.org/HEARTORG/GettingHealthy/Diet-and-Lifestyle-Recommendations_UCM_305855_Article.jsp
4. American Heart Association (AHA) (2013). Dietary Recommendations for Children. Retrieved December 6, 2013 from: http://www.heart.org/HEARTORG/GettingHealthy/NutritionCenter/Dietary-Recommendations-for-Healthy-Children_UCM_303886_Article.jsp
5. Anderzhanova, E. et al. (2007) Altered basal and stimulated accumbens dopamine release in obese OLETF rats as a function of age and diabetes status. Am. J Physiol. Regul. Integr. Comp Physiol. 293; R603-R611).
6. Aylin P, Williams S, Bottle A: (2005)Obesity and type 2 diabetes in children, 1996–7 to 2003–4. BMJ 331:1167
7a. Bissonnette, DJ. (2010) Obesity in America: A National Crisis. Mankato, MN: St-Jude Nutrition Medical Communications: run time 2hr 36 min. Distributed by Films for the Humanities and Sciences since 2011
7b. Bissonnette, DJ (© 2014) The Diabetes Epidemic: A Medical Catastrophe. DVD documentary; run time: 77 minutes. Mankato, MN: St-Jude Nutrition Medical Communications.
7b. Bleich et al. (2015). The complex relationship between diet and health. Health Affairs, 34(11), 1813-12A. http://dx.doi.org.ezproxy.mnsu.edu/10.1377/hlthaff.2015.0606
8. Boseley, S. (2013) Smoothies and fruit juices are a new risk to health, US scientists warn. The Guardian Friday September 6
9. Bray, GA (2009) Obesity: Science to Practice Edited by Gareth Williams and Gema Frühbeck, New York: John Wiley & Sons: 3-18
10. Bray, GA (1997). Progress in understanding the genetics of obesity. J. Nutr 127:940S-942S
11. Brown, JE. (2008). Nutrition through the Life Cycle. Belmont CA: Thompson Higher Education p: 104.
11b. Burgess-Champoux TL, Larson N, Neumark-Sztainer D, Hannan PJ, Story M. (2009) Are family meal patterns associated with overall diet quality during the transition from early to middle adolescence?. J Nutr Educ Behav;41(2):79-86. doi:10.1016/j.jneb.2008.03.113
12. Burke, BS (1945). Nutrition and its Relationship to the Complications of Pregnancy and the Survival of the Infant. Amer. J. Publ. Health, 35:334-339. Retrieved October 16, 2013 from: http://ajph.aphapublications.org/doi/pdf/10.2105/AJPH.35.4.334
13. Carmona R.H. (2005). US Surgeon General Releases Advisory on Alcohol use during Pregnancy. Health and Human Services Press Office February 21, 2005. Retrieved on October 16, 2013 from: http://www.surgeongeneral.gov/news/2005/02/sg02222005.html
14. CDC. National Centers for Health Statistics. Births: Final Data 2011. National Vital Statistics Report. Vol: 62 No 1. Retrieved October 16, 2013 from: http://www.cdc.gov/nchs/data/nvsr/nvsr62/nvsr62_01_tables.pdf
14b. CDC (2019) - Childhood Obesity Facts. Retrieved from the CDC webpage on July 29, 2020. URL: https://www.cdc.gov/obesity/data/childhood.html
15. Center for Disease Control and Prevention. Healthy Weigh-It's not a Diet, It's a Lifestyle! About BMI for Children and Teens. Retrieved October 18, 2013 from:

http://www.cdc.gov/healthyweight/assessing/bmi/childrens_bmi/about_childrens_bmi.html

16. CDC/ Nutrition, Physical Activity and Obesity: School Health Guidelines to Promote Healthy Eating and Physical Activity. Retrieved May 14, 2012: http://www.cdc.gov/healthyyouth/npao/strategies.htm.

17a. CDC: A Growing Problem. Retrieved May 15, 2012: http://www.cdc.gov/obesity/childhood/problem.html

17b. CDC: Safer Healthier People (2000). Overview of the CDC Growth Charts; Retrieved December 9, 2013 from: http://www.cdc.gov/nccdphp/dnpa/growthcharts/training/modules/module2/text/module2print.pdf

17b. Chaparro, M. P., Harrison, G. G., Pebley, A. R., & Wang, M. (2014). The relationship between obesity and participation in the supplemental nutrition assistance program (SNAP): Is mental health a mediator? Journal of Hunger & Environmental Nutrition, 9(4), 512-522.

17c. DeBono, N. L., Ross, N. A., & Berrang-Ford, L. (2012). Does the food stamp program cause obesity? A realist review and a call for place-based research. Health & Place, 18(4), 747-756.

18. Drake AJ, Smith A, Betts PR, Crowne EC, Shield JP(2002) Type-2 Diabetes in Obese White Children. Arch Dis Child. 86:207–208

19. Driscoll CD et al (1990) Prenatal alcohol exposure. Comparability of effects in humans and animal models. Neurotoxicol. Teratol. 12: 307-314.

20. Dunn, HD (1940) Vital Statistics of the United States 1938. Bureau of the Census, United States Department of Commerce. Retrieved October 16, 2013 from: http://www.cdc.gov/nchs/data/vsus/VSUS_1938_1.pdf

21. Eckardt, MJ et al (1998) Effects of moderate alcohol consumption on the central nervous system. Alcoholism. Clin & Exp Res 22 (5): 998-1040.

22. El-Bastawissi et al (2007) Effect of the Washington Special Supplemental Nutrition Program for Women, Infants and Children (WIC) on Pregnancy Outcomes Matern Child Health J.11:611–621.

23. Ehtisham S, Barrett TG, Shaw NJ (2000):Type-2 Diabetes in Children: An Emerging Problem. *Diabet Mel.* 17:867–871.

23b. Feldman S, Eisenberg ME, Neumark-Sztainer D, Story M. Associations between watching TV during family meals and dietary intake among adolescents. *J Nutr Educ Behav.* 2007;39(5):257-263. doi:10.1016/j.jneb.2007.04.181

24. Field, A. E., Austin, S. B., et. al. (2003). Relation between dieting and weight change among preadolescents and adolescents. *Pediatrics, 112,* 900–906.

24b. Finkelstein, E. A., Khavjou, O. A., Thompson, H., Trogdon, J. G., Pan, L., Sherry, B., & Dietz, W. (2012). Obesity and severe obesity forecasts through 2030. American Journal of Preventive Medicine, 42(6), 563-570. 10.1016/j.amepre.2011.10.026

25. Flegal, K et al. (2002) Weight-for-stature compared with body mass index–for-age growth charts for the United States from the Centers for Disease Control and Prevention. Am.J.Clin.Nutr.75(4): 761-766 Retrieved October 18, 2013 from: http://ajcn.nutrition.org/content/75/4/761.full

25b. Franck, C., M.Sc, Grandi, S. M., M.Sc, & Eisenberg, Mark J,M.D., M.P.H. (2013). Taxing junk food to counter obesity. American Journal of Public Health, 103(11), 1949-1953.

25c. Franklin, B., Jones, A., Love, D., Puckett, S., Macklin, J., & White-Means, S. (2012;2011;). Exploring mediators of food insecurity and obesity: A review of recent literature. Journal of Community Health, 37(1), 253-264.

26. Gamble, S.B. et al.(2005) Abortion Surveillance—United States. Division of Reproductive Health, National Center for Chronic Disease Prevention and Health Promotion. 57; SS-13: 1-33.

27. Gibson, RS. (1990) Principles of Nutritional Assessment. New York: Oxford University Press, 691pp

28. Goldblight SA and Maynard JA. (1964) An anthology of food science:milestones in nutrition. Vol 2. Westport, Connecticut: The Avi Publishing Co, Inc.

29. Gomez, F. et al. (1956) Mortality in second and third degree malnutrition. J of Trop. Pediatrics 2:77-83

29.b Griffin, J. (2002, January 17). Practice Nurse, 23(1), 26+

30. Grove, RD, and Hetzel, AM. (1968). Vital Statistic Rates in the United States 1940-1960. United States Department of Health, Education & Welfare. Washington DC: Public Health Service. National Center of Health Statistics. Retrieved October 16, 2013 from: http://www.cdc.gov/nchs/data/vsus/vsrates1940_60.pdf

31. Haine, L et al. (2007) Rising incidence of type-2 diabetes in children in the UK. Diabetes Care 30(5): 1097-1101

32. Harnack, et al. (1999). Soft drink consumption among US children and adolescents: nutritional consequences. J. Am.Diet.Assoc. 99:436-441

32b. Harling, G., Subramanian, S., Bärnighausen, T., & Kawachi, I. (2013). Socioeconomic disparities in sexually transmitted infections among young adults in the United States: examining the interaction between income and race/ethnicity. *Sexually transmitted diseases*, *40*(7), 575–581. https://doi.org/10.1097/OLQ.0b013e31829529cf

32c. Harris, J. L., Bargh, J. A., & Brownell, K. D. (2009). Priming effects of television food advertising on eating behavior. *Health Psychology, 28*(4), 404-413.

32d. Haslam, D. (2016), Weight management in obesity – past and present. Int J Clin Pract, 70: 206–217. doi:10.1111/ijcp.12771

33. Health and Human Services, United States Government, ASPE Research Brief: Childhood obesity. Retrieved May 17 2012 http://aspe.hhs.gov/health/reports/child_obesity/.

34. Henriksen, T. (2006) Nutrition and Pregnancy Outcome. Nutr Rev. May;64(5 Pt 2):19-23.

34b. Hilton JM, and Devall EL(1998). Comparison of parenting and children's behavior in single-mother, single-father, and intact families. Journal of Divorce & Remarriage; 29:23–54.

35. Institute of Medicine (2009). Weight Gain during Pregnancy: Reexamining the Guidelines. Rasmussen, KM (Chair) Report Brief May 2009

35b. Jilcott et al. (2011). Associations between Food Insecurity, Supplemental Nutrition Assistance Program (SNAP) Benefits, and Body Mass Index among Adult Females. Journal of the American Dietetic Association, 111(11), 1741-1745.

35c. Katz, D. L. (2014). Childhood Obesity, 10(6), 443-444;

35d. Kenny, P. J., (2011) Common cellular and molecular mechanisms in obesity and drug addiction. Nature Reviews Neuroscience, 12(11), 638-651

36. Kerri N, B., Jayne A, F., Dianne, N., Mary, S., & Simone A, F. (2007). Fast food for family meals: relationships with parent and adolescent food intake, home food availability and weight status. Public Health Nutrition, 10(1), 16-23.

37. Kramer, MS. (1998) Maternal Nutrition, Pregnancy Outcome and Public Health Policy. Canadian Medical Association Journal 159(6): 663-665.

37b. Krebs-Smith, S.M et al. (2010). Americans do not meet federal dietary recommendations. J Nutr. 2010 Oct;140(10):1832-8. URL: https://www.ncbi.nlm.nih.gov/pubmed/20702750/

38. Lai, HC et al. (1998) Growth status in children with cystic fibrosis based on the National Cystic Fibrosis Patient Registry data: evaluation of various criteria used to identify malnutrition. J Pediatr. 132(3 Pt 1):478-85.

39. Ledikwe, Jenny H; Julia A Ello-Martin, & Barbara J Rolls. (2005). Portion Sizes and the Obesity Epidemic1,2. The Journal of Nutrition, 135(4), 905-9.

40. Lee, RD and Nieman, DC. (1996). Nutritional Assessment. Boston: Mosby 2nd edition p:454

41. Lewis DD., Woods, SE.(1994) Fetal Alcohol Syndrome. Amer. Family Phys 1994; 50(5)1025-32, 1035-6.

42. Lustig, RH (2010) Fructose: metabolic, hedonic, and societal parallels with ethanol J Am Diet Assoc. 110 (9):1307-21

43. Malek, K. (2013) Planned Parenthood Ignores 71 Studies Linking Abortions, Breast Cancer January 22 LifeNews.com. Retrieved October 16, 2013 from: http://www.lifenews.com/2013/01/22/planned-parenthood-ignores-71-studies-linking-abortion-breast-cancer/

44. Mann, T. et al. (2007) Medicare's Search for Effective Obesity Treatments. American Psychologists; 62(3): 220-233

45. Martin, JA et al (2012) Birth: Final Data for 2010. In: National Vital Statistics Reports; vol 61 (1). US Department of Health Statistics

46. Martin, JA et al (2010) Birth: Final Data for 2008. In: National Vital Statistics Reports; vol 59(1). US Department of Health Statistics

47. Martin, JA et al (2002). Births: Final Data for 2000. In: National Vital Statistics Reports; vol 50(5). US Department of Health Statistics. Retrieved October 16, 2013 from: http://www.cdc.gov/nchs/data/nvsr/nvsr50/nvsr50_05.pdf

48. Martin, Andrew. (2004) USDA Frozen Fries are fresh veggies. June 15, 2004 by the Los Angeles Times. < http://articles.latimes.com/2004/jun/15/nation/na-fries15 >

49. Martorell, R. (2005) Diabetes and Mexicans: Why the two are linked. Prev Chronic Dis [serial online] [*Retrieved Dec 3, 2013*]. Available from: URL: http://www.cdc.gov/pcd/issues/2005/jan/04_0100.htm.

50. May, PA and Gossage, JP. (2001) Estimating the prevalence of FAS. A summary. Alcohol Research & Health 25 (3):159-167.

51. Mattson, SN and Riley, FP. (1996) Brain abnormalities in fetal alcohol syndrome. In: Abnormalities of Fetal Alcohol Syndrome: From Mechanism to Prevention. CRC Press, Boca Raton p: 51-68.

51b. McDonnell, C. J., & Garbers, S. V. (2018). Adverse childhood experiences and obesity: Systematic review of behavioral interventions for women. *Psychological Trauma: Theory, Research, Practice, and Policy, 10*(4), 387–395. https://doi.org/10.1037/tra0000313

51c. McGuire, S. (2011). *The Impact of Food Away from Home on Adult Diet Quality*. ERR-90, U.S. Department of Agriculture, Econ. Res. Serv., February 2010. **URL: https://www.ncbi.nlm.nih.gov/pmc/articles/PMC3183595/**

52. Meguid, MM. et al (2000) Hypothalamic dopamine and serotonin in the regulation of food intake. Nutrition. 16:843–857.

53. Murphy, TF. (1931) Births, Stillbirths and Infant Mortality Statistics, 17th Annual Report. Department of Commerce, Bureau of the Census. Retrieved October 16, 2013 from: http://www.cdc.gov/nchs/data/vsushistorical/birthstat_1931.pdf

54. NIH (2000) National Institute of Health; National Heart Lung and Blood Institute: Obesity Education Initiative. Retrieved October 21, 2013 from: http://www.nhlbi.nih.gov/guidelines/obesity/prctgd_c.pdf

55. NIH (2020). National Institutes of Health; National Heart Lung and Blood Institute. How are overweight and obesity diagnosed? Retrieved October 21, 2013: https://www.nhlbi.nih.gov/health-topics/high-blood-pressure

55b. NIH (2017). How dietary factors influence disease risk. Retrieved from the National Institutes of Health NIH Research Matters website. URL: https://www.nih.gov/news-events/nih-research-matters/how-dietary-factors-influence-disease-risk

56. National Health & Nutrition Examination Survey (NHANES) (1999-2000). CDC. Retrieved October 18, 2013: http://www.cdc.gov/nchs/data/nhanes/databriefs/adultweight.pdf

57. National Institute on Alcohol Abuse and Alcoholism. (2002) NIH publ. # 00-1583 Dept. of & Human Services p: 283-338.
58. Nativity Statistics, www.cdc.gov/nchs/births/htm. Accessed April 30, 2012.
59. National Center for Health Statistics. Breast Feeding Report Card: United States 2011. Retrieved May 10 2012: http://www.cdc.gov/breastfeeding/data/reportcard.htm.
60. National Diabetes Facts Sheet (2011) published by the Center for Disease Control and Prevention. Retrieved March http://www.cdc.gov/diabetes/pubs/factsheet11.htm.Pediatric Nursing 2007; 19(4):4)
61. Nestle, M. (2007) Eating Made Simple. Scientific American. 297(3): 60-69

61b. Nguyen, Linh T. "Would you like tax exemptions with that? How food exemptions under state sales tax are not reaching lower income communities in food deserts." Journal of Gender, Race and Justice, Winter 2017, p. 187+. Opposing Viewpoints in Context, http://link.galegroup.com.ezproxy.mnsu.edu/apps/doc/A486712066/OVIC?u=mnamsumank&xid=95662d24.

62. Ogden CL, Carroll MD, Curtin LR, McDowell MA, Tabak CJ, Flegal KM.(2006) Prevalence of overweight and obesity in the United States, 1999-2004. JAMA 295:1549-55.
63. Ogden CL, Flegal KM, Carroll MD, Johnson CL. (2002) Prevalence and trends in overweight among U.S. children and adolescents, 1999-2000. JAMA 288:1728-32.
64. Ogden CL, Carroll MD, Curtin LR, Lamb MM, Flegal KM. (2010) Prevalence of high body mass index in U.S. children and adolescents, 2007-2008. JAMA 303(3):242-9.
65. Olney, JW et al. (2002) The enigma of fetal alcohol neurotoxicity. Annals of Medicine 35(2):109-119.
66. Palmer, S. (2006) Adolescent Bariatric Surgery: Too much too soon? Today's Dietitian 8(1): 30-35.
67. Pew Research Center (2012). Pew Social and Demographic Trends. US Birth rate falls to a record low: Decline is Greatest Among Immigrants. Washington DC: Retrieved October 16, 2013 from: http://www.pewsocialtrends.org/files/2012/11/Birth_Rate_Final.pdf
68. Pinhas-Hamiel O, Zeitler P. (2005) The global spread of type 2 diabetes mellitus in children and adolescents. J. Pediatr 146:693-700
69. Pinhas-Hamiel J. et al. (1996) Increased incidence of non-insulin dependent diabetes mellitus among adolescents. Pediatrics; 128:608-615.
70. Planned Parenthood Federation of American (2008) Income Tax Returns. Available at: <http://www.plannedparenthood.org/files/PPFA/PPFA_FY09_Form_990_Copy_for_Public_Inspection.PDF>.
71. Planned Parenthood Annual Financial Report 2010-2011 and Planned Parenthood Annual Report 2011-2012 are available at: <http://www.plannedparenthood.org/about-us/annual-report-4661.htm>.
72. Planned Parenthood Annual Report 2009-2010 is available at: <http://www.plannedparenthood.org/files/PPFA/PP_Services.pdf>.

73. Popkin, B.M. The World is Fat (2007). Scientific American. 297 (3): 88-95
74. Position of the American Dietetic Association (2005): Promoting and Supporting Breast Feeding. J. Am. Diet Assoc. 105:810-818.
75. Randall, CL (2001) Alcohol and Pregnancy: Highlights from three decades of Research. J. of Studies on Alcohol. 62(5): 554-61.
76. Rhodes, L. Moorman, JE, Redd, SC, DM Mannino, (2003) Self-reported asthma prevalence and control among adults—United States 200 Division of Environmental Hazards and Health Effects, National Center for Environmental Health, CDC 52(17): 381-384.
77. Rosenbloom AL, Joe JR, Young RS, Winter WE (1999) The emerging epidemic of type 2 diabetes mellitus in youth: *Diabetes Care*; 22:345–354.
78. Sandler, L. (2013). Having It All Without Children. In: TIME: The Child Free Life. August 12 issue. Retrieved October 15, 2013 from: http://content.time.com/time/magazine/article/0,9171,2148636,00.html
79. Schlosser, E. (2002). Fast Food Nation New York: Harper Perrenial, 383pp
80. Shultz, LO. et al. (2006). Effects of traditional and Western environments on prevalence of type 2 diabetes in Pima Indians in Mexico and the U.S. Diabetes Care 29(8): 1866-1871
81. Schwartz, MB.,Vartanian, LR., Wharton, C.M., Brownell, KD. (2008). Examining the nutritional quality of breakfast cereals marketed to children. JADA 108(4): 702-705.

81b. Senguttuvan, U., Whiteman, S. D., & Jensen, A. C. (2014). Family Relationships and Adolescents Health Attitudes and Weight: The Understudied Role of Sibling Relationships. *Family Relations, 63*(3), 384-396.

81c. Shannon, C. L., & Klausner, J. D. (2018). The growing epidemic of sexually transmitted infections in adolescents: a neglected population. *Current opinion in pediatrics*, *30*(1), 137–143. https://doi.org/10.1097/MOP.0000000000000578

82. Shirazian, T and Raghavan, S. (2009) Obesity and pregnancy: Implications and Management Strategies for Providers. Mount Sinai Journal of Medicine 76:539-545.
82b. Shook SE, Jones DJ, Forehand R, Dorsey S, Brody G. (2010). The mother-coparent relationship and youth adjustment: a study of African American single-mother families.J Fam Psychol; 24(3):243-51.
83. Shutz, Y and Jequier, E. (1998) Resting Energy Expenditure, Thermic Effect of Food, and Total Energy Expenditure. In: Handbook of Obesity, Bray, GA, Bouchard, C. James (Eds). New York: Marcel Dekker Publishing: 443-455.
83b. Smith, L. P., Ng, S. W., & Popkin, B. M. (2013). Trends in US home food preparation and consumption: Analysis of national nutrition surveys and time use studies from 1965-1966 to 2007-2008. *Nutrition Journal, 12*(1), 45. https://search.proquest.com/docview/1347666476?pq-origsite=summon&accountid=12259

84. Song WO, Chun OK, Kerver JM, Cho SC, Chung CE, and Chung S. Breakfast read to-eat cereal consumption enhances milk and calcium intake in the U.S. population. J Am Diet Assoc. 2006 Nov;106 (11):1783-1789
85. Sood, B et al. (2001). Prenatal exposure and childhood behavior at age 6 to 7 years: I. Dose-response effect. Pediatrics 108 (2): E35.
86. Stephenson, J. Bader, D. (2012) Health Checks: Carbohydrate, Fat and Calorie Guide. Appletree Press, Mankato MN pp 139.
87. Stice, E., Cameron, R. P. (1999). Naturalistic weight reduction efforts prospectively predict growth in relative weight and onset of obesity among female adolescents Journal of Consulting and Clinical Psychology, 67, 967–974.
87a. Stone, A (2014) Multipurpose prevention technologies for reproductive and sexual health, Reproductive Health Matters, 22:44, 213-217, DOI: 10.1016/S0968-8080(14)44801-8

87.b. Stone, L. (2020). The Global Fertility Crisis. Retrieved from the National Review magazine website on July 29, 2020. URL: https://www.nationalreview.com/magazine/2020/01/27/the-global-fertility-crisis/
88. Story, M. et al. (2008). Creating healthy foods and eating environments: Policy and environmental approaches Ann. Rev. Public Health 29:253–72
88b. Sung CJ, Sung MK, Choi MK, Kang YL, Kwon SJ, Kim MH, et al. (2001). An ecological study of food and nutrition in elementary school children in Korea. Kor J Community Nutr, 6(2): 150–61

89. Sutton, PD et al. (2011) Recent Declines in Birth in the United States, 2007-2009. National Center for Health Statistics Data Briefs no 60.

89b. Tartar, A., Recht, H., Qiu, Y. (2019). The Global Fertility Crash: As birthrates fall countries will be forced to adapt or fall behind. Bloomberg Business Week. Retrieved July 29, 2020. URL: https://www.bloomberg.com/graphics/2019-global-fertility-crash/
90. The National Diabetes Information Clearinghouse is a service of the National Institute of Diabetes and Digestive and Kidney Diseases, National Institutes of Health. Retrieved April 30, 2012 http://diabetes.niddk.nih.gov/dm/pubs/statistics/#Gestational

90b. Thorp, A. A., Mcnaughton, S. A., Owen, N., & Dunstan, D. W. (2013). Independent and joint associations of TV viewing time and snack food consumption with the metabolic syndrome and its components; a cross-sectional study in Australian adults. *International Journal of Behavioral Nutrition and Physical Activity, 10*(1), 96.

91. Tobias, D et al.(2011) Physical Activity Before and During Pregnancy and Risk of Gestational Diabetes Mellitus.Diabetes care 34: 223-229.
92. Twenge, J. (2012) Millennials: The Greatest Generation or the most Narcissistic. The Atlantic May 2. Retrieved October 15, 2013 from: http://www.theatlantic.com/national/archive/2012/05/millennials-the-greatest-generation-or-the-most-narcissistic/256638/
93. United States Department of Health and Human Services. (n.d.). Childhood obesity. Washington, DC: Retrieved May 19, 2012, from http://aspe.hhs.gov/health/reports/child_obesity/.
94. United States Department of Health and Human Services (2008). Physical Activity Guidelines for Americans: Chapter 3 Active Children and Adolescents. Retrieved December 6, 2013 from: http://www.health.gov/paguidelines/guidelines/chapter3.aspx
95. Viljoen, DL et al (2001). Alcohol dehydrogenase-2*2 allele is associated with decrease prevalence of fetal alcohol syndrome in the mixed ancestry population… South Africa. Alcoholism, Clin & Experimental Research; 25(12): 1719-22.
96. Wasson, Walter L., M.D.(1913).Vermont Eugenics: A Documentary History. This document is: *"Alcoholism and Eugenics"Vermont Medical Monthly*, August 15.
97. Waterlow, JC (1972) Classification and definition of protein-calorie-malnutrition. British Med. J. 3: 566-569
98. Wilson, D. and Roberts, J.(2012) Reuters: Special Report: How Washington went soft on childhood obesity. Washington DC, April 27, 2012
99. Wolfe, JF.(2003). Low Breast Feeding Rates and Public Health in the United States. American Journal of Public Health 93(12): 1-11.

99b. Zagorsky, J. L., & Smith, P. K. (2009). Does the U.S. food stamp program contribute to adult weight gain? Economics and Human Biology, 7(2), 246-258.

100. Zhang, CC et al.. (2006) A Prospective Study of Dietary Patterns, Meat Intake, and the Risk of Gestational Diabetes Mellitus. Diabetologia 49.11 : 2604-2613.
101. Zimmer, C. (*March* 15, 2010) Answers begin to emerge on how thalidomide caused defects *New York Times,*). Retrieved 2010-03-21 http://www.nytimes.com/2010/03/16/science/16limb.html?ref=science&pagewanted=all

CHAPTER 6

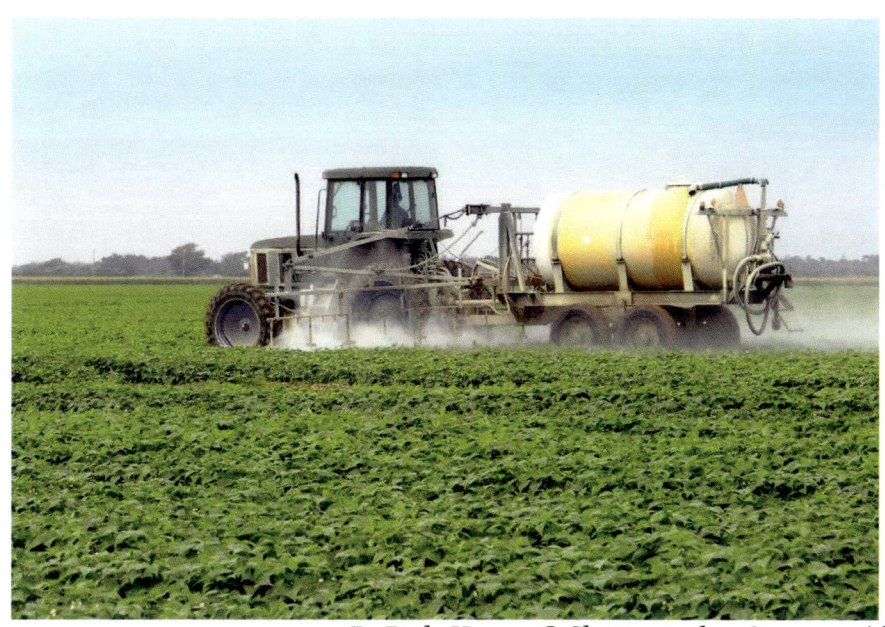

FOOD SAFETY—MODERN CHALLENGE & CUMBERSOME NIGHTMARE

6.1 The Forging of a Safe Food Supply

The United States has been acclaimed as having possibly one of the safest food systems in the world. However, this did not come to be without trial and tribulation. The first U.S. regulation of the food industry began when President Abraham Lincoln founded the U.S. Department of Agriculture (USDA) through an Act of Congress in 1862. But it was the USDA's Division of Chemistry, which was assigned the task, under the leadership of chief chemist of Dr. Harvey W. Wiley, to control food adulteration at the national level, by establishing food processing standards. He campaigned strongly in support of passing the **Pure Food & Drug Act**, which was often referred to as the Wiley Act.[56]

The Division of Chemistry soon was renamed the **Bureau of Chemistry** under the tutelage of Charles M. Whetherill in 1901. The Federal government's goal with this act was to monitor the purity of the food supply, which, at that point, was a welcomed involvement as many impurities were contaminating the U.S. food supply. In fact, it was not uncommon, in the 1800s, to find pieces of metal, sand, rock, and organic material, such as bugs, rotting and diseased meat, in food products. In England, during that same time period, the problem of food adulteration was a reality as well, that finally was exposed by Thomas Accum's book titled: *Treatise on the Adulteration of Foods and Culinary Poisons*, published in 1820. As a chemist, Accum was able to accurately describe practices that shocked the nation. He documented the practice of using alum in wheat flour, in addition to lead and copper salts in beer brewing. Although he was run out of the country by food industry leaders, for his scathing description of the food industry, other books followed that were equally condemning of food manufacturing practices.

> **In the early 19th century, the impurity of the US food supply was well known to consumers, as refrigeration and sanitary practices were not widely used.**

Likewise, in the U.S., the impurity of the food supply was a well-known reality in the early 19th century, as refrigeration and sanitary practices were not well known.

By 1880, greater urbanization took place with more rural farm workers gravitating to the cities for work. This coincided with technological advancements that permitted the establishment of large-scale urban manufacturing. Food production changed dramatically to accommodate the large population base, now conglomerating in the cities, and that needed to be fed. It was in this context that numerous food vendors began popping up everywhere to make money.

The industrial production and distribution scale of milk, prompted deceptive practices among some farmers and dairy producers. They would frequently dilute milk with water in order to artificially and deceptively boost volumes, thus increasing sales. Unfortunately, the incidence of food poisonings jumped noticeably as volume rather than quality of food produced, became the priority. Several historians claim that there was a public uneasiness surrounding the consumption of manufactured food because of the perceived deceptions wielded by many of the food distributors. According to Petrick:[37]

As historians James Harvey Young, Nancy Tomes and Lorine Swainston Goodwin have all illustrated, the urbanizing process made acquiring and consuming all manners of food (from meat to milk to apples, flour and canned goods) an anxiety-provoking process, especially for the women who were largely responsible for purchasing and cooking the family's meals.

The period of 1870 to 1930 favored the development of the canning industry, which gradually contributed toward making the food supply safer, but there were problems or birthing pains, as it were, associated with canning at such a wide scale. For instance, chemists early on, discovered that by adding small doses of sodium benzoate to food, they could extend the holding time of vegetables significantly after harvest, thus allowing year-around canning to take place.

The Bureau of Chemistry's Harvey Wiley discovered, however, that even in small doses, sodium benzoate caused some gastrointestinal distress.[56] The H.J Heinz Company, hearing about the additive, publicized their refusal to use sodium benzoate in their pure foods. Also, acid foods such as tomatoes would cause the lead solder in cans to leach into tomatoes, thus increasing the risk of lead poisoning.

The young and the elderly, according to historians, would commonly succumb to foodborne illnesses; it was dangerous to eat as there were no preparation standards governing the industry until the Pure Food and Drug Act of 1906. It has been argued that infant mortality, during that time, was elevated because of foodborne illnesses. Indeed, poisonings from poor canning practices put the public health at risk of botulism poisoning. Even as the 20th century began, scandals of food adulteration and chemical contaminations frequently made newspaper headlines.

Petrick makes the case that the problem was very pervasive. She writes:[37]

Nancy Tomes argues, 'that more and more American consumers, particularly women, really believed that foodstuffs could bring illness and death into their homes was evidenced by their willingness to pay higher prices for special sanitary packaging,' like glass bottles and tin cans.

The H.J. Heinz Company, founded in 1876 was one of the first companies in the late 19th century, along with National Biscuit Company (NABISCO), Quaker Oats, Kellogg's, and the Campbell Food company to introduce, into the market place, very high quality food preparation standards the public was craving for.

Their pricing was often twice that of unbranded foods, but yet the public, perturbed by the industry's nefarious practices, was willing to pay for pure products. Hence began the powerful U.S. food corporations that were soon going to establish a world presence. In fact, H. J. Heinz had expanded, by 1919, to 16 factories located around in the U.S., with some in Canada, Britain and Spain. It had become the biggest food producer in the world.

At Henry Heinz's death, his son Howard took over the company. As a trained chemist he was able to improve the purity, flavor and safety of the food through scientific methods. He introduced the safety can, double-seamed can, and large steam retorts in order to bring commercial canning to the highest level of safety by 1920. Using water filtration and pasteurization, Howard Heinz significantly cut foodborne illnesses, thus reassuring the public that the food was at last safe.[37]

> **By using water filtration and pasteurization, Howard Heinz significantly cut foodborne illnesses in the early 1920s.**

By the 1850s, in the U.S., it was known that imported animals were a source of disease. Insistence by USDA secretary, Isaac Newton, led to the establishment of legislation, requiring the quarantine of foreign imported animals, in order to prevent the spread of animal disease in the U.S. By 1865, legislation was passed, quarantining foreign animals, but because responsibility came under the Department of the Treasury, little if any action was taken to contain foreign animals and so, disease continued to spread.[37]

In 1884, responsibility for those quarantine stations was transferred to the USDA's **Bureau of Animal Industry** (BAI). It then proceeded to organize a network of quarantine units in New York, Boston, Baltimore and Philadelphia, as well as custom offices on both the Canadian and Mexican borders. The goal was to shield the U.S. against foreign animal disease. But protecting the health of domestic animals was only part of the problem, if the U.S. was going to become a world economy with an impressive agricultural export. The U.S. needed to demonstrate that it had a system of quality that could ensure the export of safe meats to other countries.

In 1890, President Benjamin Harrison signed the first law, requiring the inspection of salted pork and bacon, prior to foreign export. In doing so, he set the stage for the U.S. as a major meat exporter. Ensuring safe exports was only the tip of the iceberg for the U.S. government, as the real challenge was guaranteeing a massive domestic distribution of millions of pounds of safe meat and food to the American public.

Advances in technology, during the 1800s, permitted the food industry to reach higher standards of quality. A pure food supply was not just a dream of unreachable idealism, but was becoming enforceable with the railway expansion across the continental U.S., which used refrigeration cars, thanks to electricity. Indeed, these innovative changes ensured year-around safe transportation of meat and other perishable foods. This was an astonishing achievement since concerns, about the food supply, near the end of the 19th century, had expanded to encompass food poisonings.

In England, the Welbeck Abbey incident, in which 72 people became ill and 4 died from having eaten American-imported ham, became historically noteworthy; it was the first time that meat had been sent to a microbiologist for testing and confirmation of food poisoning. The incidence served as a reminder of the dangers of foodborne illnesses.

In the U.S., the meat industry, whether at the level of slaughter houses or packing plants, was unsanitary and dangerous. Immigrant workers gravitated there because the work was so repugnant that the industry had trouble hiring U.S.-born workers (**Figure 6.1**).

However, in 1906, author Upton Sinclair, wrote: *The Jungle*, a novel that gave a scathing depiction of the meat packing industry as it existed in the U.S., at the beginning of the twentieth century. Sinclair recounts the abuses of the paid slave laborers, who worked long hours in such filthy working conditions, that meat packing became known as the most dangerous occupation in the U.S. *The Jungle* shocked the U.S. public by its vivid description of that filth as it existed in packing and slaughter houses. Even today that reputation still remains, according to Eric Schlosser's *Fast Food Nation*.

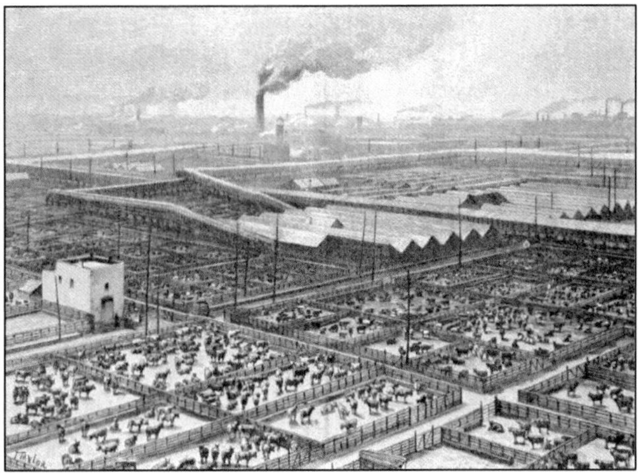

Figure 6.1 Central slaughterhouse in Chicago. Engraving was by Maynar, from picture by painter Taylor. Published in magazine "Niva", publishing house A.F. Marx, St. Petersburg, Russia, 1893 © Oleg Golovnev

Sinclair describes horrific scenes of workers accidently falling into meat grinders only to have their remains incorporated into the meat products and shipped to merchants for distribution in stores.

Though he initially mistrusted Sinclair's depiction of the meat industry, President Theodor Roosevelt, became convinced of the accuracy of Sinclair's description after he sent trusted Labor Commissioner, Charles P. Neill and social worker James Bronson Reynolds, to conduct surprise audits of the American meat packing industry. Even with the schedule of audit visits leaked to the plants ahead of time—plants had time at least to do some cleaning—the Neil-Reynold's report to the president confirmed that Upton Sinclair had indeed written an accurate portrayal of the industry.[37]

As a result, President Roosevelt presented the report to congress in 1906, which, along with public pressure arising from Sinclair's novel, facilitated the enactment of the **Federal Meat Inspection Act (FMIA) and the Pure Food and Drug Act** in 1906.[50] Two decades later, concerns about the poultry industry, specifically, lead to the passing of the USDAs Federal Poultry Inspection Service (FPIS) in 1926.[37]

There was a sense in Washington that much needed to be done to ensure food safety at a national level; the country's geography was immense and the opportunities to accidently distribute adulterated and bacteria-infested food was significant, given the country's complex distribution network.

Shortly after, in 1927, the USDA's Bureau of Chemistry was renamed the Food, Drug and Insecticide Administration. In 1930 it finally became the Food and Drug Administration (FDA). This was an important organizational manoeuver that created the FDA as an entity that was to be separate from the USDA. Consequently, food safety received budgetary backing and executive powers to oversee the safety of the American food supply. And so by 1938, Americans witness the passing of the **Federal Food Drug & Cosmetic Act**,[50] which authorized the Federal government to set up specific food standards that would govern the food industry.[37]

After the WWII, both interstate commerce, and the meat processing industry, significantly grew as the government began to build a massive and complex interstate highway system that facilitated the efficient transport of products. Suddenly, the demand for dressed, ready-to-cook and processed chicken and meats increased. And so, in 1946, the Agricultural Marketing Act authorized the Federal government to grade meat on the basis of animal class, in addition to the condition and quality of meat. Americans could now consider the purchase of meat that was either, prime, choice, good, standard, commercial, utility, cutter or canner. The grade was based on the age of the animal, in addition to juiciness, flavor, and marbling.

Chicken and turkey, by the 1950s, was a staple of the American home. The production levels of poultry meats and products rose to phenomenal heights, through the 50s and 60s, in the wake of the growing numbers of baby boomers. Consequently, poultry needed to be more closely scrutinized. In 1957, the **Poultry Products Inspection Act (PPIA)**[50] ensured that poultry would be continuously inspected before and after slaughter, and just prior to processing. The problem was the increased prevalence of food poisonings that were being documented by the CDC. Salmonellosis was one of the big problems to emerge from a poultry industry that grew so large, that it began to house chickens in tightly confined quarters.

In the 1950s, the food industry began using sophisticated technologies and additives, and was manip-

In 1958, the FDA deemed sugar, salt, vitamins, spices and monosodium glutamate as Generally Regarded as Safe (GRAS).

ulating food to create a broad assortment of processed by-products. Suspicion that the newer food additives represented potential health risks, began to trouble the public. In the early fall of 1950, orange Halloween candy, made from FD&C orange dye # 1, was linked to a cluster of children who had become seriously ill from eating the candy. Around that same time, a series of hearings, chaired by U.S. House of Representative, James Delaney, spurred by worries of the carcinogenecity of pesticide residues and food additives, were being held in Washington D.C. The press coverage drew public alarm, and the phones of House and Senate representatives were ringing off the hook. In response to the abundant non-regulated use of additives, the Food Drug and Cosmetic Act of 1938, was amended with the Food Additive Amendment, in 1960. The amendment successfully passed only after several investigations revealed that many more coloring agents and additives caused harmful effects and were delisted from the FDA's list of permitted additives.

By 1960, the Delaney clause, which was part of the Color Additive Amendment to the 1938 Federal Food and Drug Cosmetic Act, was also passed in congress. This legislation forbade the FDA from approving any additives demonstrated to cause cancer in laboratory animals or man, following reasonable exposure.[55] At that time, hamburgers, hotdogs, French fries, and an array of colorful milkshakes, ice cream sundaes and sodas were beginning to invade the market place. The public was also witnessing the appearance of strange-colored items such as maraschino cherries, multi-colored marshmallows, and colorful varieties of candies. The 200 color additives that were used by the food industry, by the 1950s, were given a provisional status pending further investigation. Not long after 1960, approximately half of the accepted coloring agents were removed from the FDA's list of safe ingredients. It was the responsibility of the food manufacturers to demonstrate that the ingredients they were using were Generally Regarded as Safe (GRAS). Sugar, salt, vitamins, spices, and monosodium glutamate, were grandfathered into the GRAS listing. The government wanted to ensure that those new ingredients, added to food, in addition to drug and pesticide residues, detected in products, were in amounts considered safe for consumption. The FDA established a two-tier food additive classification system to ensure the safety of the national food inventory: first, those additives requiring FDA certification, and second, those exempt from certification requirements. If an additive is derived from either plants or minerals, it would be exempt. The only exception to that rule is the cochineal extract from an insect, from which is derived the "carmine" pigment, which received full approval for use in food. For exempt additives, the FDA places the onus on food companies to prove that the additive, submitted for approval, complies with the FDA's definitions and with purity standards. Additives, requiring FDA certification, fall under the category, synthetic organic dyes. Traditionally, color additives that have required certification were coal-tar colors. Today, coloring agents currently being submitted for certification, are synthesized from petroleum-based compounds.[55] The FDA does have executive powers to enforce its regulations. It has, more recently, issued several warnings to food manufacturers for not declaring the use of certain coloring agents, used in their products, notably: FD&C Yellow No. 6 in dehydrated papaya, FD&C Red No. 40 and FD&C Yellow No. 6 in bakery products, and for FD&C Blue No. 1 and FD&C Yellow No. 5 in noodle products, and for the presence of the unapproved color additive, Ponceau 4R in strawberry filling.[55]

Also, the food distribution network, that was rapidly expanding, to accommodate the voracious appetites of the growing baby boomer families of the 1950s to 1970s, was at risk of experiencing food poisoning incidents. Hence, under President Eisenhower's administration, the USDA received a facelift in order to better address the increasing concerns regarding the wholesomeness of food. And so the Bureau of Animal Industry and the Bureau of Dairy Industry were fused together in order to create the USDA Agricultural Research Service.[50] This move certainly gave a scientific tone to agriculture, as food scientists were now ensuring the integrity of the food supply. By the 1960s, as the fast food industry began growing in leaps and bounds, more emphasis needed to be placed on ensuring the wholesomeness of meat and poultry, which was being massively consumed.

In the years 1967 and 1968, the Wholesome Meat Act and the Wholesome Poultry Act were passed by Congress, to ensure that at the
State level, meat and poultry inspections were at least meeting federal standards stipulated in the FMIA and the PPIA. The government continued to monitor other sectors of food production such as eggs with the Eggs Products Inspection Act of 1970.[50]

6.2 A Nation's Unhealthy Food

As epidemiologists began, during the late 1970s and 80s, to establish strong correlations between eating habits and disease rates, scientists were understanding that foods could provide protection against diseases like atherosclerosis and some cancers, which were now at much higher rates than in previously decades.[49] Breast cancer and other malignant neoplasms were still increasing despite good progress in reducing rates of other cancers. And while death rates from heart disease had gone down, the incidence of coronary artery disease risk factors was still increasing.

The notion of disease prevention was slowly filtering into the collective unconscious. By the late 70s the Department of Health Education and Welfare had already identified health promotion and disease prevention as priorities.

In 1979, *Healthy People*: The Surgeon General's Report on Health Promotion and Disease Prevention, was completed. It set the ground work for improving the nation's health with Healthy People 1990 goals.[53]

This first national health initiative, prioritized decreasing mortality rates in different age groups, notably infant mortality, and identified 15 nutrition objectives. The most important ones are noted here:[52]

1. decreasing iron deficiency anemias in pregnancy
2. preventing child growth abnormalities
3. containing the numbers of overweight adults, especially women of child-bearing age
4. increasing the number of overweight adults initiating weight loss diets
5. controlling excessive sodium consumption,
6. heightening the population's awareness of the link between food and diseases such as, hypertension, heart disease, dental caries and cancer.

The intent was to educate the public about ways to prevent the numerous secondary diseases that arose from obesity. Foods high in fiber, low in calories and sodium, to name a few, were being promoted as preventative. The objectives made sense in light of rising rates of obesity by 1974.

The nutritional quality of the American diet had become a liability; excessive amounts of sugar, sodium and fat were being consumed through sodas, fast foods and frequent snacking. The movie "**Supersize Me**" provided the public with a shocking account of the physical problems that can arise from frequent fast food consumption. People were able to relate to this movie because of their own personal experiences of not feeling quite right, after consuming the high calorie and fat loads of a Big Mac, medium fries, and an M&M McFlurry.

The public was becoming ill at a fast enough pace that health care costs were swelling inordinately by the mid-1990s. In fact, morbidity and mortality costs, associated with cardiovascular disease (CVD), were estimated to be $286.5 billion by 1999, according to the American Heart Association estimates.[2]

The suspicion that our diet as a nation was making us sick, certainly began with the early books of Adelle Davis, who became the most famous nutritionist in the early to mid-20th century. She introduced the idea that individual diets needed to contain ample vitamins and minerals; that there were strategies for eating healthy.

She was the author of four best-selling books published in the 30s, 40s, 50s and 60s: *Let's Cook It Right, Let's Have Healthy Children, Let's Get Well*, and *Let's Eat Right To Keep Fit*. She sold millions of copies throughout the U.S., and set the foundation for the natural food movement that was to sweep the U.S. market around the time of her death in the 1970s.

It was likely, however, William Dufty's 1975 best seller book: *Sugar Blues* that drew national attention to the high sugar content of the U.S. diet, and to the rather nefarious consequences of excessive sugar on human health.

Because Dufty was the husband of Hollywood legend, Gloria Swanson, who crusaded against the impoverished American diet, the book got the spotlight it needed to sell like hotcakes. Although the book reached best seller status, it was seen as promoting quackery with no real science to support the claims.

Nevertheless, the seed of doubt was planted and began to spread, encompassing a growing segment of a potentially very lucrative market that wanted better quality food. Food companies like General Nutrition Company (GNC) began selling natural unprocessed foods that were advertised as protective against a whole array of conditions, such as arthritis, diabetes, high cholesterol, indigestion, and various types of cancers.

A minority of the market became regular customers that were willing to pay more to get natural unprocessed foods that contained minimal or no additives; whole grains, in addition to the healthy oils were greatly sought after. Marginalized in the 1970s, as conspiracy theorists that believed the food supply was impoverished by a rogue food industry, natural foodists grew in numbers. They caused the growth in the sale of natural food to reach $11.1 billion by 2003. They would regularly purchase odd foods and compounds such as brewer's yeast for its natural vitamin B content, lecithin, a phospholipid extracted from soybean oil for improved memory and cognition, natural cranberries to fight off bladder infections, and St. John's wort to treat mild depression. They also purchased foods with no added sugar, and ingested a full arsenal of vitamin and mineral supplements at the crack of dawn every day. These products were advertised as having curative and preventative actions that were unsubstantiated by any research. Nevertheless, personal testimonials, tied to certain products, impacted sales significantly.

> **Natural foods began to mean foods that were minimally processed and without artificial additives.**

The public was slowly awakening to the idea that the U.S. food habits were actually making the nation sick. Larger numbers of consumers began, at the turn of the millennium, to purchase more unprocessed foods, whole grain products and foods that contained less sugar. In response to the growing market, the government attempted to regulate the use of the term "natural" on food labels in order to protect the consumers from fraudulent foods.[40]

In 2006 the Food Safety and Inspection Service (FSIS) of the USDA began public hearings to better define what was meant by **natural**. Though a regulatory definition had not yet been established, food labelers—guided by FSIS policies—began to add "natural" to the label of foods that were minimally processed. They could not contain: artificial sweeteners, colors, flavors and other artificial additives; nor could they be grown by hormones, or contain antibiotic residues, hydrogenated oils, stabilizers, and emulsifiers, according to FSIS guidelines.[53b]

It took 20 years before the U.S. government was able to garner enough epidemiological information, on the U.S. population health status, before putting together a broad national public health program aimed at containing and decreasing disease rates.

It had become clear that the Westernized diet, bolstered by $32 billion per year in aggressive and sophisticated marketing campaigns, had managed to bring the American populace to the brink. So then, in 1990 the U.S. established the Healthy People 2000 program. Health objectives were established by the U.S. Public- Health Service, which came under the authority of the much larger department of Health & Human Services.[53]

Exercise, nutrition and tobacco use were identified as the top three areas of concern for the decade 1990-2000. There was clear evidence, that diet-related diseases were either killing or physically and mentally compromising the American people.[49]

6.3 Natural Foods to Super Foods: Making the U.S. Diet Healthy

New natural food companies began to appear, and sectors of the food industry quickly reconfigured production, and developed natural food lines in the 1970s, and then nutraceuticals and functional foods by the mid to late 1990s. The term, "nutraceutical," was coined in 1989 by Dr. Stephen DeFelice MD, chairman of the Foundation for Innovative Medicine. He derived the term by combining the words nutrition and pharmaceutics. The concept hit home for many individuals who were ready to use food in a medicinal way. Doctor DeFelice defines nutraceuticals as follows:[10]

A nutraceutical is any substance that is a food or a part of a food and provides medical or health benefits, including the prevention and treatment of disease. Such products may range from isolated nutrients, dietary supplements and specific diets to genetically engineered designer foods, herbal products, and processed foods such as cereals, soups and beverages.

The nutraceutical industry exploded in the last decade because of the public's growing desire to prevent disease through nutrition. Soon big players like Monsanto, American Home Products, Dupont, Abbott Laboratories, Johnson & Johnson, and Novartis, became involved in what soon would be a very profitable industry.
In fact, in 2011, the global sales of nutraceuticals reached $142 billion, and is estimated to surpass $250 billion by 2018, according to Bourne Partners, a North Caroline-based management consulting firm.[4] At the moment, U.S. sales are currently estimated at $86 billion per year and it is expected to grow to $90 billion by 2015. Nutraceuticals are really made up of three important sectors: **nutraceutical ingredients, dietary supplements** and **functional foods**. Health Canada, defines functional foods as normal food products that have the ability to reduce the likelihood of developing chronic disease. They write:[30]

A functional food is similar in appearance to, or may be, a conventional food, is consumed as part of a usual diet, and is demonstrated to have physiological benefits and/or reduce the risk of chronic disease beyond basic nutritional functions.

In Japan, for foods to be labeled as functional, three criteria must be met: first, the food cannot be in capsule, tablet or in powder form; second, it must be consumed daily as part of a normal diet; and third, it must regulate biological processes in order to prevent or control disease.

The Academy of Nutrition and Dietetics is less narrow in its definition. The Academy's position is that:[38]

*"...although all foods provide some level of physiological function, the term functional foods is defined as whole foods along with fortified, enriched, or enhanced foods that have a potentially beneficial effect on health when consumed as part of a varied diet on a regular basis at effective levels based on significant standards of evidence.
The Academy supports
The Food and Drug Administration's approved health claims on food labels when based on rigorous scientific substantiation.*

In that sense then, any food enriched or fortified with vitamins, minerals, or phytochemicals can be called functional. For instance, this means that margarine with added phytosterol becomes a functional food because of the cholesterol lowering ability of that plant stanol. It means that milk fortified with vitamin D is, by definition, a functional food, as it can prevent or help treat rickets. In a similar manner, if a food manufacturer were to include vitamin E in a soup, it would become a functional food, if it could be shown that regular consumption of the soup reversed atherosclerosis.[10]

Pressured by some in the food industry, who wanted to cash in on the lucrative business of selling healthy foods, and by the American Dietetic Association and consumer groups, who wanted product transparency, the FDA enacted in 1990 the Nutrition Labeling and Education Act (NLEA), which was an amendment to the Federal Food Drug and Cosmetic Act of 1938.[54]

It required by 1994, that food manufacturers comply with strict labeling guidelines pertaining to the nutrient content of food. Manufacturers were now obligated to list the nutrient content on a specifically formatted label—known as the nutrition facts panel—located on the package.[54] It also authorized the FDA to control any health claims that might appear on packaged food.

For a product to feature a **health claim** on the front label, the manufacturer must submit a request to the FDA with proof that the health claim is supported by evidence-based studies. It must demonstrate that the product, when regularly consumed, can decrease the risk of the disease.

The label becomes a platform to either showcase the nutrients contained in the product or to force food companies to consider enriching their food so as to be more competitive. As long term prospective studies began to identify trans-fatty acids, as potentially dangerous fats that doubled the atherogenicity risk, the FDA required, by an Act of congress in 2003, that the content of trans-fats be included on the labels of all food products by no later than 2006 (**Figure 6.2**).[15]

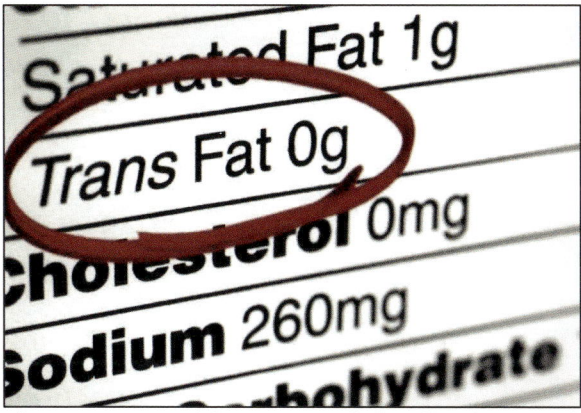

Figure 6.2 Nutrition Facts Label Indicating 0g of Trans Fats © Jonathan Vasata.

This move forced companies to rid their products of trans-fats as soon as they were able, and to find a workable alternative.

In 2004, because of documented increases in the prevalence of people reacting to allergens, in a variety of foods, congress enacted the **Food Allergen Labeling and Consumer Protection Act,** forcing manufacturers to list any of the key 8 allergens, if present in the food: wheat, milk, eggs, peanuts, shellfish, tree nuts, fish, and soy. The legislation forced food companies to come clean with ingredients and with the nutritional quality of foods.[44]

At the same time, General Foods' crystal orange soft drink, Tang® was being fortified to meet 100% of vitamin C's RDA. Originally created by General Foods, Tang® is now owned by Kraft Foods. Ads previously claimed that it had more vitamin C than even a natural orange. Tang® is currently fortified with some vitamin B, A, and iron. By today's standard, this synthetic drink (**Figure 6.3**), that contains not even a single orange ingredient, can feature on its label, content claims that can mislead many ill-informed consumers. The customer has such a trusting nature that he has been manipulated, by sophisticated marketing strategies, into believing that there is likely some orange content in the drink, or that it may even be superior to an orange.

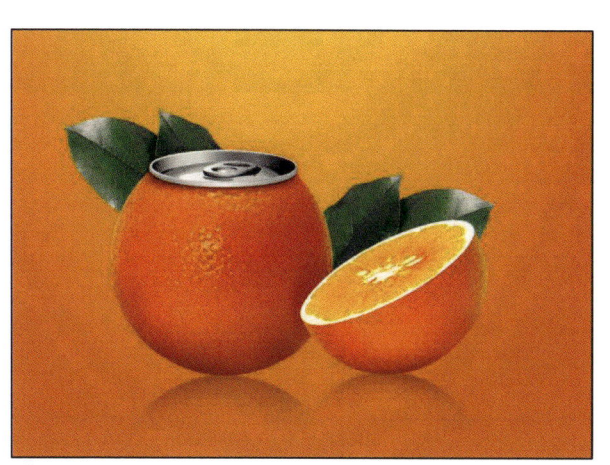

Figure 6.3 Orange Can and Half Orange © Designs Stock.

Other companies were doing it right, by creating probiotics. *Lactobacillus Rhamnosus,* added to yogurt, produces a probiotic food that encourages the proliferation of friendly intestinal bacteria. The hypothesis is that when consumed frequently, the lactobacillus displaces out of the gut any nefarious bacteria that can increase the risks of developing intestinal diseases.

Danone's Activia yogurt became a strong front runner in the probiotic craze, here in the U.S., with $130 million in sales registered for 2006. By adding *Bifidus regularis* to the yogurt, clinical trials were able to demonstrate increased regularity in subjects that consumed the yogurt daily, which was a clear health benefit for a population plagued by gastrointestinal disorders and especially constipation. Gastrointestinal diseases account for 7% of all hospitalizations in the U.S. and carried a hefty price of $20.1 billion in 2004.[35]

Despite improved personal hygiene and food safety training programs for foodservice employees such as ServSafe®, the CDC estimates that between 62 and 106 million Americans a year suffer from acute gastroenteritis caused by foodborne illnesses. The impact of food poisonings on the population is devastating as it results in 325,000 hospitalizations and 5,000 deaths annually, and costs between $10 and $83 billion per year in direct and indirect medical expenses.[34]

The most recognized bacterial pathogen is *salmonella* because of numerous outbreaks in the 1970s and 80s associated with undercooked chicken and raw eggs. Recent zero tolerance legislation for visible fecal contamination of poultry, has cleaned up the industry considerably and brought down the incidence of *salmonella* outbreaks. There are, however, less wider-known pathogens such as *Clostridium perfringens*, *Bacillus cereus*, and *Staphylococcus aureus* that yearly sicken scores of individuals.[34]

Between 1903 and 2011, outbreaks with large fatalities were not numerous, however, there are notable incidences of outbreaks, listed among the 10 deadliest in U.S. history, from which government agencies have learned vital information.[18] The deadliest foodborne illness on record, transpired in Long Island, New York, between 1924 and 1925. The problem occurred when polluted waters from Long Island, New York were used to hold oysters, resulting in fifteen hundred people from New York to Chicago and Washington DC falling ill from typhoid fever, which lead to 150 deaths.

The second deadliest outbreak was in 1903 in Ithaca, New York. The Six Mile Creek dam was being constructed using, what some health officials suspect, were Italian workers who were carriers of *Salmonella typhi*. The Ithaca water company decided to expedite the construction of the dam, by not installing a water filtration system until the dam was completed. Many of the workers used the river rather than the outhouses, leading to the coliform contamination of the water supply. A total of 1350 people fell ill to typhoid fever, which resulted in 82 deaths among whom were 29 Cornell University students.

Third on the list is the 1911 *Streptococcus* infestation of raw unpasteurized milk. It was delivered to Boston area homes, where a total of 48 people re-

> Food poisoning results in approximately 325,000 hospitalizations and 5,000 deaths annually.

portedly died from the outbreak.

For the fourth deadliest outbreak, we have to jump ahead to a 2011 *Listeria* outbreak of Rocky Ford

> Annually, *E. coli* 0157:H7 causes approximately 62,000 human infections with an alarming 55% death rate.

cantaloupes in Colorado. In this case, at least 146 people, spread over 28 states, became sickened, and 36 succumbed.

In fifth place was a 1985 *Listeria* infestation of Mexican cheese, causing the death 28 Hispanic women. This most serious foodborne outbreak affected mostly pregnant women.

The sixth case took place with the 1922 *Streptococcus* contamination of raw milk, delivered to Portland Oregon residences, causing 22 deaths.

In 1998, ballpark hotdogs and Sara Lee deli meats were recalled after 21 people died from listeriosis. Health officials traced the 7th worse infestation back to a Michigan meat processing plant.

In 1919, a total of 19 people died in three states, as a result of botulism poisoning, traced to canned ripe olives that were manufactured in California; this was the eighth worst U.S. outbreak.

In 2008-2009, nine died from *Salmonella typhi* found in peanut butter and peanut paste; the incident infected a total of 714 people in 46 states, making it the ninth worst outbreak. And finally, in 2002, Listeria struck again, affecting Pilgrims

Pride's sliced turkey, which killed 8 people in an outbreak that hit several states.

The 1990s was the decade of the deadliest *E. coli* 0157:H7 poisonings from undercooked hamburger in U.S. history. The most famous case occurred in 1993, when a Jack-in-the-Box restaurant undercooked their hamburger to 150F rather than 155F. This incident caused 500 customers to become ill, and killed 4.[8, 18]

Annually, the CDC estimates that there are 62,000 human infections from *E coli* 0157:H7 with a 0.55 death rate. Approximately 17% of those illnesses are serious enough to require hospitalization, primarily because of diarrhea and kidney failure.[45] It was these outbreaks of E coli 0157:H7 that led the U.S. government to develop a program of quality control called: Hazard Analysis Critical Control Points (HACCP), which greatly improved sanitary practices. It ensured a closer monitoring of high risk food products, during storage, preparation, cooling, reheating and serving.

Foodborne disease outbreaks are regularly monitored by an active surveillance system called Food-Net. It is used to coordinate the CDC, and 10 state and local health departments, thus representing a catchment of 38 million people. The system is set up to collect data on seven bacteria that are associated with high morbidity and mortality, most notably *Campylobacter* species, *E. coli* O157:H7, *Listeria monocytogenes*, *Salmonella*, *Shigella*, *Vibrio parahaemolyticus*, *Yersinia enterocolitica*. In addition, it monitors two parasites: *Cryptosporidium parvum*, and *Cyclospora cayetanensis*.[34] Although the monitoring list of pathogens is relatively narrow, the most numerous cases of food related gastroenteritis, reported between 1996 and 2000, were either ill-defined intestinal infections or gastroenteritis of a non-infectious origin. This means that of the estimated 250-350 million cases of gastroenteritis reported in the U.S., on an annual basis, roughly 60 to 84% are of an unknown origin; some sources have even ventured to estimate that 90% of a probable 267 million cases of gastroenteritis, reported annually, are likely of viral origin. The difficulty here is that viruses, unlike bacteria, are very difficult to detect in food. Interestingly, the most significant cause of viral foodborne illnesses are of the Noro or Norwalk-like type originating from the *Caliciviridae* family. These are essentially spread by the fecal-oral route.[34] This means that if someone goes to the washroom but does not wash his hands, and then touches a surface, the virus can be transmitted to another who touches that same surface. Other vectors of transmission include vomit, food, and water.

However, taking viral transmission as a whole, public health officials have estimated that about 39% of Norovirus outbreaks were food-related. The elderly are particularly vulnerable to a viral outbreak, primarily because of their weaker immune system, and they tend to reside in large groups like nursing homes, which account for about 30% of Noro-virus outbreaks.

The most frequent cause of foodborne illness is improper handling of cold or hot foods.

Cruise ships have been historically the preferred location for the largest Norovirus outbreaks reported so far. Beverly McCabe-Sellers and Samuel Beattie have reported, in their review of food safety,[34] that between 1993 and 1997, the most significant cause of foodborne outbreaks in the U.S. was attributed, by far, to improper holding of cold or hot foods. A distant second was **poor personal hygiene**, and thirdly **cross-contamination**. Inadequate cooking and unsafe food sources were in fourth and fifth positions respectively.

Generally, health officials will suspect either *Bacillus cereus* or *Clostridium perfringens*, when there is temperature abuse of food that involve, improper holding temperatures. For instance, *C. perfringens* is often tied to improper holding temperatures of meats or poultry. When a chef leaves a cooked chicken on the counter at room temperature for over 6 hours, and then refrigerates it overnight in a temperature over 45F°, he commits a temperature-holding mistake. Hot food should be cooled from 135 to 70F° within 2 hours, and then from 70 to 41F° within 4 hours according to National Restaurant Association (NRA) guidelines. This can be accomplished by promptly placing food in the refrigerator after allowing a short time (~15 minutes) for the food to cool down on the counter. A general rule is to wait for steam or noticeable heat release to subside before covering and refrigerating.

Likewise, after cooking, should chicken be placed in a cafeteria line that is heated to a hot-holding temperature of only 128F° and held for over 6 hours, there would be a clear temperature abuse incident. This improper holding condition heightens the chances of a *C. perfringens* infestation. Ideally, hot-held food should be maintained at a temperature ≥ 135F°. The patients' main symptom, following a C. perfringens infection, shows up as mild gastroenteritis that often does not get reported to health officials. What make these bacteria particularly nefarious are the heat-resistant spores they produce. The spores are formed during temperature abuses such as poor refrigeration and long exposure to room temperatures. These abuses make reheating practices, using adequately high temperature treatments, completely ineffectual in producing safe food. This is because of those heat-resistant spores formed during poor holding temperatures. Some strains of *Clostridium perfringens* can produce a nasty enterotoxin that causes diarrhea and abdominal cramps that lasts 48 hours.

Bacillus cereus infestations are also tied to meats, cooked milk and dairy products even after pasteurization, cooked vegetables, rice and pasta. Noroviruses, on the other hand, tend to be more associated with foodservice workers practicing poor personal hygiene.

Public health officials almost always suspect *Campylobacter* contamination when raw meat cross-contaminate a raw lettuce cutting surface. More recently, *Campylobacter* has been identified as a potential trigger for Guillain-Barre Syndrome, a powerfully debilitating neurological disease that strikes suddenly.[34]

The most frequently diagnosed bacterial infections are featured in **Table-6.1** along with the bacteria and the general conditions that are favorable to an infection.

TABLE 6.1 Bacterial foodborne illnesses and the conditions leading to the infestations.

Bacteria	Illnesses	Conditions
Salmonella typhi	Typhoid	
Staphylococcus aureus	Staphylococcal food poisoning	Found in nasal passages, skin and throats of people and animals. It is caused by the poor hygiene practices of food handlers in combination with poor temperature control (remaining between 41 and 135F° for extended periods.
Clostridium botulinum	Botulism	Rare but very dangerous. Occurs in home canning of low acidity foods, and baked potato wrapped in aluminum foil
Listeria monocytogenes	Listeriosis	Bacteria found primarily in soil and water; it can contaminate poultry, cattle and raw milk. It can be a problem in meat processing plants. Can contaminate foods that are not heat treated such as: processed meats, smoked sea foods, and soft cheeses like brie and feta
Salmonella spp	Salmonellosis	Caused by undercooked eggs, ground beef, poultry and unpasteurized milk
Clostridium perfringens	Clostridium perfringens infection; spore producing. One of the most frequent causes of food poisoning.	Batch food production kept <135F° Associated with cafeterias, hospitals, prisons, nursing homes, and catering
Campylobacter jejuni	Campylobacteriosis	It is recognized as the most common cause of food poisoning in

| | | | the U.S. It occurs from undercooked or raw poultry, contaminated water and unpasteurized milk. |

Source: Food Poisonings from www.Food Safety.gov which is a gateway used by the U.S Federal Government to communicate food safety information to the public. The webpage is a collaborative effort of the FDA, USDA, CDC, NIH, U.S. Department of Health and Human Services, and the White House.

Food poisonings are widespread throughout the United States, and health officials have been trying to educate the public about the specific dangers associated with improper food preparation techniques. The National Restaurant Association's Education Foundation established strict food safety criteria and rules that are taught, through their ServSafe® foodservice training, to workers and managers.

First, they teach that hot food should be held at a temperature ≥ 135F° just prior to service. The temperature must not drop under 135F° for longer than 2 hours, otherwise strict safety standards dictate discarding the food.

Second, cooling methods dictate that hot food temperatures must travel through the danger zone quickly (135F° to 41F°). ServSafe® guidelines state that hot food must move from 135F° to 70F° within 2 hours, and that an additional 6 hours is permitted to allow the temperature to cool from 70F down to 41F.

Third, cooks must prevent the cross-contamination of food from occurring, while physically manipulating high risk foods such as pork, hamburger, fish and poultry. Some foodservice operations have developed a system of color-coded cutting boards, which ensure that only meats are cut on the red boards, and only green cutting boards are utilized for fresh produce.

Fourth, foods need to be cooked until their internal temperatures reach desired temperatures for a minimum of 15 seconds. Safety guidelines require that hamburger reach an internal temperature of 155F°; fish can be cooked until the temperature attains 145F°. Poultry can carry so many pathogens, and so officials require an internal temperature of 165F° for 15 seconds. Pork, veal, beef and lamb must all be cooked to at least 145F° before serving.

Despite valiant programs that ensure the proper training of foodservice personnel, food poisoning incidences are still increasing. Troubled by an estimated 4000 foodborne illnesses from major outbreaks reported between 2006 and 2010, and a shocking 4200 product recalls, the Obama administration signed into law in 2011, the United States **FDA Food Safety & Modernization Act**.[19] It provides the FDA with new enforcement authority that will hopefully increase compliance to food safety rules. Under this Act, hazard analysis becomes mandatory. The earlier food hazard analysis system called, HACCP was replaced by the Hazard Analysis Preventive Control Plan (HAPCP).

6.4 Food Poisonings on the Rise: Consequence of Globalization and Eating Away From Home

6.5 Food & the Contamination of the Environment

6.5.1 The use of Pesticides
Historically, pests have always threatened, to some degree, agricultural yields, and humans had to learn to contain their impact on crop production. Records from Roman times, confirm that burning sulfur controlled pests, and salt application was successful to some degree in weed management.

In the 1600s, ant infestations were eradicated with the use of arsenic mixed with honey. But, it was not until the late 19th century's chemical revolution, that crude chemical compounds such as calcium arsenate, nicotine sulfate, and sulfur were spread over crops by farmers, but only with mild successes.

The true beginning of chemical pesticide use, really only took root in the U.S. after WWII, as more complex and efficacious chemical treatments were being developed by a post-war chemical industry.

In the 1950s and onwards, farmers began utilizing DDT, BHC, aldrin, dieldrin, endrin, and 2,4-D. Controlled and regulated by the Environmental Protection Agency (EPA), pesticides were promptly perceived as safe and necessary by the general population. These chemical compounds were assuredly seen as opening up new frontiers and opportunities, and so the population confidently supported their use.

In many instances, farmers liberally sprayed these pesticides on their crops causing unforeseen residues to appear on the plants, water and soil (**Figure-6.4**). However, the population's trust in pesticides was quickly shattered, with the publication of Rachel Carson's best seller: *Silent Spring*. Published in 1962, the book described the rather worrisome environmental consequences that could arise from careless applications of pesticides—a practice that had already begun. Hence, by the 1960s, Americans mistrusted the pesticides, insecticides and herbicides that were being sprayed on agricultural fields around the country. Were there enough residues, on fruits and vegetables, to warrant the alarm bells that were being set off by zealous environmentalists?

The United States has progressively used significant amounts of pesticides between 1988 and 2000, going from 1.19 billion pounds annually to 1.23 billion pounds in 2000, and costing $11.165 billion in annual user expenditure, according to the Environmental Protection Agency (EPA).[27] However, between 2001 and 2007, the EPA reports a more or less steady 13% decline in the pounds used. Nevertheless, the U.S. still spayed 1.13 billion pounds of pesticides in 2007, causing environmental groups to contest the ongoing poisoning of the environment. Studies have shown that pesticide residues can leach into ground water, creating serious environmental problems; also children, because of their lower body weights, can be at higher risk of neurological damage from residues left on fruits. The evidence became so strong that children's health was at risk, because of the use of specific pesticides, that the EPA imposed new restrictions on methyl parathion (also known as Penncap-M) and azinphosmethyl. There was convincing evidence emerging that these pesticides could cause brain and neurological damage, especially to children.[14]

These pesticides were also widely used on products heavily consumed by toddlers such as apples, peaches, wheat, rice, pears, sugar beets and cotton.

Keith Delaplane,[11] an assistant professor of entomology at the University of Georgia, claims that residues are not very high. He argues that banning the use of all pesticides would most certainly be counterproductive, as crop yields from wheat, corn and soybeans would be expected to drop as much as 73%. This, he continues, would cause prices to soar, and thus destabilize the market; U.S. agriculture

> **Questions remain about whether the risks associated with pesticide use outweigh the benefits.**

would become less competitive on the world market, and the vacuum, created by less U.S. agricultural production, would be quickly filled by imports from countries with less pesticide control legislation. This would leave the door wide open for crops with illegal pesticide residues to enter the country.

He also points out that U.S. agricultural production is a real paradox. Whereas 95% of the population, in developing countries, produce food to feed themselves and the other 5% of the population, by contrast, within the North American context, only 3 to 5% of the population produces food for the other 95 to 97%. The reality, then, of North American agricultural production, is that it greatly relies on technology and pesticides to ensure that few farmers are able to grow and harvest large yields in relatively little time.

In our rather diseased-free western world, we tend to forget that pesticides have been instrumental, in keeping out of our environment, yellow fever, encephalitis, plague, typhoid fever, malaria, dog heartworms, and Rocky Mountain spotted fever. Furthermore, insecticides have also improved the sanitation of our homes by successfully eradicating ticks, cockroaches, flies and fleas. In the end, the question of whether pesticides should be used in U.S. agriculture, given their known impact on environmental pollution, can only be answered using the **risk: benefit ratio**. Scientists can determine if the risks associated with pesticide use outweighs the benefits that can be achieved from their use. The first issue surrounding pesticides are the residue levels detected on food. Understanding residue levels will be helpful in conceptualizing risks.

In the 1950s, residue levels were detected in parts per million (ppm). By the 1960s, parts per billion (ppb) was the new measurement standard for residues, whereas by 1975, measurements were improved enough to be able to detect residues in parts per trillion (ppt), and then, parts per quadrillion (ppq) in 2012. However, because our detection instruments are now very sophisticated and sensitive, scientists are more likely to find infinitely minuscule concentrations of residues in crops that would have previously gone undetected.

This raises an important conceptual problem: does finding 4 parts per quadrillion constitute a toxic level of pesticide? Should we be concerned that any residue at all is found on food? To help visually capture how small these residue levels really are, imagine one grain of salt dropped into an Olympic-size swimming pool; that would be the equivalent to a concentration of one part per trillion. So then, it only becomes possible to comprehend the biological burden of a residue, by establishing what toxicologists refer to as the lethal dose necessary to kill 50% of the test rats (LD_{50}) in a specific laboratory test. Hence, the lower the LD_{50} is, the more dangerous the poison. This annotation is not reserved only for deadly chemical compounds. In fact, table salt has an LD_{50} for adults (3g/Kg body weight) and for children (2 Tablespoons). Once the LD_{50} is determined, then toxicologists need to determine the No Observable Effect Level (NOEL). This value is the concentration of pesticide, used in animal experiments, for which no biological effect was observed. This value is then divided by a number between 100 and 1000, in order to establish an **Acceptable Daily Intake** (ADI). The ADI is regarded by the EPA as a safe amount to regularly consume. When establishing this amount, the EPA also considers the residue normally detected on specific fruits and vegetables. However, by monitoring the National Disappearance data of specific foods, it must factor in the frequency and amount of produce consumed by the population, as well as the various consumer age groups that consume specific produce. This means that in order to establish pesticide intakes from watermelon, the EPA refers to National Disappearance data to see, on average, the estimated watermelon consumption per capita. Scientists then can conclude, using the normal eating patterns of Americans, whether there is a high probability of ingesting concerning levels of pesticides from watermelon, for instance,[11, 13] given its normal seasonal use.

To ensure that pesticide residues are remaining below EPA safety thresholds, the FDA samples between 12,000 and 14,000 foods from randomly selected grocery stores nationwide for residue levels. Although the sample could be considered suboptimal, considering the size of the nation's grocery store food inventory, the findings from these tests have still been revealing. In 1987, after measuring 14,492 food samples, produced domestically and imported from 79 countries, the FDA found pesticide residues on 50% of the samples, and less than 1 percent had residue levels that exceeded EPA legal tolerance limits. While very few samples exceeded EPA restrictions, it is nevertheless concerning that pesticides are frequently consumed, albeit at low concentrations.

The second issue, pertaining to the impact of pesticides on the body's biological system, is the type of toxicity. There is **acute toxicity**, which involves one very high dose of pesticide that exceeds the body burden's upper limit, causing the person to experience acute illness.

There is also, **chronic toxicity**, which involves incremental increases in the body's burden over a prolonged intake of lower concentrations of pesticide. Toxicologists refer to this as a bioaccumulation of pesticide residue in the body. This is precisely the problem with frequent ingestion of low concentrations of pesticides: though they do not cause acute toxic effects, they can nevertheless lead to more serious and concerning illnesses because of the fat solubility of these compounds. This means they are stored in the adipose tissue of the body, and are not promptly evacuated.

The third consequence of environmental pesticides is the toxic effect of applying pesticides through spraying. Indeed, aerosolized pesticides can drift with the wind, potentially becoming toxic for individuals who may inhale the vapors. In fact, pesticide drifts have been shown to cause sickness among the workers that apply the pesticides, and among those individuals inhaling the drifts at a distance. Lee and colleagues,[28] working under the direction of the National Institute for Occupational Safety and Health, Centers for Disease Control and Prevention, in Cincinnati, reported that agricultural spraying even affected individuals away from the application site. Between 1998 and 2006, there were 2,945 cases of illnesses resulting from this kind of outdoor pesticide drift. Lee concludes:[28]
14–24% of occupational pesticide poisoning may be attributed to off-target drift from agricultural applications.

Data collected from California, confirms that individuals, living in agricultural areas, will tend to be exposed to pesticide drifts at rates that are 69 times greater than in non-agricultural regions. The extent of the drift will vary with whether applied by truck or with aerial spraying.

The fourth pesticide issue is the impact on children. This is significant, as their body weights are small and consequently, pesticide body burden, expressed on a Kg body weight basis, indicates some worrisome concerns. Lu and colleagues,[31] from the Center for Food Safety and Nutrition, found that:

Although none of the pesticide residues, measured in the CPES, exceeded the U.S. EPA's tolerances, the frequent consumption of certain food commodities with episodic presence of pesticides, that are known to cause developmental and neurological effects in young children, underlies the need for further mitigation and should be monitored routinely by PDP"

Apples, peaches, grapes, carrots, lettuce, strawberries, pears and spinach are the foods most contaminated with pesticide residues in children's diets.

According to Shopper's Guide 2009, apples, peaches, grapes, carrots, and lettuce, in addition to strawberries, pears and spinach were identified as among the most contaminated foods consumed by children in the U.S.[31]

To more fully understand the potential extent of the environmental damage, ensuing from pesticide application, consider that in the 48 U.S. states surveyed, there is a total of 117 million acres of pasture, 405 million acres of rangeland, and 368 million acres of cropland. Now, at least 99% of that territory is sprayed with pesticides that leach into the surface and ground waters, thus contaminating the drinking water.

The problem gets accentuated by the livestock's nitrate-rich waste, as it destabilizes the ecosystem, and poses a threat to human health, along with the parasites like *Cryptosporidium* and *Giardia*, which make their way into the surface water.

It is clear that, whether environmental contaminations by pollutants are from industrial hazardous wastes or agricultural pesticide and herbicide residues, the food systems that are contaminated, can greatly affect the health of the populations living in these areas.

In the 1960s, there was awareness that our lakes and rivers were becoming polluted, and it did not take long for ecologists to make the link between polluted waters and poisoned food supplies and wildlife. The U.S. government responded in 1970, with the **Clean Water Act**. It regulated polluted runoffs from farm lands, and protected wetlands. Subsequently, the **Safe Water Drinking Act**, intended to ensure the purity and safety of the drinking water, was passed in 1974.

However, the more pronounced and reoccurring problems appear to be tied to occupational exposures to pesticides, especially among women and young farmers. Environmentally, there is no doubt that pesticides are poisons, and therefore workers need to exercise caution in their preparation and applications. Lee and colleagues,[28] in their study of pesticide drifts in the U.S. between 1998 and 2006 wrote: *Our findings show that the risk of illness resulting from drift exposure is largely borne by agricultural workers, and the incidence (114.3/million worker-years) was 145 times greater than that for all other workers.*

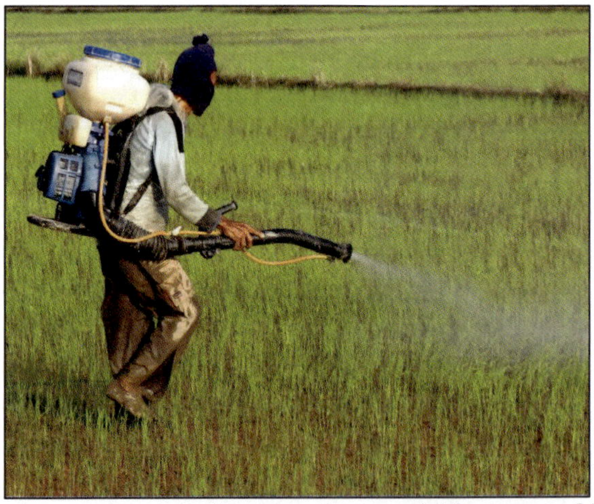

Figure 6.4: Worker spraying pesticide on a paddy field while unprotected © Raisman

More recently, efforts were made to orient pesticide research in the direction of more environmentally friendly compounds that mimic the chemical makeup of natural pesticides with narrow targets.

For instance, the pesticide, "pyrethroid," was created to mimic the natural plant poisons called, Pyrethrins, which have been used for hundreds of years. Also, the development of Insect-Growth-Regulators (IGRs) illustrates the industry's efforts at producing compounds that mimic insect hormones that limit growth, rather than nefarious chemicals that contaminate and kill. The most impressive advances in pesticide development in recent years are called **biorational pesticides**. These are among the most enviro-friendly techniques, which consist of using bacteria, viruses and other insects that predatorily compromise the invading pest.

6.5.2 The Use of GMOs in Food

Genetically Modified (GM) crops were introduced into U.S. agriculture in 1995, and by 1999 they occupied approximately 81 million acres (32 million Hectares) spread across the U.S. and Canada, representing 81% of the world's GM crop production. There were only an additional 19 million acres of GM crops cultivated around the world at that time.[48] This is, in part, because the Europeans maintained a staunch opposition to GM crops, based on highly emotional fears that were steeped in safety issues. In fact, in 1990 the European Council adopted precautionary Directive 90/220/EEC on the deliberate release of Genetically Modified Organisms (GMOs). This manoeuver made the process of either importing or growing GMOs very cumbersome and difficult. Christopher J. M. Whitty, chief scientific adviser at the UK Department for International Development (DFID) in London, and professor of international health at the London School of Hygiene and Tropical Medicine writes:[57]

European opposition to GM crops, although couched solely as worries about safety, also stems from concerns about the effect of large-scale farming on small-scale farmers, and the potential for biotech companies to create monopolies.

This reality would eventually surface within the U.S. agricultural sphere. In a May 13, 2013 New York Times article, Adam Liptak comments on a U.S. Supreme Court ruling that favored the patentability of GM seeds. He writes: [30] *Farmers who buy Monsanto's patented seeds must generally sign a contract promising not to save seeds from the resulting crop, which means they must buy new seeds every year. The seeds are valuable because they are resistant to the herbicide Roundup, itself a Monsanto product.* In this case, Indiana farmer, Vernon Hugh Bowman, was found guilty of purchasing seeds, contaminated with Monsanto GM seeds, from the owner of a local grain elevator. He planted the mixed seeds, and then kept the seeds from the harvest, a move, according to Judge Elena Kagan, that was in violation of the Monsanto contract. He had to pay $84,000 in restitution to Monsanto. The aggressive legal pursuits, by Monsanto, were consequential to their promise to put an end to the "suicide seed" research that they had been working on, in the late 1990s. This would have created seedless plants with no reproductive capabilities, thus arguably putting third world farmers at a financial disadvantage, since they would not have been able to reuse seeds from GMO plants. In reality, the impact of "patented seeds" is the same as "suicide seeds," since the latter requires a contract, with Biotech companies such as Monsanto, that makes the purchase of new GM seeds every year, mandatory. These seed patents create such a dependency on one supplier that it becomes questionable whether a farmer could ever legally terminate a contract without having to pay large sums of dollars in restitution.

The principle of genetically modifying a plant gene is very different than causing Mendelian cross pollination breeding between plants. Farmers have been cross-pollinating for a hundred years by, for instance, recognizing the superior yield quality of one plant and crossing it with a plant that might be more resistant to certain pests; the technique was imprecise, lengthy, and difficult to control. Ever since the 1920s, mutation breeding using X-rays was popularized, and by 1945, gamma rays, neutrons, alpha and beta particles were popularly used to generate plant mutations that were much faster, but still subject to imprecisions. GM crops, in contrast, are produced by trans-genetically introducing foreign DNA into plant genes at precise locations. For one thing, Whitty[57] advances that genetic engineering is much faster in introducing genetic alterations to a specific plant, compared to more traditional pollination techniques. Whitty clarifies the technique with an example that flaunts its clear benefits at a production level:[57] *by crossing the Bt toxin gene into local cowpea varieties, researchers in Nigeria have produced resistance* [to the Maruca pod borer] *in 95% of plants in confined field trials. In principle, Bt cowpea could increase yields throughout Africa by about 70%.*

Whitty is talking about trans-genetically inserting the toxin gene, of the bacterium *Bacillus thuringiensis,* into a cowpea gene. A net advantage is achieved with this manoeuver, as the cowpea can then naturally kill the Maruca pod borer (*Maruca vitrata*), an insect that destroys yearly many cowpea crops in Nigeria.[57] This type of GM crop produces its own natural pesticide, in the form of crystal proteins, that kill larvae. The expectation is an eventual overall decrease in the use of pesticides; this is referred to as a first generation GM plant.[23] The question of whether GM crops were actually able to reduce the use of pesticides was investigated in 2000. The results were mixed. Though increased yields and reduced pesticides usage were reported, in GM soybean crops in Tennessee and Mississippi, no yield benefits were seen in Missouri and Arkansas, and nor was there decreased pesticide use in the Mississippi Portal, according to a USDA report. In fact, since the introduction of GM crops, overall pesticide usage in the U.S. climbed to between 2-6.5% by the year 2000.[14,16] There has been, however, a gradual 8.2% decline in overall pesticide usage between 2000 and 2007.[14]

Second generational GM foods, are those that are genetically engineered to increase crop yields, vitamin, mineral, and fatty acid contents, and to control levels of phytates, lignins, and allergenic compounds. First and second generation GM crops are intended for food or animal feed, and, as such, have been engineered to improve pest resistance, herbicide tolerance, disease resistance, cold and drought tolerance, and nutritional content. Second generation GMOs for example, would be for "*bio-fortification*", whereby a specific nutrient is genetically encoded to be synthesized by a plant that normally does not contain the nutrient. The example of "*golden rice*"—a transgenic rice, rich in provitamin A (beta carotene)—nicely represents a second generation GM food. Created by inserting daffodil and bacteria DNA into the rice genome, the rice became a rich source of beta-carotene, a precursor to vitamin A. The procedure created rice that was capable of finally eradicating vitamin A deficiency-derived blindness in several regions around the world. The patent was licensed to an Agribusiness company named Syngenta, with the clear indication that Golden-Rice be made freely available to third world developing countries.[22] Unfortunately, writes Whitty, the wide distribution of "*golden rice*" has not been sanctioned by any country yet. Nevertheless, the Bill and Melinda Gates Foundation underwrite its continued development; the foundation is also funding the creation of GM bananas high in iron, and cassava, resistant to viruses that can be cultivated in Sub-Saharan Africa. The focus is really the elimination of hunger throughout the world.[24] In contrast, third generational GM crops are tagged for either pharmaceutical purposes or industrial molecules. The main goal of a 3rd generation pharmaceutical GM plant would be to synthesize therapeutic drugs such as insulin, gastric lipase enzyme, in addition to plant-derived vaccines for hepatitis B, rabies and Norwalk virus, which are currently undergoing clinical trials.[23] Monsanto, the world's largest producer of genetically modified seeds, is strongly lobbying government with a consistent message that describes the clear benefits associated GM plants. Though there are no catastrophic incidences, tied to the use of GM plants, so far in the world,[12] the main concern, according to Dr. Domingo and colleagues[12] from Rovira I Virgili University's School of Medicine in San Lorenzo, Spain, is the scant research on the safety of GMOs. Dr. Javed Akhter,[1] a researcher from King Faisal Specialist Hospital and Research Centre in Riyadh, Saudi Arabia, is raising concerns and setting off alarm bells, that this kind of genetic manipulation is potentially dangerous. He writes:

Genetic engineering can destabilize the way DNA replicates, transcribes and recombines.

He continues:
As a result of altered regulatory functions, genetically modified organisms (GMOs) may exhibit increased allergenic tendencies, toxicity, or altered nutritional value. They may also exhibit mutations, which are errors that can occur in the sequences or reading of the DNA within the cell. Altering regulatory functions may create new components or alter levels of existing components of an organism. One concern often expressed is that this may create antibiotic-resistant bacteria.[1]

The non-intentional error could have devastating and uncontrollable consequences, since the DNA insertion technique cannot really control how regulatory mechanisms in the cell might be impacted. The more immediate effects could be heightened allergenicity, greater toxicity and disruption in the nutrient content of the food. The real uncertainty is when the GMO is taken out of the controlled lab environment or test field, and released into the natural environment. Akhter writes:[1]

The interaction of GMOs with humans or natural ecosystems cannot be anticipated or tested before commercial release. This complexity makes it difficult to determine the short- and long-term effects of genetic modification.

It is this uncertainty that caused a split in the U.S. and European Union (EU) policies governing the

GM development. Whereas the EU requires that GM foods be properly labeled so that consumers can make informed decisions, Monsanto and other Biotech companies are petitioning the U.S. government to wave the labeling requirement for GM foods,[1] on the basis that they are no different than their natural counterpart—a position now held by the FDA. It is, in fact, this hands-off position that has many worried since the FDA has moved away from its role as watchdog, and taken a more passive position that relies on industry to ensure the safety of its GMOs.[32] It was the FDA's 1994 investigation of Calgene, Inc.'s FLAVR SAVRTM tomato that caused a major shift in strategy. It found the GM tomato to be no different than the non-GM counterpart, thus greatly decreasing the need for high vigilance on the part of the FDA. Domingo and colleagues write[12]: *An important problem seems to be related to the safety assessment of new GM foods, which is initially based on the use of the concept of "substantial equivalence." This concept is based on the following principle: "if a new food is found to be substantially equivalent in composition and nutritional characteristics to an existing food, it can be regarded as being as safe as the conventional food.*

Domingo also noted the flagrant absence of peer-review scientific studies examining the safety of GMOs. Indeed, if the scientific community is not vetting the corporate research of GM foods, then maybe there should be alarm about the less vigilant reviews of their safety, here in the U.S. Despite numerous groups in the U.S. opposing the full acceptance of GMOs into the marketplace, corporate lobbying of government has caused numerous bills, aimed at forcing labeling requirements on GM foods, to fail. It had become clear that identifying GMOs on labels would deter consumers from purchasing them. Despite the divisive stances, there are nevertheless clear indications that the number of GM plants is increasing. In 2010, there were about 202 GM crop events, in the U.S., that were registered with the *International Service for the Acquisition of Agri-Biotech Applications (ISAAA)*. By contrast, in Europe, only seven GMO Herbicide-resistant plants have been approved and they include: soybeans, rapeseed, sugar beet, maize, potato, cotton and carnations. Worldwide, since 2011, GMOs occupy an estimated 395 million acres, with the most significant growth occurring in developing countries such as Brazil, Argentina, India, and Paraguay. The EU eventually became less resistant to the import of U.S. GM-Os because of the European Commission's 1996 ruling, permitting the marketing of Swiss genetically engineered corn. This more or less forced the European Parliament to specifically challenge that decision to import GMO corn from Switzerland and not the U.S. The Americans were screaming unfair trade practices, and threatening to level trade barriers against the EU. The Commission was cornered into having to review its import policies of GMOs more carefully, and apply them more consistently. This decision eventually led to the European Parliament and the Council of Ministers, provisionally agreeing to market U.S. GMO corn. Although the EU became less resistant to the import of U.S. GMOs, it is specifically the trade association, Euro-Comm-erce, along with European food retailers that demanded that GMO-containing foods be clearly identified and separated from the non-GMO products. In 1996, a compromise was reached with the establishment of the Novel Foods Regulations. It stated that all novel GM foods, for which genetic manipulations did not change the food characteristics or properties, do not require a label. However, for the GM corn and soybeans, already previously accepted into Europe, the EU parliament voted in 1997 to require that GM corn and soybeans be packaged with a label that stated "Genetically Modified". This was a hard position that confirmed the EU's reticence at freely accepting GM crops.[32] Public opinion in Europe rose against GM crops with protests becoming more prevalent. There was uneasiness, among Europeans, regarding such a manipulation of their food supply. The U.S. had forgotten the importance Europeans had long given to a pure food supply. Lynch and Vogel accurately capture the turmoil erupting on the European continent in the late 1990s. They write:[32] *Monsanto, the American based firm which is the major supplier of genetically modified seeds in the United States and thus, potentially, of genetically modified foods sold in Europe bore the brunt of public opposition to GMOs. British newspapers called Monsanto the "Frankenstein food giant" and the "biotech bully boy." To redeem its public image and that of genetically-engineered food, Monsanto began a $1.6 million advertising campaign in the UK and France in 1998. In the UK, the campaign backfired: before the campaign began, 44% of British consumers surveyed had negative opinions of GMOs while after the campaign's conclusion 51% did so. In France, the number of consumers who said they would not buy foods containing GMOs also rose during the campaign, though by a smaller margin. Monsanto also became the target of a number of demonstrations.*

Nevertheless, GMO research and development continued to be strong with countless numbers of new GM plants tested and marketed since the new

Millennium. Internationally, it seemed that European opinion was clearly being ignored for two main reasons: first, the issues of malnutrition, that plague developing countries and underprivileged areas, are not a European problem, and so many felt that only those countries, who could benefit greatly from bio-fortified GM plants, should make the decision of whether or not to adopt GM-based agriculture; second, since only 10% of the world's population will come from Europe by the end of this century—the consequence of demographic winter—many advance that Europe's position on GM foods is of no consequence over the long term, and should not impact those countries able to benefit from the bio-fortification of crops.[32]

6.6 The Organic Food Movement

The organic movement originated from the public's concern that the environment and the food supply were becoming so contaminated, and nutritionally impoverished, that they endangered population health. Modern agriculture and livestock have been damaging the soil structure of our crop and pasture lands, through extensive tilling and irrigation, the use of heavy equipment, and the overgrazing practices of livestock. These have all contributed towards an annual loss of 2.7 tons of top soil/acre/year in 2007,[53c] and have led to a slow impoverishment of the mineral soil content.[53d] In response, relatively large pockets of the population began to embrace more enviro-friendly and health-minded consumer practices. Purchasing food, not laced with pesticide residues that could potentially sicken children, was perceived as a wise shopping alternative by the late 1970s. The idea that the environment and diet could lead to chronic forms of debilitating illnesses,—originally seen as radical environmentalism—quickly became a growing mainstream consumer preoccupation by the early 1990s, and a very profitable market for farmers, food producers and distributors, interested in the sale of wholesome organic foods.

> Modern agricultural and livestock raising methods are damaging the soil structure and contribute to an annual loss of 1.7 tons of topsoil.

Foods had been marketed, prior to 1990, as organic without any clear guidelines stipulating what the term actually meant. That changed in 1990, when the U.S. congress passed the **Organic Foods Production Act**. Organic farmers, now regulated by the **USDA's National Organic Program** (NOP)[36] since 2002, only occupied 2.20 million acres of cropland and pasture nationwide in 2003, but saw dedicated acreage use almost double to 4.05 million acres in 2005 and by 2011, 5.4 million acres were being farmed organic.[53a] Despite using a very small fraction of available arable land mass, organic farmers posted $12.6 billion in annual sales of organic foods and beverages that year, and an impressive 67.5% jump to $21.1 billion by 2008.[6, 53b] The magnitude of growth in the organic food industry, can be better visualized by stepping back and broadly looking at the astounding 455.5% increase in organic food sales between 1997 and 2007.[53b] The impressive growth was facilitated by the many grocery stores that began selling organic and natural foods. According to Grocery Shopper Trends 2008, about 82% of retail stores sold natural and organic foods.[35b]

Worldwide, the organic movement represents a $60 to $90 billion dollar industry. These sale values are nothing to scoff at, and so restaurants have been developing eco-friendly menus that feature locally grown and organic foods. Surveys conducted by the American Culinary Federation member chefs in 2009, and the National Restaurant Association in 2008, revealed that "organic" and "locally grown" were going to be the hottest menu trends of the future.[35b]

The NOP requires organic farming systems to strictly utilize crop residues and animal manure as fertilizers, and to conduct crop rotations and cover cropping, in order to prevent soil erosion. Organic farming ensures continued and sustained soil fertility in addition to greater biodiversity, and has been gaining in popularity in the last decade. This is because organic foods are marketed as more enviro-friendly and healthier,[6] among baby boomers and generations X and Y, who make up between 69 and 72% of the consumers. Annual revenues from the sales of organic foods topped $12.6 billion in 2001, because of the public's perception that personal health can be improved if the foods consumed are natural and pesticide free.[53b]

Natural foods and **organic foods** are not exactly the same things. Foods defined as, **natural** do not generally come under government controls, except they must comply with standards pertinent to the health code. However, poultry and meats, marketed as "natural," are regulated by the Food Safety and Inspection Service of the USDA, and as such, must be minimally processed; additionally, they cannot contain synthetic preservatives, artificial colors, sweeteners or flavors; nor should hydrogenated oils, emulsifiers, or stabilizers be part of the ingredients. Moreover, methods of agricultural production are not regulated either.[53b] In the end, consumers have to be wary of foods labeled as "natural".

Organic foods are however, natural, and the consumer can be assured that, if the farm is certified as an organic agriculture system by the USDA, and follows the NOP, it does not use any of the following compounds in its agricultural practices: synthetic pesticides, bioengineered genes, petroleum-based fertilizers and sewage sludge-based fertilizers, and irradiation. Live-stock ranches can also receive the ORGANIC label if they show their cattle can roam and graze outside, and are not administered hormones or antibiotics.[53e]

Studies have shown that the soil of organically grown foods is richer in minerals, and therefore the food harvested from these soils is more nutrient-rich. Organic foods also contain more phytonutrients like carotenoids, flavonoids and other kinds of polyphenols compared to non-organic foods.[6]

Organic farmers nevertheless still fight an ongoing battle to preserve authentic organic crops, as chemical insecticide mists, from neighboring farms, do drift over and contaminate organic farms. The other problem is that insecticide residues that may have been used on soils, prior to being zoned organic, remain in that soil. However, given the difficulty controlling the integrity of organic soils, only 2.6% of organic crops tend to have lingering insecticide residues, compared to 26% of crops harvested from non-organic fields.[28]

For a food to receive the USDA approved **100% ORGANIC** seal, the food must contain only organic ingredients, whereas the **ORGANIC** seal requires that the food contain at least 95% organic ingredients. Some foods can post on the label: **Made with Organic Ingredients** if between 70 to 95% organic ingredients are found in the food. Products containing less than 70% organic material are not eligible to use either the ORGANIC seal or to refer to organic ingredients on its label.

The problem is that organic products are more expensive than conventional foods, and tend to be purchased by more educated higher income earners. This leaves the poor and lower class with conventional non-organic foods as their dietary base. This certainly screams out injustice, as the lower social classes appear to get stuck with the raw end of the deal. Strategies certainly exist that can assist financially struggling single mothers and low income households. They can purchase from:
1. farmer's markets;
2. cooperative food stores;
3. community gardens;
4. healthy fresh produce sections in corner and convenience stores.

Federal, state and local governments need to also change the nature of the food inventory that is making up the food banks, so that the poor can access healthy food choices. Items such as mac & cheese, candies, cakes, and sodas need to be restricted.

Locally grown produce and raised livestock, for instance, are new concepts that support the growth of local economies, and encourage the production of diverse agriculture. Key advantages are potentially better freshness and, if grown organically, there is the assurance of no pesticides.[36] As good as that seems, local governments have been attempting to regulate locally grown agriculture with what has been perceived as cumbersome regulations. As a result, local small farms have trouble complying with these heavy regulatory standards as they simply do not have the technology or the staff.[27]

Regulations governing what could be called "locally grown" are non-existent, but there are general rules. Locally grown farms:

1. should be reachable without involving more than one day of travel;
2. should not be greater than 100 miles away from a regional town or city;

The lack of a consensus and the generally higher prices paid for locally grown has not deterred consumers, who are willing to pay premium prices for what they perceive as healthy.[33, 39, 46, 47]

6.6.1. Creating a Healthy Diet that Prevents Disease

If our farmers are implementing agricultural practices that impoverish the soil, and indeed leaving us with pesticide residues and soil erosion, then they are producing contaminated foods of poor nutrient content.[53d] In that sense, our current agriculture becomes unsustainable over the long term. It is here, then, that the organic movement, in addition to the efforts to create locally grown produce and raise grass grazing livestock, that are not routinely given antibiotics and growth hormones, become a viable solution to an impoverished and troubling diet. Walter Crinnion, in a 2010 review of the literature, concluded that pesticide residues, consumed from a conventional North American diet, were leaching into the blood stream of children. The research he reviewed convincingly pointed to a problem with the North American food supply. He writes:[6]

Children eating organic foods had a six-fold lower level of organophosphate pesticide residues in their urines than those who ate more conventionally. The research group tested preschoolers before and after changing their diets from conventionally grown organic foods. When the shift was made to organic diets the urinary levels of malathion and chlorpyrifos became undetectable until their conventional diets were restored.

The notion that the environment plays a significant role is particularly convincing in light of a December 11, 2013 L.A Times article that captured public attention. Journalist David Pierson described an FDA plan to rein in the non-medical use of antibiotics on farm animals. Pierson reported on the worrisome increase in antibiotic-resistant pathogens that were killing an estimated 99,000 souls every year. Michael Taylor, FDA deputy Commissioner for Food and Veterinary Medicine, is calling on pharmaceutical companies to voluntarily cease the marketing of antibiotics and other drugs, used in treating humans, as growth promoters in farm animals. In the future, the goal is to require a veterinarian prescription for the use of antibiotics, on farm animals. Public health officials are decrying that the FDA is only calling on voluntary cooperation of the pharmaceutical and meat industries. At this point, many feel that a strong legislative bite is needed to squelch, what New York Congresswoman, Louise Slaughter described as:

...the overuse of antibiotics in corporate agriculture,...

As a legislator, she sees that more intervention is needed to repair decades of damage. Her criticism is an indictment of American agriculture. In commenting about FDA measures, she continues:

...and it falls woefully short of what is needed to address a public health crisis.

These findings and others intimate that the food we consume and the environment in which our food is grown, contribute towards rising incidences of disease.

Dr Mary Story, a University of Minnesota nutrition professor, captures a more integrated understanding of this environment using broad and meaningful brush strokes that zero in on the environment as a major vector for our societal health woes. Dr. Story advances that for individuals to purposely and concretely make health food and lifestyle choices, they must be supported by wholesome environments that foster good and sound decisions.[49] Many of the environments that parents and children live, play and work in have become compromised, and so it is in the schools, child care, workplaces, homes, retail food stores and restaurants that corrective action is needed. At a macro-social level, agricultural policies and food marketing by corporations need also to be revised, and quickly. So many disparities in accessing healthy foods currently exist, placing lower socioeconomic and minority groups at a clear disadvantage. The reality is that grocery stores, and specialty food shops are almost non-existent in lower income urban neighborhoods, whereas abundant fast food outlets and corner stores with processed and snack foods inventories are peppered everywhere in these environments.[49]

Right now the research is not conclusive that expanding a locally grown food system would impart better health to the overall community. However, elevated prevalence rates of cancer, cardiovascular disease, orthodontic problems, dental caries, diabetes, attention deficit hyperactivity disorders, food allergies and intolerances, all point in the direction of fundamental problems in lifestyle, the environment, diet or all three, as important influences.[33, 49]

6.7 Food Allergies & Intolerances

The American Academy of Allergy, Asthma and Immunology reports that, between 40 to 50 million Americans suffer from allergy diseases, and that as many as 54.6% of U.S. citizens positively react to one or more allergen.[44]

But when it comes to food there are three red flags that catch the attention of health experts: First, 3-4% of adults and 8% of children suffer specifically from a food allergy, a percent that overshadows the considerably lower international prevalence rates found among children in Denmark (2.3%), Germany (4.6%) and the United Kingdom (6%).

Second, although it is worrisome enough that 35% to 50% of all cases of anaphylaxis come from reactions to food allergens,—between 50 to 62% of fatal food anaphylaxis are caused by peanuts—epidemiologists are particularly intrigued by the 142.86% increase in the incidences of food anaphylaxis, between 1999 and 2008, that was reported by the Mayo Clinic in Minnesota.[3]

Third, what is troubling is the 18% increase in the prevalence of pediatric food allergies between 1997 and 2007. The question is: why are children developing allergic reactions to foods at such a rate of increase—almost a 2% increase per year.[21]

The public outcry, over this prevalence in those under 18, raised some red flags in Washington, especially since the percent deviated upwards from the European average. The National Institute of Allergy and Infectious Diseases formed an expert committee to help establish guidelines for the diagnosis of food allergies.

They determined that an allergy refers to an adverse bodily reaction to a specific immune-mediated response, occurring reproducibly when exposed to a given food. Adverse food reactions can thus be classified as either immune-mediated (food allergies, celiac disease) or non-immune-mediated (food intolerances).[5]

There are in total, an estimated 12 million Americans suffering from food allergies in the U.S. according to the Food Allergy and Anaphylaxis Network. This number has been growing in size, and commanding legislative action in Washington.

In January 2006, the Food Allergen and Consumer Protection Act, forced food manufacturers to identify, in the ingredient list, the top 8 allergens that affect Americans if present in the foods.
Celiac disease, which causes an immune-mediated response to the wheat protein, gluten, has been on the rise.[42] Again, nobody is able to pin point the cause for the increase. Compared to the 1950s, Americans today are four and a half times more vulnerable to contracting celiac disease.[42] Consequently, the demand for gluten-free products has skyrocketed in the last 10 years, and many restaurants are now introducing allergy and gluten-friendly menu items to appease the celiac customer, who cannot properly digest grains that contain the gluten protein such as: wheat, durum, semolina, spelt, rye, barley and more. They can, by contrast, consume oats and rice without any difficulties.[7]

The foodservice industry, in the U.S., is phenomenally large. With projected annual gross sales of $580 billion per year, foodservice operators are all too eager to cash in on the new sales from celiac and allergic patrons, who have normally stayed away from restaurants.[5, 29] But the gripping background question is: why are there greater numbers of adults and children developing allergies?

DISCUSSION QUESTIONS

1. Explain the impact of greater urbanization, near the end of the 1800s, on food production and food safety.

2. How important was the Pure Food & Drug Act of 1906 for the safety of the American food supply? Explain.

3. Discuss the historical importance of H.J Heinz Company's contribution to the American food industry.
4. Explain how Upton Sinclair's, *The Jungle*, changed the meat packing industry in the early 20th century.
5. Explain the facelift the USDA received, under President Eisenhower's administration, and the impact on the U.S. food supply.
6. Explain the difference between Natural and Organic foods, as discussed in this textbook.
7. Make the case for why pesticides need to be used in U.S. agriculture.
8. Defend the argument that current herbicide and pesticide use in U.S. agriculture needs to be contained and even limited.
9. Discuss the more encouraging changes to pest control that have taken place over the last 10 year. Explain why these advances are significant.
10. Discuss why food safety practices in the food industry need to be monitored very closely.
11. Explain the key areas of food safety that tend to be responsible for the most significant numbers of foodborne illness outbreaks in the U.S.

Rererences

1. Akhter, J. et al. (2001) Editorial: Genetically Modified Foods: Health and Safety Issues. Annals of Saudi Medicine; 21 (3-4): 161-164 Retrieved October 29, 2013 from: http://www.kfshrc.edu.sa/annals/Old/213_214/01-032.pdf
2. American Heart Association. Heart and stroke statistical 2013 update. Dallas, Texas: American Heart Association. Retrieved December 18, 2013 from: http://circ.ahajournals.org/content/127/1/e6
3. Bailey, S. A. (2011). Restaraunt staff's knowledge of anaphylaxis and dietary care of people with allergies. *Clinical & Experimental Allergy*, 41 (5): 713-717.
4. Bourne Partners (April 2013). Sector Report: Nutraceuticals. Connecticut, USA. Retrieved October 25, 2013 from: http://bourne-partners.com/content/media/articles/38.pdf
5. Boyce, B. (2011). Making Menus Friendly: Marketing Your Food Intolerance Expertise. *Journal of the American Dietetic Association*, 111 (12): 1809-1812.
6. Crinnion, W. J. (2010). Organic Foods Contain Higher Levels of Certain Nutrients, Lower Levels of Pesticides, and May Provide Health Benefits for the Consumer. Alternative Medicine Review, 15(1), 4-12.
7. Cureton, P. (2006). Gluten-free dining out: Is it safe? *Practical Gastroenterology*, 29: 61-68.
8. Davis, M. plus et al. (1993). Update: Multistate outbreak of Escherichia coli O157:H7 infections from hamburgers -- Western United States, 1992-1993, Morb. Mort. Weekly Rep. 42(14):258-263.
9. Darmon, N., & Drewnowski, A. (2005). Food choices and diet costs: An economic analysis. Retrieved March 10, 2012 from http://jn.nutrition.org/content/135/4/900.short
10. DeFelice, SL (1992). Foundation for Innovative Medicine. Nutraceuticals—Opportunites in an Emerging Market. *Reprinted from* Scrip Magazine, *September 1992*. Retrieved October 25, 2013 from: http://www.fimdefelice.org/p2463.html
11. Delaplane, K. Pesticide usage in the United States: History, benefits, risks and trends. Cooperative Extension Service; University of Georgia. Retrieved June 25, 2012 from: http://ipm.ncsu.edu/safety/factsheets/pestuse.pdf
12. Domingo, JL. (2007). Toxicity Studies of Genetically Modified Plants: A Review of the Published Literature Critical Reviews in Food Science and Nutrition, 47:721–733
13. Draper, A and Green, J. (2002) Food safety and consumers: Constructions of choice and risk. Social Policy & Administration 36(6): 610-625.
14. .EPA to Limit Use of Toxic Pesticides CNN. com. Retrieved August13, 1999. http://www.cnn.com/NATURE/9908/02/pesticide.risk/
15. Federal Register (2003). 68 FR 41433 July 11, 2003: Food Labeling; Trans Fatty Acids in Nutrition Labeling Act. Retrieved October 13, 2013 from: http://www.fda.gov/Food/GuidanceRegulation/FoodFacilityRegistration/ucm081637.htm
16. Fernandez-Cornejo, J., and W.D. McBride. (April 2000) Genetically Engineered Crops for Pest Management in U.S. Agriculture: Farm-Level Effects. AER No. 786, U.S. Department of Agriculture, Economic Research Service. http://www.ers.usda.gov/publications/aer786/aer786.pdf
17. Fernandez-Carnejo, J and W.D McBride. (May 2002) Adoption of Bioengineered Crops. AER No. 810, U.S. Department of Agriculture, Economic Research Service. Retrieved June 15, 2012 http://www.ers.usda.gov/publications/aer810/aer810.pdf
18. Flynn, D. The 10 deadliest Outbreaks in US History. Food Safety News. Retrieved June 22, 2012 from: http://www.foodsafetynews.com/2012/04/the-ten-deadliest-outbreaks-in-history-revisited/
19. Fortin, ND (2011). The United States FDA Food Safety Modernization Act: The Key New Requirements. European Food & Feed Law Review, 5: 260-268
20. Glanz, K., Resnicow, K., Seymour, J., Hoy, K., Stewart, H., Lyons, M. (2007). How Major Restaurant Chains Plan Their Menus The Role of Profit, Demand, and Health. *American Journal of Prventive Medicine*, 32: 383- 388.
21. Gupta, R, et al. (2011) The Prevalence, Severity and Distribution of Childhood Food Allergy in the United States. Pediatrics 10.1542/ ped.2011-0204
22. Harmon, A. (August 24, 2013) Golden Rice Life Saver? New York Times. Retrieved November 1, 2013 from: http://www.nytimes.com/2013/08/25/sunday-review/golden-rice-lifesaver.html?pagewanted=2
23. Hoffman-Sommergruber, K. and Dorsch-Häsler. (2012) National Research Program (NRP) #59: Benefits and

Risks of the Deliberate Release of Genetically Modified Plants: Review of the International Literature. Zurich: Swiss National Science Foundation

24. James, C. (2011). Global Status of Commercialized Biotech/GM Crops: 2011. ISAAA Brief No. 43. ISAAA: Ithaca, NY

25. Jang, Y., Kim, W., & Bonn, M. (2011). Generation Y consumers' selection attributes and behaviors intentions concering green restaurants. International Journal of Hospitality Management, 30: 803-811

26. Kashima, T. M. (2010). Feasibility of integrated menu recommendation and self-order system for small-scale restaurants. *American Institute of Physics*, 1285 (1), 132-144.

27. Kiely, T., Donaldson, D. Grube, A. (May 2004) Pesticides, Industry Sales and Usage: 2000 and 2001 Market Estimates. Biological and Economic Analysis Division Office of Pesticide Programs Office of Prevention, Pesticides, and Toxic Substances U.S. Environmental Protection Agency Washington, DC 20460. Retrieved October 26, 2013 from: http://www.epa.gov/opp00001/pestsales/01pestsales/market_estimates2001.pdf

28. Lee, S. J et al. Acute Pesticide Illnesses Associated with Off-Target Pesticide Drift.
Agricultural Applications: 11 States, 1998–2006. Environ Health Perspect 2001; 119:1162–1169.

29. Leftwich, J. B. (2011). The challenges for nut-allergic consumers of eating out. *Clinical & Experimental Allergy*, 41 (2): 243-249.

30. Liptak, A. (May 13, 2013). Supreme Court Supports Monsanto in Seed-Replication Case. New York Times. Retrieved November 1, 2013 from: http://www.nytimes.com/2013/05/14/business/monsanto-victorious-in-genetic-seed-case.html?ref=geneticallymodifiedfood&_r=0

31. Lu, C et al (2010) Assessing Children's Dietary Pesticide Exposure: Direct Measurement of Pesticide Residues in 24-Hr Duplicate Food Samples. Environ Health Perspective. 118:1625–1630

32. Lynch, D and Vogel, D. (April 5, 2001). The Regulations of GMOs in Europe and the United States: A Case Study of Contemporary European Regulatory Politics. Council on Foreign Relations.

33. Martinez, S., Hand, M., Pra, M., Pollack, S., Ralston, K., Smith, T., et al. (2010). Local Food Systems Concepts, Impacts, and Issues. Washington D.C.: USDA. Economic Research Report (ERR no 97) 87 pp.

34. McCabe-Sellers, B & Beattie, S.E. (2004) Food Safety: Emerging trends in foodborne illness surveillance and Prevention. J.A.D.A 104: 1708-1717

35. Milenkovick, M. et al. (2004). Health Care Costs & Utilization Project. Hospital Stays for Gastrointestinal Diseases 2004
http://www.hcupus.ahrq.gov/reports/statbriefs/sb12.pdf. Retrieved June 21, 2012

36. National Organic Program USDA http://www.ams.usda.gov/AMSv1.0/NOPConsumers retrieved June 27, 2012

37. Petrick, GB. (2011). 'Purity as life': H.J. Heinz, religious sentiment, and the beginning of the industrial diet. *History and Technology*. 27(1): 37–64

38. Position Paper of the Academy of Nutrition and Dietetics (2013) Functional Foods. J. Academy of Nutr. & Diet. 113 (8):1096-1103

39. Position paper of the Position of the American Dietetic Association (2007): Food and Nutrition Professionals Can Implement Practices to Conserve Natural Resources and Support Ecological Sustainability. Journal of the Amer. Dietetic Association; 107(6): 1033-1043.

40. Pusztai, A. et al. (2003) Genetically Modified Foods: Potential Human Health Effects. In: Food Safety: Contaminants and Toxins (ed. JPF D'Mello) pp. 347-372. CAB International, Wallingford Oxon, UK

41. Roberto, C. A., Larsen, P. D., Agnew, H., Baik, J., & Brownell, K. D. (2010). Evaluating the Impact of Menu Labeling on Food Choices and Intake. American Journal Of Public Health, 100(2): 312-318.

42. Rubio-Tapia, A., Kyle, R. A., Kaplan, E. L., Johnson, D. R., Page, W., Erdtmann, F., et al. (2009). Increased Prevalence and Mortality in Undiagnosed Celiac Disease. Gastroentero-logy, 137 (1): 88-93.

43. Shoshanah, I., Sharp, J., Moore, R., & Stinner, D. (2009). Restaurants, chefs and local foods: insights drawn from application of a diffusion of innovation framework. Agriculture and Human Values, 26: 177-191.

44. Skypala, I. (2011). Adverse Food Reactions--An Emerging Issue for Adults. Journal of the American Dietetic Association, 111 (12): 1877-1891.

45. Slutsker, L., A.A. Ries, K. Maloney, J.G. Wells, K.D. Greene, and P.M. Griffin. (1998). A nationwide case-control study of Escherichia coli O157:H7 infection in the United States, J. Infect. Dis. 177:962-966.

46. Starr, A. (2010). Local Food: A Social Movement? *Cultural Studies and Critical Methodologies*, 10: 479-490.

47. Starr, A., Card, A., Benepe, C., Auld, G., Lamm, D., Smith, K., et al. (2003). Sustaining local agriculture: Barriers and opportunities to direct marketing between farms and restaurants in Colorado. *Agriculture and Human Values*, 20:301-321.

48. Stewart, CN Jr, Richards, HA 4th, Halfhill, MD. (2000) Transgenic plants and biosafety: science, misconceptions and public perceptions. Biotechniques.(4):832-6, 838-43

49. Story, K., Kaphings, K.M., Robinson-O'Brien, R., Glanz, K. (2008). Creating Healthy Foods and Eating Environments: Policy and Environmental Approaches. Ann. Rev. Public Health; 29:253–72. Retrieved October 24, 2013 from: http://www.med.upenn.edu/chbr/documents/2008-Story-CreatingHealthyFoodEatingEnviro.pdf

50. USDA Food Safety & Inspection Service. FSIS History. Retrieved October 24, 2013 from: http://www.fsis.usda.gov/wps/portal/informational/aboutfsis/history

51. US Department of Health and Human Services, Public Health Service: Cancer Control Objectives for the Nation, 1985-2000. Bethesda, MD: National Institutes of Health, National Cancer Institute, 1986 (drafts).

52. US Department of Health Education and Welfare (1979): Healthy People: The Surgeon General's Report on Health Promotion and Disease Prevention. DHEW Pub. No. (PHS) 795507. Washington, DC: Gov. Printing Office.

53. US Department of Agriculture (USDA), US Department of Health and Human Services⊗1985) Nutrition and Your Health, Dietary Guidelines for Americans, 2d Ed. Home and Garden Bull No. 232. Washington, DC: Gov. Printing Office.

53a. US Department of Agriculture (USDA). Economic Research Service (October 2013). Growth Patterns of the US Organic Industry. Retrieved December 17, 2013 from:

http://www.ers.usda.gov/amber-waves/2013-october/growth-patterns-in-the-us-organic-industry.aspx

53b. US Department of Agriculture (USDA), National Agricultural Library. Natural and Organic Foods. Food Marketing Institute. Retrieved December 11, 2013 from: http://www.fmi.org/docs/media-backgrounder/natural_organic_foods.pdf?sfvrsn=2

53c. US Department of Agriculture (USDA). National Research Conservation Service Soil Erosion on Cropland 2007. Retrieved December 17, 2013 from: http://www.nrcs.usda.gov/wps/portal/nrcs/detail/national/technical/nra/nri/?cid=stelprdb1041887

53d. US Department of Agriculture (USDA) National Research Conservation Service. Soil Degradation. Retrieved December 17, 2013 from: http://www.nrcs.usda.gov/Internet/FSE_DOCUMENTS/nrcs142p2_053174.pdf

53e. US Environmental Protection Agency (EPA). Organic Farming (Updated June 27, 2012). Retrieved December 17, 2013 from http://www.epa.gov/oecaagct/torg.html

54. US Food and Drug Administration (FDA). (2013) Labeling and Nutrition Guidance Documents and Regulatory Information Guidance for Industry. Updated July 31, 2013. Retrieved December 10, 2013 from: http://www.fda.gov/Food/GuidanceRegulation/GuidanceDocumentsRegulatoryInformation/LabelingNutrition/default.htm

55. US Food and Drug Administration (FDA). (October/November 2003 issue). Color Additives: FDA's Regulatory Process and Historical Perspectives Reprinted from Food Safety Magazine. Retrieved December 10, 2013 from: http://www.fda.gov/ForIndustry/ColorAdditives/RegulatoryProcessHistoricalPerspectives/

56. Wiley, H.W. (1929). The History of a Crime against the Food Law. Washington DC: Harvey W. Wiley MD Publisher. 413pp

57. Whitty, C.J.M. et al. (2013) Comment: Biotechnology: Africa and Asia Need a Rational Debate on GM Foods. Nature; 497:31-33

CHAPTER 7

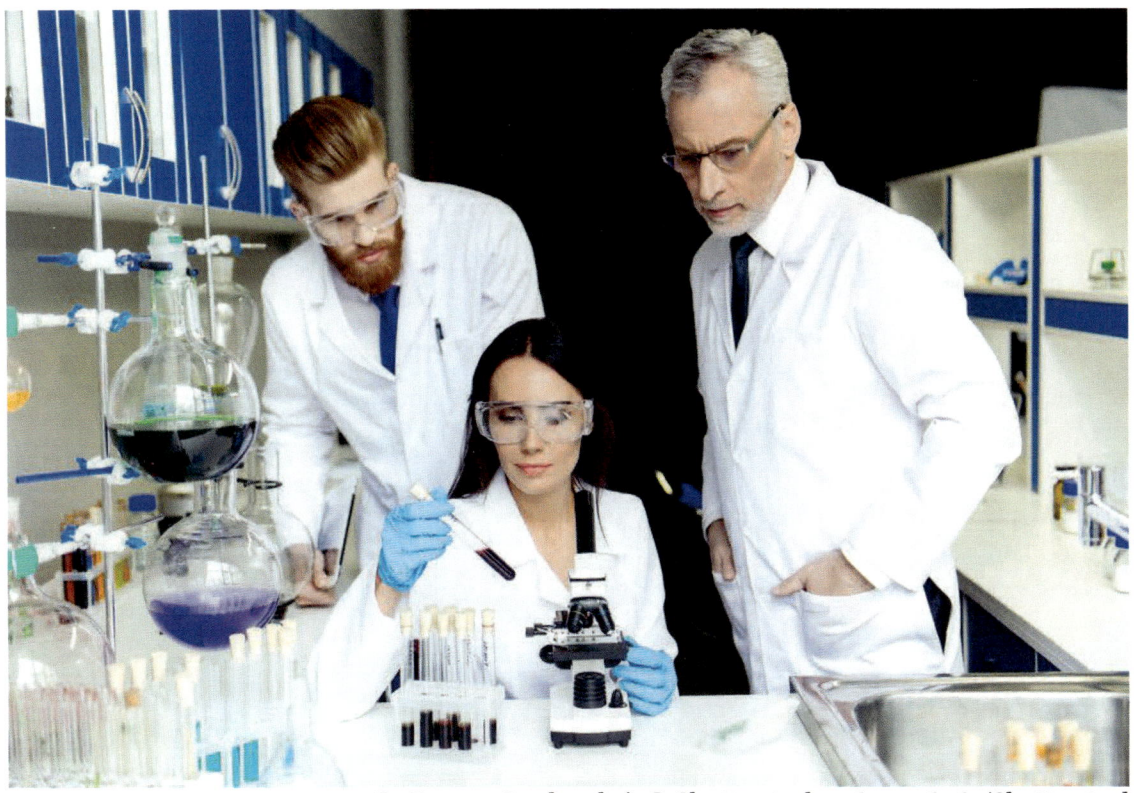

NUTRITION RESEARCH IN THE MODERN AGE: PRINCIPLES OF EPIDEMIOLOGY & CLINICAL TRIALS

7.1 What is Research?

Understanding the idea of research is vital in the science formation of a student. Research is a method of inquiry that assists the individual in uncovering the truth; in the end, it is identifying truth that is the ultimate goal, and as such, the method of inquiry needs to be the most objective and controlled.

Research always begins with an **observation** that raises questions. For instance, a nutrition researcher observes that those patients, followed over many years, who consumed more than 5 fruits and vegetables per day, tend to have less heart disease and cancer.

Next the **question**: Can fruits and vegetables prevent disease? This question, if answered properly through a legitimate path of inquiry, will allow the researcher to formulate valuable and truthful conclusions that can help physicians better manage their patients. But first, the researcher must be fully able to answer the question. He does this by searching the literature to verify if any studies have previously documented protective effects of fruits and vegetables. At this point he must search in peer-reviewed journals that are dedicated to the fields of nutrition, heart disease and cancer.

There are several nutrition journals that can be consulted using **PubMed, Medline** or **Academic Search Premier**. These are excellent databases that provide access to a large number of online peer-reviewed journal articles. In reviewing the literature, the scientist looks for previously published studies that have documented protective roles of nutrition against heart disease or cancer. If the area of inquiry has been studied extensively, it is best to look for review articles that comprehensively summarize the research findings over the last decade, for instance. Nutrition Reviews and Annual Review of Nutrition are among the most consulted review journals. The impact of genetics on heart disease is an area that has been extensively studied. Look for the 1989 Annual Reviews of Nutrition scientific paper titled: Human Genetics and Human Coronary Heart Disease: A Public Health Perspective (volume: 9 pages: 303–345). This review has over 50 references, and will provide the scientist with the most complete understanding of that field. This article will also serve as an excellent model for a review paper.

Illustrated in **table-7.1,** are the key nutrition and medical peer-reviewed journals that can be consulted. At this stage, two things can happen: first, the literature may show that there hasn't been any previous documentation of the relationship between nutrition, heart disease and cancer. The researcher confirms then that his question is novel, and he needs to formulate a theory using closely related literature and his own intuitions.

Second, he finds that previous literature does indeed document some aspects of the diet that can protect against chronic diseases. At this point, the investigator needs to formulate a theory using relevant scientific information pertinent to the link existing between nutrition and the disease in question. A theory is the description of a mechanism that can explain the relationship between fruits and vegetables and heart disease. Defined by Marian Webster, a theory *is a principle set to explain phenomena already supported by data. Theories will pull together experimental results to provide full explanations such as "The Big Bang Theory."*

As an example, *in vitro* studies may confirm that cruciferous vegetables contain phenolic compounds that inhibit genetic cancer mutations. In remaining consistent with this example, the scientist could formulate the following theory: *Vegetables of the cruciferous type consumed with fruits provide sufficient phenolic compounds to protect the epithelium of the colon from free radical attacks that potentially destroy the epithelial cells and cause DN mutations leading to cancer.*

Once a clear theory is formulated with the help of the literature, a hypothesis can then be devised.

TABLE 7.1 Nutrition and Medical Peer-reviewed Journals

TOPIC	Peer-reviewed Journal
Nutrition	Am. J. of Clinical Nutrition
	Journal of Nutrition
	J. Am. College of Nutrition
	Nutrition Research
	Euro. J. of Nutrition
	J. of Academy of Nut. & Diet.
	Can. J. of Diet. Practice & Res.
	Annual Rev. of Nutrition
	Nutrition Reviews
Cancer Medicine	Cancer
	Cancer Journal
	Am J. Clinical Oncology
	Annals of Oncology
CVD Medicine	Circulation
	Circulation Research
	Hypertension
	Stroke
	J. Am. Heart Assoc.
	J. of the Am. Med Assoc.

*CVD: Cardio-vascular disease

Again, Marian Webster defines hypothesis as *an assumption made before any research has been completed for the sake of testing*. The hypothesis must be verifiable and in that sense measurement need to be specified with sufficient clarity so as to be repeatable. Once the hypothesis is formulated, the research team needs to create a study design that will confirm their hypothesis.

Here is an example of a hypothesis: *Vegetables of the cruciferous type, consumed in excess of 3 cups per day in addition to fruits ingested in excess of 2 cups per day, will protect adults ages 18 to 65 years of age against colon cancer over a 20 year period.*
Take note that the hypothesis has specific quantity limits of fruits and vegetables; it also specifies the ages of the subjects and over what period of time measurements will be taken. In that sense, the hypothesis can be tested several times.

The team will need to decide whether the research question requires an **epidemiological** or an **experimental study**. The former is a method that permits the researcher to establish a relationship between disease and lifestyle in a population. The latter is a form of study that experiments with various treatments, frequency of treatments, doses of medications, causative and preventative agents that are applied to cells in a petri dish, laboratory animals or humans. For humans specifically, if the question is: what is the most efficacious treatment for a specific human disease? Then the method of inquiry requires a **clinical trial**, because it has to do with the treatment of disease.[2]

In wondering about the protective features of vegetables—in the previous example—the scientist is asking the question: can fruits and cruciferous vegetables prevent or protect against disease? This hypothesis, formulated earlier, really pertains to prevention rather than the treatment of disease. If determining prevention or causation is the goal, then the disease is studied using an epidemiological framework. The first step for this kind of endeavor requires determining the extent of the occurrence of disease, which is measured through the prevalence. Rothman writes:[5]

The fundamental task in epidemiologic research is thus to quantify the occurrence of illness.

The high prevalence of a disease justifies efforts aimed at understanding its cause and finding a treatment. Afterwards, epidemiologists study what, in the environment, is contributing to the surge in disease prevalence. It is at this point, that they formulate a hypothesis, about what might be causing the disease. The goal, Rothman goes on to write "*is to evaluate hypotheses about causation of illness and its sequelae and to relate disease occurrence to characteristics of people and their environment.*

In this case what, in the population diet, environment or lifestyle, is causing the disease? And a second meaningful question would be: what do people need to eat, to prevent it?

On the other hand, if the investigator is attempting to establish the causative mechanism of the disease, then he must consider an experiment, at the cellular level, using a petri dish, or at the biological level, using experimental animals or humans. If the possible mechanism, explaining the protection given by vegetables, is known, but the ingested quantities, necessary for true positive and observable cancer protection, are unknown, then, again an epidemiological design would be advantageous. In this context, researchers may determine that those populations, consuming upwards of 8 servings of cruciferous vegetables per week, have significantly less cancers over a 20 year period, than those who consume less than 3 servings per week.

7.2 Epidemiologic Research

The first step in epidemiological research is the identification of a population problem. The clinician working in family practice may see many obese patients, and could think America is getting fat, but could not legitimately conclude this unless a measurement, at the population level, was taken.

The **Cross-sectional epidemiological** design, allows the investigator to measure a randomly selected representative sample of the population, and in it, the number of subjects who are obese or who suffer from cancer. This kind of research design asks the question: how many people have the disease? It is an important one because it allows the researchers to confirm that there is indeed an obesity problem or cancer epidemic, and thus legitimizes any effort at finding a cure or treatment.

The cross-sectional design permits the researchers to determine the **prevalence** of a disease or condition, which is expressed as the percent of people that have the disease relative to those at risk of getting the disease.

A prevalence study, then, would determine the percent of people suffering from obesity, diabetes or heart disease. This design allows a random cross-sectional sample of the population to be selected, as indicated by the pie chart in **Figure 7.1**. The assumption is that, although it is a smaller sample, because the selection is random, it still represents the correct distribution of race, gender, age and professionals normally found in the larger population. The CDC obesity prevalence data collected between 1980 and 2011 is compiled through a succession of cross-sectional studies.

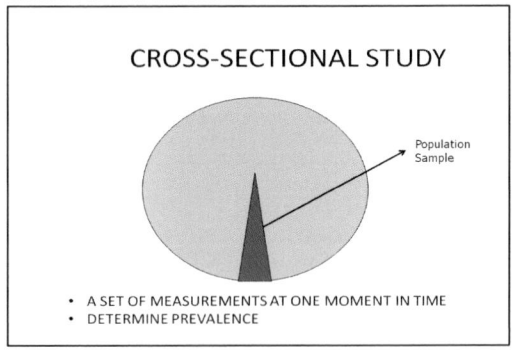

Figure 7.1 Cross-sectional design

One of the most frequently quoted studies in the popular media is the **Case-Control study** design. This is the quick and easy epidemiological technique, aimed at establishing if there is a likelihood of a relationship between the dependent variable (the disease) and the independent variable (lifestyle, diet or environmental factor). The design consists of identifying a control group that does not have the disease, and a disease group that has contracted the illness of interest **(Figure 7.2)**.

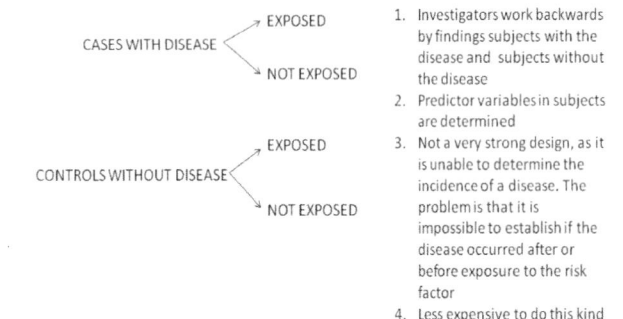

Figure 7.2 Case-Control study design

The goal of the design is to ultimately determine whether those who have the disease were exposed, to a greater degree, to some kind of independent variable such as lifestyle, diet or an environmental agent, compared to the control group that did not have the disease.

The problem with the design is that the information is gathered retrospectively. This means that all the subjects are questioned by the investigators about their lifestyles. Those with the disease begin to ponder what agents in their past may have contributed towards the development of the disease. The limitation here is the **recall bias**; what exactly is the subject remembering? How accurate is it? Subjects afflicted with a disease tend to remember more details (accurate and inaccurate) compared to subjects who are healthy. The danger in this rather weak design is that the investigator can establish weak or completely false associations.

For instance, in verifying how people may have developed cancer, in a cluster of the population with alarmingly high rates of lung cancer, the strength of the case control design can only be as good as the hypothesis, the questions asked and the subjects recruited. If it is the expert's suspicion that frequent aftershave use causes lung cancer in men from the daily exposure to the fumes, then the controls, if properly recruited, should correct for any false positives, since the men in the control group also likely used aftershave, but did not develop cancer.

In this manner, the control group prevents the investigator from erroneously concluding that aftershaves are the cause because all the diseased men used daily application of the after-shave. However, the control group may not help all that much, if the suspected causative agent was a confounder or in other words an external variable that correlates with both the independent (true causing agent) and dependent variable (cancer). For instance, coffee may be suspected in causing cancer, but the truth is that smoking is the real cause; none of the investigators suspect the cigarettes, so their questions revolve around frequency of coffee intake, strength of coffee and types of coffee. They find that those in the disease group consumed stronger coffee and greater amounts compared to the control. They erroneously conclude that coffee causes bladder cancer.

This actually occurred in the 1980s.[3] So coffee, the confounder, correlated with smoking and with the cancer, for indeed, those who drank a lot of coffee did develop more cancer. The problem the epidemiologists did not catch was that smokers tend to be heavy coffee drinkers. This is because they metabolize caffeine faster than non-smokers. The consequence is more frequent ingestion of coffee in order to maintain the coffee high. Hence, because the investigators had a bias belief that coffee was a culprit, they eventually found a correlation with coffee though it was fallacious. It should be evident why case-control studies have, in the past, erroneously correlated milk consumption with greater risk of heart disease, and high fiber diets with greater incidences of colonic cancers.

Epidemiological cohort studies are by far the most accurate design when attempting to establish true correlations that are indeed accurate. Cohort studies can either be retrospective or prospective cohorts **(Figure 7.3)**.

A **prospective cohort** is a large group of individuals that is followed over time, and for which **incidences** of diseases are documented, and lifestyles, body composition and dietary practices are reported. The size of the cohort often equals tens of thousands of people, and sometimes hundreds of thousands. The large number of subjects allows investigators to document the incidences of a disease or in other words the rate of appearance of the disease, and correlate the disease with lifestyle determinants and dietary practices for instance.

A **positive correlation** is calculated when the dependent and independent variables move in the same direction. To help visualize this, the example of dietary fat and serum cholesterol could be useful; when dietary fat intake is elevated (independent variable) serum cholesterol (dependent variable) tends to also be elevated; this is a positive correlation. By contrast, a **negative correlation** occurs when the dependent variable moves in a direction that is opposite to the independent variable; hence, when dietary soluble fiber increases in the diet, serum LDL cholesterol tends to decrease. This is a negative correlation.

The closer the correlation is numerically to the number one, the more causative that relationship is likely to be. In medical research, **causation** is very rarely established, but rather because the correlations are close to, but still less than one, clinicians are able to conclude that there is a risk of developing the disease. A high correlation signifies a high risk, whereas a low correlation generally means a low risk of contracting the condition.

In medical science there are only four medical conditions, for which very high correlations, hinting on causation, have actually been established:
1. Epstein-Barr virus and infectious mononucleosis
2. asbestos and mesothelioma of the lung
3. cigarette smoking and lung cancer
4. HIV virus and AIDS.

Aside from these four conditions, correlations only help to establish risk. Some may want to make the case for peptic ulcers and Helicobacter Pylori. While reasonable, this relationship remains weak overall, as only a little more than 50% of peptic ulcers are related to H. Pylori.[7] Moreover, this particular correlation could also signify that peptic ulcers cause H. Pylori infestation.[8]

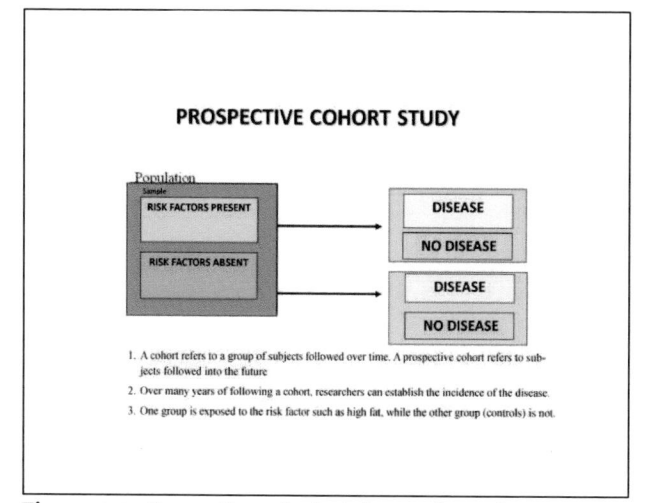

Figure 7.3: Prospective cohort study can detect the incidence of disease

When a prospective cohort study is terminated, and investigators cease to monitor and follow subjects, the collected information is in fact stored. Investigators, reexamining the stored archived data, are conducting a **retrospective cohort**. In other words, they are re-examining the data of a prospective cohort that has been terminated.

The weakness of this design is that no new measurements can actually be made, but the strength is that it's much less financially prohibitive than the prospective cohort, since a large team of investigators is no longer needed to keep track of the large cohort. The size of the cohort provides a statistical advantage, thus allowing strong conclusions to be made even though the study has ended.[2]

7.3 Experiment Research
7.3.1 Lab-Based In Vitro Studies

Understanding what agents may be responsible for causing gene mutations that eventually become cancerous, requires a lab-based environment that controls the conditions to such a degree, that it permits a systematic testing of various agents or stimulants. These controlled conditions, permit the identification of chemical compounds, enzymes, and metabolites involved in specific structural changes. Knowing what is going on at the cellular and sub cellular levels is important in establishing a mechanism for causation.

7.3.2 Lab-Based Animals Studies

Laboratory animals allow researchers to study whether or not there is of biological base to the disease mechanism. If the animal model emulates the human biological system very well, then it increases the likelihood that the mechanism may be applicable to humans. Findings that are made in animal studies can never fully be extrapolated to humans. Scientists must talk about the likelihood, the possibility and the risks that might occur in humans. The animal model does allow a more thorough physical look at the cellular, tissue, organ, vascular and neurological systems—something that would not be permitted ethically in human studies. Animal studies do need to be organized following experimental conventions that are applicable to human experimentation. Thus, lab rat studies always require a control group and a treatment/exposure group, depending on the goal of the study.

If the hypothesis is that high protein intake in rats (1.75 g/Kg) leads to increased muscle mass, then the control group, receiving the usual rat lab chow containing 0.65 g/Kg, should help the investigators measure the extent to which protein above the usual amount, synthesized additional muscle mass in the rats.

If researchers wanted to determine if fluoride, in the diet, is dangerous, they would need to set up the following experimental groups: (1) A control group receiving a minimum dose of fluoride that is below accepted ppm cut-off concentration; (2) a first test group-1, receiving a concentration of fluoride that is 25% greater than in the controls; (3) and finally a 2nd test group with 50% greater levels of fluoride than in test group-1. The stratification of the doses, from low to high, allows the researchers to determine whether or not there is a dose dependent effect of fluoride on the neurological, cardiovascular, lungs and brain systems, for instance (**Figure 7.4**).

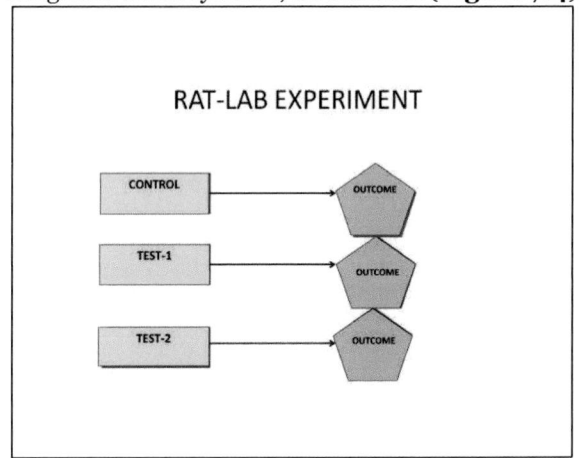

Figure 7.4 Animal lab-based experiment

7.3.3 Human Intervention Trials

Clinical trials are solely intended to measure the effectiveness of a treatment modality on disease outcomes.[5] An accurate interpretation, of the treatment's therapeutic effect, is dependent on the control group.

Control Group Design—the control group design, that controls for no treatment of any kind, contrasts with the exposed or treatment test groups. Following this design, the subjects, in the control group, are generally matched for age, gender, and body weight with those subjects in the treatment groups. The control group is essentially controlling for the effect of no treatment, while the treatment group receives the agent, medication, or dietary factor.

In **Figure 7.5**, the maneuver consists of exposing one group to a treatment, while the other one receives no treatment. The experimenters are interested in the outcome of the treatment.

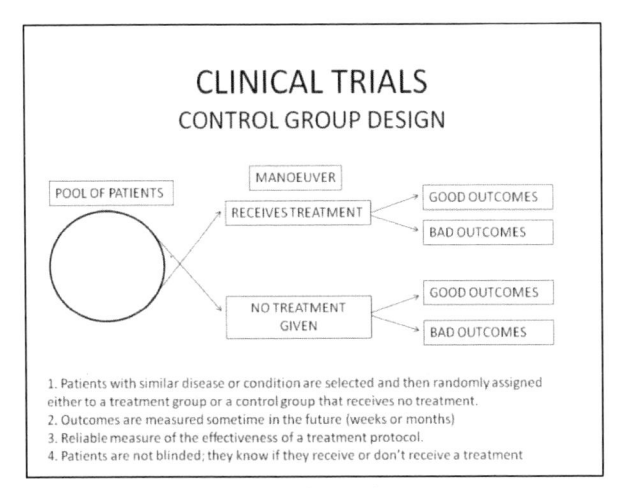

Figure 7.5 Control group trial design

If the treatment is a vitamin C supplement, and the patients are afflicted with colds, for instance, then those subjects receiving the vitamin would be expected to recover more quickly than if they never received one. In clinical trials the subjects that are selected, should ideally all have a condition or a disease that needs treatment.

Another example would be patients with high blood triglycerides and LDL cholesterol. The treatment given to test group 1 could be a standard North American diet plus omega-3 fatty acids in the form of EPA and DHA. The control group, by contrast, could be eating a normal North American diet with no supplement. The outcomes in the controls would either involve further increases in triglycerides and LDL cholesterol, over a three-month period, or ongoing maintenance of these markers at their current levels. The treatment group that receives the EPA & DHA capsules should experience a significant decline in serum triglyceride concentrations, and perhaps a modest downward shift in the LDL cholesterol levels.

In this design, the main weakness is that the controls know that they are receiving no treatment whereas the treatment group is actually aware of the treatments it is receiving. In other words, because the scientists did not use a placebo pill, the study was not blinded. In a double-blind study both the researcher and the subjects are unaware of who did or did not receive the treatment. Blinding helps eliminate any bias the researcher may have in knowing who is treated and who is not treated. It also prevents the subject from acting differently, depending on whether he is treated or not treated. An athlete who knowingly receives a creatine supplement daily, as part of a trial that tests whether creatine improves performance, could very likely work much harder in his training, thus showing improved performance results. Was it his enthusiasm in training or the supplement itself which was responsible for the improved running times? Hard to say; which is why single blinded studies, at the very least, are important and necessary.

Pre-test & Post-test Design—this design is utilized when there is no control group available. It allows a quick test of whether a treatment has an effect on a pre-existing condition; subjects with hyperglycemia (elevated serum glucose values in the pretest) when treated with the medication, glyburide, should expect to see the serum glucose values decline over a specific period of time in the posttest. Researchers can conclude that there appears to be a therapeutic effect of glyburide on blood sugars, using a pretest-posttest design. The drug seems to work, however investigators remain unable to completely measure the therapeutic effects of the drug since there is no control group to compare to (**Figure 7.6**).

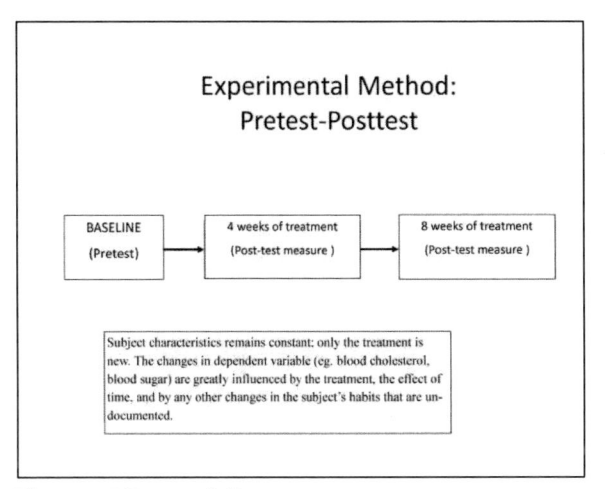

Figure 7.6 Pretest & Post-test

Case Report—this is hardly a study design, but rather a method of documenting pathophysiological, hematological, endocrinological and neurological changes on a small cluster of subjects. While statistical significance cannot be achieved, with this kind of study, by virtue of the fact that the sample size is so small (1 to 3 subjects), impressive levels of detailed data can, however, be collected and analyzed. This study design, therefore, provides a clear advantage over the clinical trials, which have larger sample sizes, but less detailed data.[2]

The case report allows, therefore, clinicians to thoroughly document the many parameters of the disease, in addition to treatments and treatment effects. The only restriction imposed on this kind of design is that the findings cannot be generalized to the general population.

Placebo-Controlled Double-Blind Clinical Trial—This very sophisticated experimental design uses a placebo that imitates the appearance of the treatment—the placebo pill looks like the treatment pill—thereby allowing the researcher to be blinded to the group that receives the actual treatment. In this manner, the investigator is prevented from showing too much interest in the treatment group at the expense of the placebo subjects. This design also precludes the researchers from conducting a favorably bias interpretation of the treatment group's outcomes, and of underreporting the clinical findings in the placebo group.

In this model, double-blind means the subjects are also blinded and thus unable to alter their physical activity, their dietary choices, and their psychological outlooks, based on whether they are receiving or not receiving the treatment. This is particularly noticeable in cancer patients who undergo clinical trials; the treatment and the placebo must be given randomly to the cancer patients in order for the treatment outcomes to be accurately interpreted. If the patients are not blinded, then they run a very high risk of experiencing depressive episodes and poor attitudes if they know they are not in the group receiving the potentially life-saving treatment. The result could be an over exaggerated estimation of the clinical effect of the treatment drug, since it is being compared to a non-placebo controlled group, whose outcome measures are likely more sub-optimal than if it had received a placebo.

The Crossover Clinical Trial Design—There is no doubt that the crossover design provides significant additional power to the clinical trial, in that it can measure the effect of treatment in addition to the effect of removing a treatment. Indeed this design allows the control group to eventually become the treatment group, and the treatment group to become the control group (**Figure 7.7**).

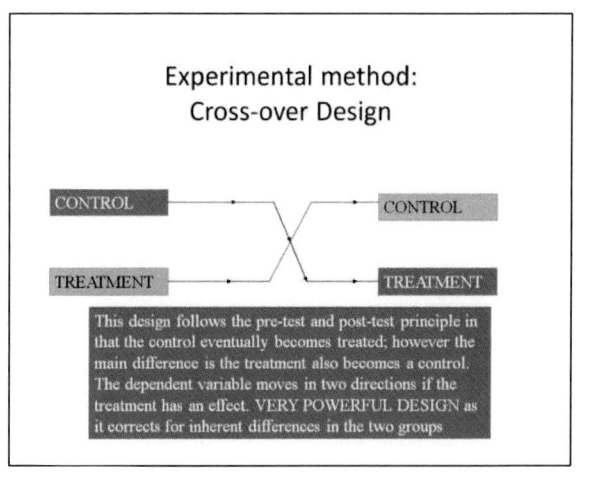

Figure 7.7: Controlled Cross-over Clinical Trial

To better understand the power of this design, it may be pedagogically preferable to provide an example. If researchers are interested in testing the effectiveness of an anti-hypertension drug, they would provide a placebo to the control and the true drug to the treatment group. Having followed the two over three months, they find that the control group, who has hypertension, but received the placebo, did not show any change in their blood pressure. On the other hand, the treatment group, that did receive the blood pressure-lowering medication, experienced, over that same period of time, a 60% drop in blood pressure. Following a two-week washout period, the control group, that was previously administered the placebo with no change in hypertension, now receives the drug with a noticeable 72% drop in blood pressure. By contrast, the treatment group, that previously showed a drop in blood pressure, is now receiving a placebo, and experiencing an increase in blood pressure compared to when the group was on the medication.

The conclusions derived from these findings are very significant, as this research design was clearly able to demonstrate that the noticeable improvements in blood pressure were solely attributed to the therapeutic effects of the drug. In fact, when the drug was removed from the treatment group, the hypertension worsened. The crossing over of the groups, demonstrates two phenomena: the effect of treatment, and the effect of no treatment. This example illustrates its remarkable power to accurately measure the treatment effect. It is for this reason that the randomized double-blind, placebo-controlled cross-over clinical trial is the most powerful clinical research design, currently used in medical research.

7.4 Hypothesis Exercise

The section on nutrition research is culminating with an exercise in formulating hypotheses. The flowchart in **Figure 7.8** provides the student with three basic steps that need to be followed in order to ensure the correct formulation of three hypotheses pertaining to a subject matter in nutrition. It all begins with an observation that is made within the food and nutrition environments. Students will have to think about food preparation within the home, food service operations regularly patronized, grocery stores regularly shopped at for weekly provisions, the food industry or some kind of nutrition and health topic.

For instance, a student may have observed, in a restaurant regularly patronized, that after eating certain foods there is a tendency to feel stuffed or even possibly slightly nauseous. This is a real observation that clearly affects the quality of life. A question that might arise from this observation would be: do I eat too many calories or too much fat when I go to a restaurant? Why do I feel nauseous after eating at a specific restaurant? Is this a problem that affects many people in American society? Do many Americans eat out frequently? Do Americans tend to over eat when they eat away from home? Is the obesity crisis in America somehow significantly tied to frequently eating in restaurants?

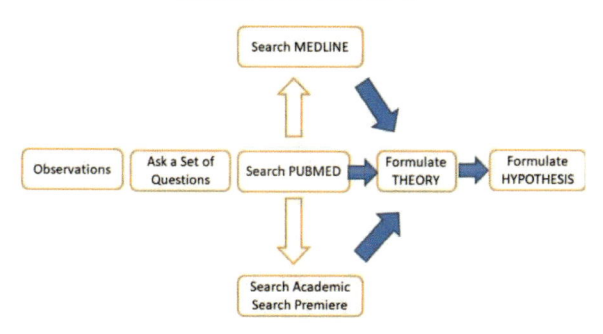

Figure 7.8 Flow chart providing steps to follow when formulating a hypothesis

In asking a set of questions, the student is defining the problem with greater clarity. Likewise, write down the questions that you wondered about. The next step is to do a literature search. There are three databases that students can access: the first is Medline, the second is PubMed, and the third is Academic Search Premier. In keeping with this set of questions, formulated above, the following are the key strategic terms that could be used in a search: **obesity, restaurants, fat intake, food service, weight gain, review, and portion size**.

What are the methods used to strategically narrow the number of articles pertinent to the search? One strategy is to request **review articles** as opposed to research papers. The advantage in reading review articles is that students can acquire a much broader understanding of the field they are reading about, because the authors are summarizing the information obtained from multiple research papers.

The review papers represent a comprehensive understanding of that specific field of research. Review papers, characteristically do not contain **method** or **result** sections, but rather, tend to be organized into multiple topical sections. Research papers by contrast, will have a hypothesis, in addition to a method and result section. Select two research papers and one review paper, and report, using the examples below, the bibliography of the three papers on a Word document.

EXAMPLES OF BIBLIOGRAPHIES
Jang, Y., Kim, W., and Bonn, M.(2011). Generation Y consumers' selection attributes and behaviors, intentions concerning green restaurants. *International Journal of Hospitality Management*, 30: 803-811

Boyce, B. (2011). Making Menus Friendly: Marketing Your Food Intolerance Expertise. *Journal of the American Dietetic Association, 111* (12): 1809-1812.

A second source of legitimate information, pertaining to the selected topic, can be government or professional websites. Here are a few professional organizations that are frequently consulted: the American Heart Association, the Academy of Nutrition and Dietetics, the American Cancer Society and the American Medical Association. The websites to these organizations represent reliable sources of information.

Look specifically for **position papers**, written by professional organizations, as they tend to provide a comprehensive review of the literature. These position papers will state very clearly the organization's professional position regarding a specific subject matter.

Please refer to the following websites:
1. Academy of Dietetics & Nutrition: www.eatright.org
2. American Society for Nutrition: http://www.nutrition.org/
3. USDA (United State Department of Agriculture) Food & Nutrition: http://www.usda.gov/wps/portal/!ut/p/_s.7_0_A/7_0_1OB?navtype=SU&navid=FOOD_NUTRITION
4. International Food Information Council Foundation (IFIC): www.ific.org
5. World Health Organization /Nutrition for Health & Development: http://www.who.int/nut/
6. American Cancer Society (ACS): Nutrition & Cancer Prevention: http://www.cancer.org/docroot/MBC/MBC_6.asp?sitearea=ETO
7. American Heart Association (AHA) Diet & Nutrition: http://www.americanheart.org/presenter.jhtml?identifier=1200010

The fourth step consists of formulating a theory that can explain the observations or answer the questions. The theory needs to contain a mechanism that explains how artificial sweeteners cause obesity, for instance. In that way the theory should consist of endocrine mechanisms, chemical and hormonal signaling, and physiological responses. Here is an example: [2b]

Artificial sweeteners affect sweet taste receptors, hormonal-signalling, notably dopamine release, reward systems and learned energy sensing perceptions in a manner that interferes with nutrient absorption, appetite control or other weight regulation mechanisms, thus causing weight gain despite the energy-free content of the sweeteners.

The final step to this exercise is to formulate three hypotheses, and write them on the word document, previously used for the three bibliographies. Here are a few examples of hypotheses that have been written in scientific papers:
1- It was hypothesized that substitution of sugar with artificial sweeteners in beverage and foods will reduce total energy intake and subsequently cause weight loss in a group of women ages 18 to 55 over a 2 year period
2- Frequent eating away from home (more than 2 days per week), will lead to increased caloric intake, body weight and fat in men and women ages 35 to 65 measured over a 3 year period.

DISCUSSION QUESTIONS

1. If you were interested in establishing whether 40g of fiber, taken in the form of three capsules per day, was effective in curing constipation, what kind of study design would you use? Explain

2. A case control study finds that those individuals, who eat plain yogurt with granola and dried fruits more than 3 times per week, are not likely to develop colon and breast cancer. Upon re-examining the data, reviewers find the conclusion, that plain yogurt prevents colon and breast, to be false. Discuss what might have gone wrong with this study.

3. Discuss why you would prefer to use a randomized controlled cross-over clinical trial to test the effect of ginger in the treatment of nausea in cancer patients.

References

1. Hayes, DP. (2005). The Protective Role of Fruits and Vegetables against Radiation-Induced Cancer. *Nutrition Reviews*; *63(9):303-311*
2. Hulley, SB and Cummings, SR (1988). Designing Clinical Research: An Epidemiological Approach; Baltimore: Williams & Wilkins, 247 pp.
2b. Mosdøl, A., Vist, G. E., Svendsen, C., Dirven, H., Lillegaard, I., Mathisen, G. H., & Husøy, T. (2018). Hypotheses and evidence related to intense sweeteners and effects on appetite and body weight changes: A scoping review of reviews. *PloS one*, *13*(7), e0199558. https://doi.org/10.1371/journal.pone.0199558
3. Nomura, A; et al. (1986) Prospective Study of Coffee Consumption and Risk of Cancer. Journal of the National Cancer Institute; 76 (4): 587-590.
4. C. Pérez-Rodrigo, J. A. Bartrina, L. S. Majem, B. Moreno, and A. D. Rubio, (2006) Epidemiology of obesity in Spain. Dietary guidelines and strategies for prevention. International Journal for Vitamin and Nutrition Research. 76(4): 163–171
5. Rothman K. (1986) Modern Epidemiology. Boston: Little Brown and Company, 358pp
6. Thagard. P. (1989) Explaining Disease: Correlations, causes and mechanisms. Minds & Machines; 8:61-78
7. U.S. Department of Health and Human Services. (October 30, 2013) National Digestive Disease Information Clearinghouse. H Pylori and Peptic Ulcers. Retrieved December 19, 2013 from: http://digestive.niddk.nih.gov/ddiseases/pubs/hpylori/#2

CHAPTER 8

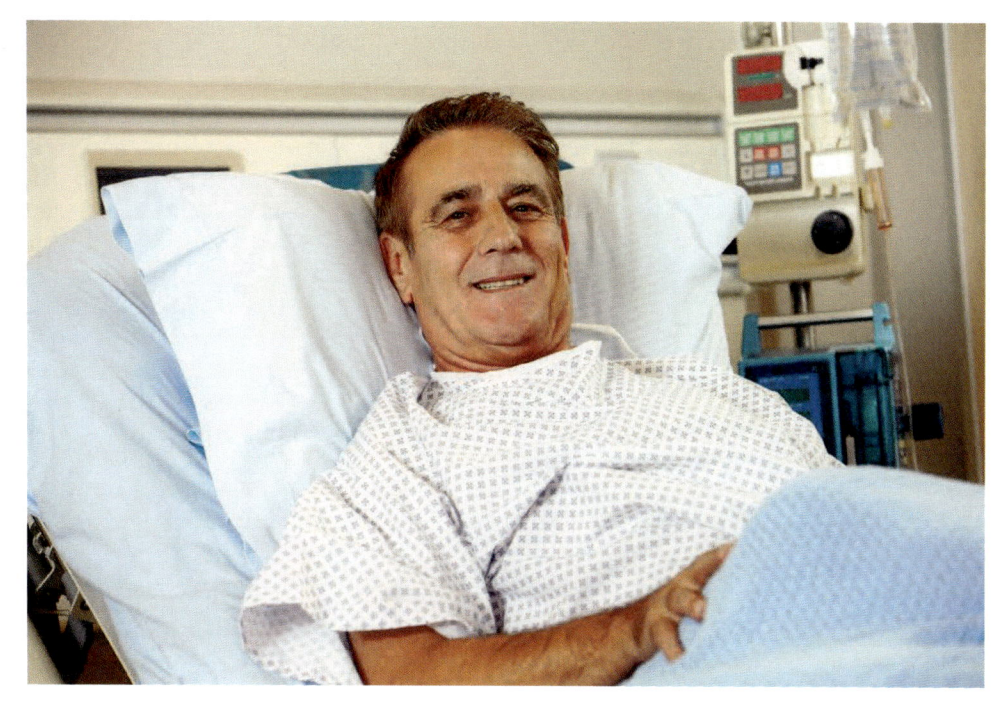

By Monkey Business Images © Shutterstock__125077229/shutterstock.com

NUTRITION AND CHRONIC DISEASE

8.1 The Prevalence of Chronic Disease in American Society

According to the CDC, national health expenditure, between 1980 and 2010, grew from $256 billion to $2.6 trillion, a jump that is so extraordinarily large that it defies the imagination.[3]

In just 30 years, health care costs increased 915% in the United States, saddling the population with a cost burden that is currently at 16.4% of the national income. Moreover, there is something more disturbing taking place that many do not yet fully comprehend.[3]

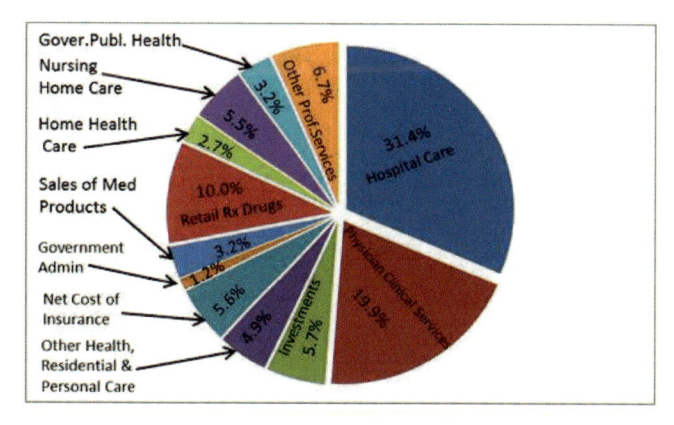

Figure 8.1 Breakdown of U.S. National Health Expenditure in 2010. Data source: Martin AB[10] and U.S. Centers for Medicare & Medicaid Services. Image created by author.

A closer examination of health costs in 2010 (**Figure 8.1**) reveals that slightly more than 50% of total health care expenditure originated from hospital care and physician/clinical services.[10] Concomitantly, employer-sponsored insurance health coverage premiums for families rose 113%, which further oppressed industry and business with daunting expenses. Coincidentally, the prevalence of chronic diseases such as heart disease, diabetes, and cancer grew at such an alarming rate, that the CDC now estimates that as much as 75% of the total health care costs are tied to chronic diseases.[2]

Since the 1980s, the most significant contributor to the epidemics of chronic diseases, now observed in American society, has been linked to the surprising surge in obesity prevalence. Obesity is indeed at the source of conditions like hypertension, atherosclerosis, gallbladder disease, sleep apnea, type II diabetes and depression. In the last 20 years, healthcare costs have increased in tandem with the complexity of the illnesses of regular patients seen in family practice.

Whereas in the early 1960s, a typical visit to the family physician would have consisted of yearly checkups, consultations for tonsillitis, pregnancy management and follow ups, high blood pressure and a persistent cough—likely from smoking,—nowadays family practice physicians regularly encounter medical train wrecks. It is common today for frontline healthcare providers to see an obese or morbidly obese 25-year-old female, who complains of lower back pain and out of control blood sugars. The patient's chart would also likely reveal that she is currently taking three antihypertensive drugs, 1-2 medications for mood disorder or depression, and at least one cholesterol-lowering drug. Her most recent history would probably reveal that urinary protein began showing up approximately 11 months ago. In a 30 to 45 minute time-slot, the physician will likely only have time to address one or two of her chronic conditions: back pain and hyperglycemia.

> **Obesity may be the fundamental cause some patients' complaints and disease, but the obesity itself will likely never be addressed by the physician.**

The other conditions will need to be addressed over multiple office visits, and will likely involve numerous billings. The truth of the matter is that, although obesity is the central cause of all of her complaints, the obesity itself will likely not be addressed by the physician. The reality is that obesity is not being solved by physicians and other frontline providers. This is because it is a public health problem, but yet, figure 64 shows very clearly that only 3.2% of the national health expenditure is dedicated to government sponsored public health.

The popular opinion that our current financial healthcare woes are the result of expensive insurance premiums may not be the complete truth. Often forgotten, in the discussion, is precisely the incredible rise in chronic diseases that is driving healthcare costs upwards. Indeed, the nature of the diseases, with which we are afflicted, are costly to manage and physically compromising.

Dr. Gary Cohen, a pediatric nephrologist, working out of New Haven, Indiana, has clearly observed an increase in obese children, suffering from hypertension, who require anti-hypertensive drugs. It is truly surprising to see increasing numbers of children under the care of pediatric nephrologists. This tends to imply that children, in greater numbers, are suffering from hypertension and diabetes, which arise from obesity. Hur and Reicks[7] have documented this rising prevalence in adolescent obesity, type-2 diabetes and cardiovascular disease.

Between 1999 and 2006, NHANES data showed that, among a national represented sample of adolescents between 12 and 19, 20.3% had abnormal lipids; among obese adolescents specifically, approximately 43% had at least one marker of hyperlipidemia.

These are symptoms that were traditionally seen in middle age men and women. In fact, the National Survey for Children's Health, confirmed that the problem was very serious with 35 to 36% of children, ages 10 to 17, being classified as overweight or obese in 2003- 2004. Contrast that finding with the

13 to 15% prevalence of overweight and obese French children, in that same age group, according to the International Obesity Task Force.

Moreover, the cost to manage obesity rose from a mere $35 million per year in the 1970s to a staggering $227 million by the year 2000. This 549% increase in health care costs becomes a harbinger for the financial storm clouds gathering in the horizon, that are about to hit our health care system.[3]

Fundamentally, there is an important question that has to be asked: what are the societal and financial implications for a society whose children are becoming profoundly ill? Critical to this discussion is the understanding of the degenerative nature of type II diabetes and heart disease, if they are not corrected by important and often times dramatic changes in eating behaviors and lifestyles. Dr. Stephen Ponder, a pediatric endocrinologist, in Corpus Christi, Texas, the fattest city in America in 2010, has been tracking the worrisome rise in the prevalence of type II diabetes in the pediatric population for several years.

He is now seeing greater numbers of children with blood sugars that are out of control. The causes are primarily attributed to poor dietary habits, and a collapsing family structure that prevents children from receiving structured care. These kids, says Ponder, need organized and disciplined care, such as blood sugar monitoring, and controlled snacks that are healthy.

Dr. Barry Popkin, is an internationally acclaimed epidemiologist and nutrition professor at the University of North Carolina at Chapel Hill. He explains that 40 years ago most people didn't get diabetes until they were 50 or 60. Presently, he explains:

We are currently seeing children, let alone adolescents in great numbers, who are either becoming pre-diabetic or diabetic.

He goes on to explain the life course of diabetes, and of the many debilitating diseases and conditions that arise from poorly controlled blood sugars. The situation is alarming when one considers that after 20 years of poorly controlled blood sugar, individuals begin to suffer from neuropathies, blindness, amputations, and chronic renal failure leading to dialysis.

> We may be witnessing the first generation of children who will not outlive their parents.

The financial repercussions are cumbersome, especially as epidemiologists are now forecasting that many of these debilitating conditions will now begin appearing in young 30-year-olds. We may now actually be looking at a generation of children who will not outlive their parents. This would in effect mean that growing numbers of children would become medically compromised by their 30s and 40s, unable to hold a steady productive job.

There are 105 million Americans who are either diabetic or at risk of becoming diabetic.[2] The problem is more accentuated among specific ethnicities such as the North American Indian, and the Asian-Pacific Islander. For instance, prior to 1900, type-2 diabetes was relatively rare in Pima Indians.[1, 4, 9]

But by the 1930s, the prevalence was at par with the U.S. population, and by the 1950s, the incidence of diabetes already surpassed that of the U.S. average.[8] When American Indian and Alaskan native children, adolescents and adults, under the age of 35, were clustered together, the number of newly diagnosed diabetics rose 71% between 1990 and 1998. The most dramatic increase in the prevalence rate of diabetes is seen in the 81% jump in males and in the 60% spike in females.[1]

These are alarming changes that do set off alarm bells at the public health level. However, there is little that can be done, even though the incidence is clearly linked to modifiable risk factors. The solution to control diabetes is rather straight forward: Increased physical activity and a changed diet that involves decreasing the high sugar and replacing it with more complex carbs, more vegetables, fruits, and less to no junk food. The problem is that poverty creates a cycle of hopelessness that is difficult to escape from, when obesity and diabetes take over. Illness invariably robs the individual of energy and ultimately vitality. Hence, meeting the financial needs of the family becomes more difficult for parents who are afflicted with diabetes and heart disease. Sharing of resources, skills and talents are less of a possibility when afflicted with chronic disease for several reasons: First, illness causes the individual to become more focused on his wounds; this is clearly observed as well in animals.

Second, chronic illness, unlike acute illness, does not resolve itself; it becomes part of daily existence, slowly eating away at vital energy that is so necessary for creative endeavors to take place, and for dreams and ambitions to fuel a deep desire to learn and to live. So then, when important segments of a population become worn down, by illnesses that never really go away, how is society, as a whole, affected? Is it, at that point, that a nation's industrial leadership and technological innovations begin to decline?

8.2 Reversing Chronic Disease, is All about Nutrition and Exercise

Is it really that simple? No it isn't. The real question that should be asked: Is it really that complicated? It is indeed a complex problem that reaches deep within the formative years of a child. It is here that the taste habituation gets encoded into the taste preferences of the youth.

If we expose our children to foods loaded with sugar, sodium and fat, throughout their formative years, they will seek those familiar foods, especially when their brains become wired to seek high taste sensations.

> Taste preferences develop habitually; the more a food is consumed, the more desire there is for that food.

If the child consumes foods that set off high secretions of dopamine, that stimulate the pleasure centers situated in the frontal lobes of the brain, then the child becomes wired for repeat food acquisition behaviors, that are set on experiencing pleasure sensations from food. Has it not always been that way? You must be saying: common, food is supposed to taste good right?

Indeed, prior to the development of a food supply, engineered by food scientists who study population taste preferences very thoroughly, the food supply was limited to foods like, dairy, fruits, vegetables, whole grains and some meats and fish.

These foods tasted very good, especially when mixed with carefully selected spices. By contrast, many of the foods we now purchase from grocery stores have been manufactured by a food industry bent on sales and increased profit margins.

In other words, the cheaper these foods are to make, the greater the profit margin, and the happier the shareholders. Here is the problem though: the purer the ingredients the more costly the food. This reality incentivizes food production companies to create foods that look, smell and taste real, but that are not real.

These nonfoods are cheap to produce and are generally very shelf stable. This means companies can mass produce these nonfoods, and ship them to grocery stores, assured of their long shelf life. Foods with a short shelf life generally translate into financial losses, because larger amounts are discarded, especially when turnover is small. The industry is clearly working to limit costly losses of this kind. So what are we left with? Next time you are in the grocery store, pay more attention to the proportion of the shelves that is dedicated to these foods with unrealistically long shelf lives. One complete grocery aisle is dedicated to sodas, and power drinks of various types; a second aisle is made up only of junk and snack foods. Here, potato chips of multiple flavors, salty pretzels, cookies of all sorts, candies, sweets, gums, tarts, and ready-to-eat cakes line the shelves at eye-level for maximum sales. The third aisle is dedicated to baking products. Except for the whole wheat, durum, rye, rice and oat flours, in addition to the yeast, baking powder, baking soda and sugar, almost everything else should be avoided, including the numerous cake baking mixes, cake and pie fillings, puddings, fake maple and chocolate syrups.

The fourth aisle is made up of breakfast cereals that are entirely processed, high in sugar, sodium and low in fiber except for the whole natural oat cereals. The processed cereals for children should be almost entirely avoided because of the taste sensations that are experienced by children who eat them. This is where the conditioning to food preferences actually begins. Aisles 1 to 4 contain the foods that have impoverished the health of our youth.

The sodas and sugar-sweetened beverages have been shown, in a review of 88 longitudinal studies, to be directly related to energy intake, and increases in body weight in children and adolescents. These are no longer debatable findings; sugar intakes from sweetened beverages are so elevated among the young, especially, that it is displacing dairy products out of the diet.

The Bogalusa Heart study has shown that between 1973 and 1994, milk intake has dropped 13.8%. During that time vegetable intake also declined nearly 9%. Despite the study showing a decrease in total fat intake, a more careful look at the data, reveals that as many as 75% of the children were still consuming amounts of total fat and saturated fat that exceeded national recommended cut-offs.[11] The study also confirmed that adiposity in the children had dramatically increased. Other studies have also reported that when milk intake declines in adolescents, specifically, body weight increases. The only real solution is a set of strategies that increase the dietary fiber content. Hur and Reicks[7] found, in compiling and analyzing data from the NHANES (National Health and Nutrition Examination Survey—1999-2004), that the intake of whole grain breakfast cereals was negatively associated with body fat in adolescent boys. They also report that when fiber was elevated so were fruits, whole grains, vegetables, carbohydrates and calories, but that meat intake, protein and fat were significantly lower. So then a set of 4 basic strategies can be established that would be most helpful in decreasing the problem of obesity and chronic disease in the U.S.

Strategy-1: Increase the fiber intake at breakfast especially. To reach this goal, almost every breakfast cereal for children needs to be removed from the home inventory. The list is so extensive, that it is best to enumerate the cereals that should be included: cooked or raw whole oats, or shredded wheat mixed with raisins or other dried fruits, such as plums, cranberries, apricots, and prunes are the best choices. There are two reasons for these choices: First, these two cereals contain no sugar, and second, there is absolutely no sodium. For those reasons alone, these cereals need to be given top priority.

This is the time to introduce fruit to enhance the taste and to cultivate the taste preferences of the young, as it is clear that they bring these forward into adulthood. Adding 2% or whole milk for children or 1 or 2% milk for adults are wholesome choices that nicely complements the cereal. Some whole grain high fiber cereals can also be included in the breakfast inventory even though there is sugar and sodium. All Bran cereals including Bran-Buds, Fiber-one, Raisin bran, Bran Flakes, and Grape Nuts cereals are good alternatives.

These choices are allowable because the fiber content is truly elevated enough, that the risk from sugar and sodium is outweighed by the benefits gained from the high fiber. Remember, that given the North American style of eating, breakfast becomes the single most important meal for fiber intake. Without fiber cereals in the morning, it is virtually impossible, for most Americans, to achieve dietary recommended intakes for fiber by the end of the day. Vegetarians and vegans are generally the exception to this rule.

Strategy-2: Eliminate sodas from the diet.
Increasingly, the evidence is pointing towards sodas as the single most significant cause of the obesity epidemic worldwide, especially among children and teenagers. It is not therapeutically accurate to recommend decreased consumption of sodas because of the highly addictive nature of these products. They pretty much have to be eliminated entirely if dietary habits are to be improved.

There appears to be a growing consensus that ongoing sugar consumption creates persistent need for sugar. Children, especially, are vulnerable to this kind of exposure. Physiologically, the argument can be made, that the immaturity of a child's brains makes it particularly vulnerable to the nefarious impact of high sugar intakes; it sets off explosive brain chemical reactions, in the hedonic center of the brain, that become addictive to vulnerable children.

Strategy-3: Increase vegetables in the diet
Increasing vegetables throughout the day will invariably mean heightening the intake of soluble and insoluble fibers. Following the Mediterranean food guide generally means an abundant consumption of vegetables whole grains, fruits, beans and nuts; overall they comprise about 75% of the pyramid (**Figure 8.2**).

Nutritionists and dietitians are now frequently seeing growing numbers of children who do not eat vegetables except for: sweetened corn from a can, and French Fries. When asked, children simply do not like the taste, and it is the competing tastes of manufactured foods that children have to distance themselves from, otherwise there is simply no hope of initiating long term wholesome eating habits.

Parents have failed to consistently introduce these vegetables into the diet, in the early childhood years. The goal here is to increase variety, for it is indeed through vegetables that the consumer can acquire a very broad intake of phytochemicals of various types. Its tastes are subtle but delicious. In lectures, I often ask students if they consume legumes. After citing a few, such as Romano beans, lentils, kidney beans, navy beans, black beans to name a few, generally less than 2% of the class admit to eating legumes.

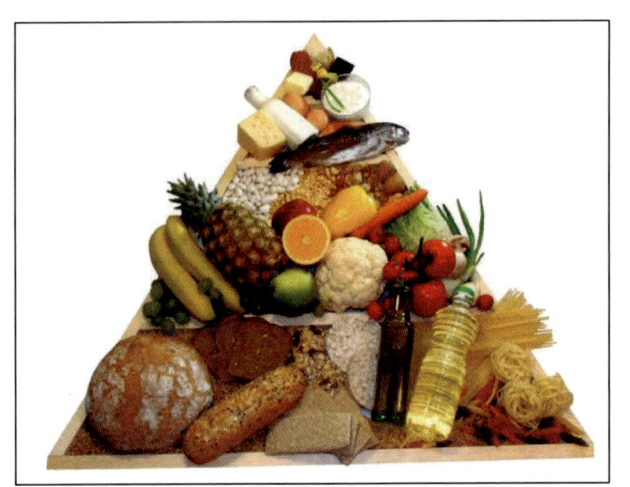

Figure 8.2: The Mediterranean Food Pyramid © Bogdan Wankowicz

This is a tragedy of monumental proportion, for legumes, rich in soluble fibers, provide vegetable protein, which when combined with grains become complete proteins. This combination decreases the need for animal proteins of high biological value; this is an important attribute since heart disease and certain cancers are highly correlated with frequent and high red meat intake. The Mediterranean diet exemplifies what it means to consume healthy foods. The pyramid (Figure 65) also emphasizes the importance of fiber intake; the base of the diet is loaded with whole grains, pastas and cereals.

> Healthy oils, including olive oil, are an important part of the Mediterranean food pyramid.

The second layer is rich in fruits, vegetables and legumes. Notice how the fish, dairy and eggs are near the top and red meats at the tip. This depiction of the relative unimportance of meat, in the overall diet, is the main feature of Mediterranean style of eating. Unlike the U.S. Food Pyramid or My Plate representations, oil is not at the tip, but rather at the base of the pyramid. The signaled importance of fat is noticeable—representing roughly 40% of the DRI calories—and contrasts greatly with the North American repugnance for fat in its idealistic vision of the healthy diet. Indeed, because of the obesity epidemic and the vilification of fat, dieting in the U.S. has been about eliminating fat from the diet—total fat tends to fall as low as 15 to 20% of DRI calories—and causing suboptimal intakes of vitamin E and essential fatty acids in many dieters.

My research, of the dietary habits of University students, has consistently shown vitamin E intake levels equal to or less than 67% of the RDA in over 70% of women, who have documented 3 day intakes. Statistically, a percent equal to or below the 67% cut-off means that students are at high risk of chronically consuming suboptimal dietary levels of vitamin E. This is based on George Beaton's probability model of dietary risk assessment.[5] Our analysis has found that the primary reason for the low levels, of this very important antioxidant, is the suboptimal intake of polyunsaturated vegetable oils. This occurs from the chronic attempts, by the young specifically, to cut back on calories for the purpose of weight loss.

Strategy-4: Increase Fruits in the diet
Fruit intake has declined in the last decade because of a successful campaign to promote fruit juices and drinks, packaged in larger portions. Many parents, feeling that fruit juice is far better than sodas, erroneously encourage the consumption of juices for hydration. The problem is that they are still delivering sugar loads that are unusually heavy, especially for a small child's body. Perceived wholesomeness, in this case, translates into a harmful practice. Three things are taking place that should not: first, the portion of juice tends to be elevated; rather than a standard 4fl-oz serving of orange juice, for instance, the mother will provide a 16fl-oz water bottle filled with juice. It sounds like a wholesome practice: all that good nutrition right at the child's fingertip. The problem is the ensuing sugar load, totaling 60g of sugar or the equivalent of 15 teaspoons, enters the blood stream. On a daily basis, this kind of sucrose intake challenges the pancreas to maintain stable blood sugar levels. It is a taxing process for the body, a sort of mild trauma to the biological system; there is also a hidden danger: many of the sweetened drinks contain high fructose corn syrup (HFCS).

In the last decade, the intake of HFCS has been steadily climbing because of the growing popularity of sodas, power drinks, and fruits drinks. Researchers are suspecting that there might be a link between the obesity crisis and the intake of HFCS.

Stephen Ponder, a pediatric endocrinologist, working in Corpus Christi, Texas, has been seeing increases in pediatric hepatic steatosis in young kids. He has tied this unusual prevalence of fatty liver in the young to high levels of HFCS intakes. Second, a 16fl-oz drink carries approximately 240 kcal, which displaces other important foods out of the diet, such as milk and fruits. Dr. Erica Holt and colleagues,[6] in studying the impact of fruits and vegetables on various markers of inflammation and oxidative stress in adolescents—they measured C-Reactive proteins, cytokines, and prostaglandins—found lower markers of oxidative stress and inflammation among those who consumed high intakes of fruits and vegetables. Dietary analysis confirmed high intakes of antioxidants, folate and various types of flavonoids.

The literature does affirm that the benefit of fruits and vegetables is real, especially for young children and adolescents who are forming their dietary habits and preferences. One of the main arguments, currently formulated against poor dietary practices in kids, is that the antioxidants consumed in healthy diets, rich in fruits and vegetables, prevent damaging free radical attacks against cell integrity.

The goal is for antioxidant intakes to at least equal the free radicals produced. Failing to achieve this balance, the fear is that low-grade inflammation and oxidative stress can, over several decades, predict a fairly high risk of chronic diseases. It is urgent that steps be taken to safeguard the children for they are but innocent spectators in a dietary free-for-all disaster.

DISCUSSION QUESTIONS

1. Discuss what you think is the most important dietary strategy that needs to be implemented, in order to greatly diminish the rate chronic disease in the U.S.

2. Looking at chronic diseases broadly in the U.S., what would be your most damning criticism of the American diet?

3. What is the main fear expressed by nutritionist, dietitians and other health care professionals about the consequence of not consuming enough antioxidants in the diet? Explain

4. Identify the 4 key dietary strategies that need to be implemented at the national level in order to decrease body fat and the risks of heart disease. Explain.

5. Identify the most significant dietary findings of the Bogalusa Heart Study between 1973 and 1994.

References

1. CDC Diabetes Public Health Resource Trends in Diabetes Prevalence among American Indian and Alaska Native Children, Adolescents and Young Adults—1990-1998. Accessed June 30, 2012 from: .http://www.cdc.gov/diabetes/pubs/factsheets/aian.htm.
2. Centers for Medicare and Medicaid Services, Office of the Actuary, National Health Statistics Group. *National Health Care Expenditures Data.* January 2012.
3. Centers for Disease Control and Prevention. Rising Health Care Costs Are Unsustainable. April 2011. Retrieved December 30, 2013 from: http://www.cdc.gov/workplacehealthpromotion/businesscase/reasons/rising.html
4. Cohen BM. Diabetes mellitus among Indians of the American Southwest: its prevalence and clinical characteristics in a hospitalized population. *Ann Intern Med.* 40:588–599, 1954.
5. Gibson, RS. (1990). Principles of Nutritional Assessment. New York: Oxford University Press, p:150
6. Holt EM, et al. Fruit and vegetable consumption and its relation to markers of inflammation and oxidative stress in adolescents. *JADA.* 2009;109:414-421.
7. Hur, I.Y and Reicks, M. Relationship between whole-grain intake, chronic disease risk indicators, and weight status among adolescents in the National Health and Nutri-tion Examination Survey, 1999-2004. JAND 2012; 112:46-55.
8. Joslin EP. The universality of diabetes. *JAMA.* 115:2033–2038, 1940.
9. Knowler WC, Pettitt DJ, Saad MF, Bennett PH. Diabetes mellitus in the Pima Indians: Incidence, risk factors, and pathogenesis. *Diabetes Metab.* Rev 6:1–27, 1990.
10. Martin AB et al, Growth in US Health Spending Remained Slow in 2010; Health Share of Gross Domestic Product was Unchanged from 2009. *Health Affairs*, 2012.
11. Nicklas TA, et al. Children's food consumption Patterns have changed over two decades (1973-1994): The Bogalusa Study. *JADA.* 2004; 104:1127-1140.
12. Pavkov, ME et al. Changing pattern of type-2 diabetes incidence among Pima Indians. *Diabetes Care.* 2007; 30(7) 1758-1763.
13. Price RA, Charles MA, Pettitt DJ, Knowler WC. Obesity in Pima Indians: large increases among post-World War II birth cohorts. *Am J Phys Anthropol.* 92:473–479, 1993.
14. Russell F. *The Pima Indians. Twenty-Sixth Annual Report of the Bureau of American Ethnology to the Secretary of the Smithsonian Institution Washington, DC.* U.S. Government Printing Office, 1908, pp. 3–389.

CHAPTER 9

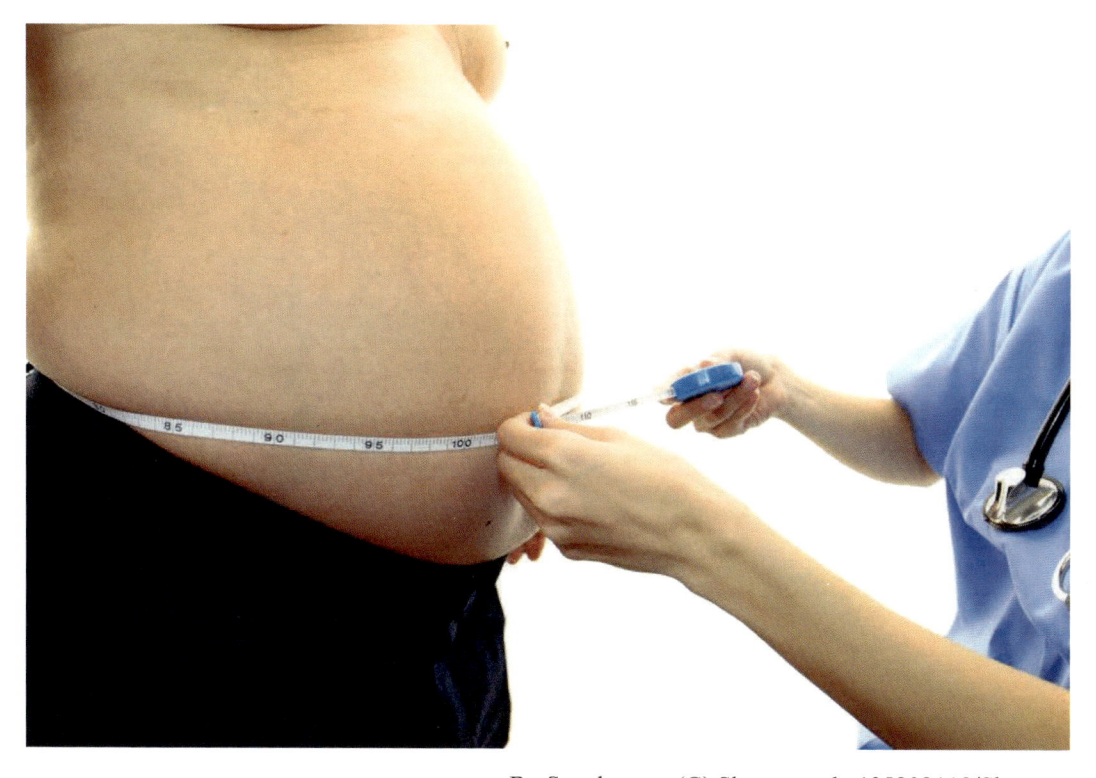

THE OBESITY CRISIS

By Sunabesyou (C) Shutterstock_135802118/Shutterstock.com

9.1 The Growing Prevalence of Obesity Worldwide & in America

There is likely no greater threat to American society than the growing prevalence of obesity among adults and children. The implications facing a society with its population succumbing to chronic diseases secondary to obesity are frightening. Currently, the CDC estimates that two thirds of American adults—that is 67%—are either overweight or obese, and that over 35% of Americans are obese, a percent epidemiologists predict will grow to 47% of the U.S. adult population by 2030 [22]

> **Currently, the CDC estimates that 70% of American adults are either overweight or obese and that over 35% of Americans are obese, a percent epidemiologists predict will grow to 47% of the US adult population by 2030.**

The obesity and overweight prevalence graph (**Figure 9.1**) describes a relatively stable overweight adult population since the 1960s; in fact, the 2008 and 1960 prevalence are identical at 32%.

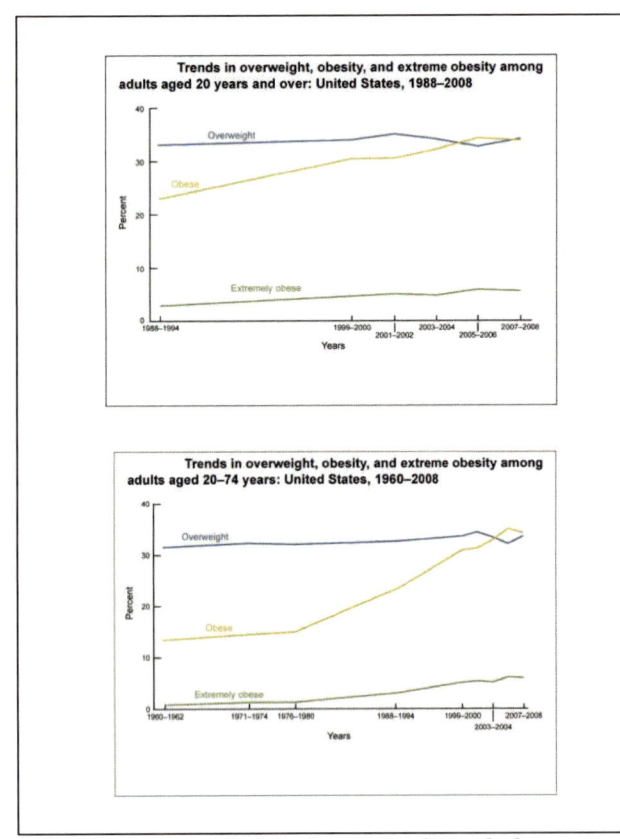

Figure 9.1: Prevalence of overweight and obese American Adults between 1960 and 2008. Source: Ogden, CL et al 2010[30]

So we haven't become dramatically more overweight, but rather, significant numbers of overweight adults have transitioned to obesity and morbid obesity, with prevalence values jumping from 13% obesity in the 1960s to 35% by 2008; this 161.5% increase in obesity has troublesome implications for the country and the economy. Despite a USA-Today article dated December 24, 2013, and featuring the headline: *Obesity levels off, but extreme cases tipping the scales*, there are concerns that the crisis is far from over. The good news is that the obesity prevalence has been relatively stable at 35% since 2010, but a steady 125% climb in morbid obesity, between 1994 and 2010, has stumped epidemiologists. They are at a loss to explain this dramatic upward shift in the numbers of adults who are at least 100lbs over their healthy weight.[30] There has to be something meaningful taking place that causes such significant hikes in body weight. It isn't the consequences of an extra 10lbs at year's end that we are looking at, but rather the devastating implications of doing nothing to abate 10lbs per year increases over an entire decade.

Obesity is also growing in other industrialized nations such as Canada, England and Greece. The top 10 countries with 30% or more obesity in the adult population are organized in **Table 9.1**.

> **There are countries struggling with a greater proportion of obese men than women, such as Canada, Greece, England, Ireland, Cyprus, Czech Republic, Spain, Australia, and Austria.**

Countries like Canada, England, New Zealand, Venezuela, and Greece are hovering around obesity rates of 25 to 27%. Mexico is right under the 30% cut-off with 29.35% of the overall population suffering from obesity; women in Mexico are particularly vulnerable as evidenced by the 35.5% adult female obesity prevalence, a value that matches up very closely to the U.S. prevalence in women.

Worldwide, the prevalence of obesity is estimated at 500 million, and the numbers that are either overweight or obese approach a shocking 1.5 billion. Epidemiologists forecast that by 2030, unless the growth rate is reversed, as many as 60% of the world population will be either overweight or obese. A closer examination of the problem reveals that obesity is growing especially in developing countries such as Mexico, Polynesia, the Middle East and some South American countries.

The Harvard School of Public Health identifies three leading factors that are fueling the obesity crisis worldwide[18] first, the food environment; second the built-environment; and third, new technologies.

Food Environment—Developing countries, once stricken with economic hardship, unemployment and poverty, experience decreased food availability. Even though a more developed agrarian society tends to be dominant in developing countries, the agricultural output is not usually sustainable. International agribusiness, more or less, dictates the cash crops that needed to be produced in order to meet the needs of the western markets.

With the globalization of the world economies, however, there is now increased access to cheap and affordable food. For instance, in the last decade, the price of beef fell an astounding 80%, and as the agricultural market broadly opened up to become more international, prices began to plummet, allowing a greater accessibility to cheap food.

Overall, weight problems are documented to be significantly more severe among women than men, in most of the nations around the world (**Table 10.1**). Contrary to what many readers might expect, it is not the U.S. that has the most obese women in the world, but rather the island of Tonga, located among the Polynesian South Pacific islands, where the International Association for the Study of Obesity (IASO) reports that as many as 70.3% of adult women are obese.

The country that holds second place for the most obese women is the island of Samoa, tucked away in the South Pacific, in between Fiji and Tonga, where 63% of adult women are obese.

The Republic of Nauru, a small Micronesian island, in the South Pacific is in third position, with 60% of women reported as obese. The U.S. is actually in 13th position worldwide, with obese adult women representing 35.8% of the adult female population. Contrary to many countries, the prevalence of obesity in the U.S. is equally distributed between the genders—there are 35.5% adult men and 35.8% of adult women classified as obese in the U.S. Likewise, in countries like England, with 26% obesity and Denmark with 11.8% obesity, the prevalence is the same between genders.

From an epidemiological perspective, the prominence of obese adult women is concerning, because of the increased risk of chronic disease tied to obese women of reproductive age, and of the devastating impact on their progeny. These obese women are paying the price of having access to greater amounts of cheap foods in the marketplace. But it's more than that, because it is not about having access to more affordable fruits, vegetables, grains and coffee, for instance. But rather, it is about developing a strong predilection for less expensive meats, dairy products and oils, that have abundantly flooded the market, and which until recently, were substantially more prohibitive in price.

One of the significant changes, that facilitated this greater accessibility to abundant and affordable food, is the appearance of mega grocery stores such as Walmart, and Carrefour. These superstores began to show up in the suburbs and the outskirts of cities. They introduced large amounts of processed foods that were calorically-dense, high in fats, sodium, sugar and low in fiber.[6]

These developing nations, saw their food traditions replaced by highly processed foods that looked and tasted good, but that was ultimately of poor nutritional quality. Indeed, the market invasion of sodas, worldwide, dramatically caused a serious upward shift in the ingestion of sugar. It is not unexpected then that soft drink consumption is the single most influential dietary contributor to the obesity crisis internationally, according to Barry Popkin, a nutrition and epidemiology professor at the University of North Carolina.[32]

Moreover, there is an additional problem in the environment that is conducive to lowering physical activity. It is the new infrastructural organization, adopted by developing nations that intend to emulate western economies, that amplifies the obesity prevalence in these countries.

The Built Environment—The changing landscape, of the ever growing urban centers, invariably leads to the appearance of malls, and to the disappearance of agricultural communities. As rural farm workers gravitate to the urban centers for the better paying factory jobs, they require cars to shop and work. The adoption of a westernized economy decreases overall physical expenditure; walking becomes less of a necessity of daily living, and overall hard physical labor is replaced by desk jobs in the financial, service and information markets. In these conditions, less energy expenditure occurs, leading to weight gain.

From an international health perspective, there is a lot more to worry about, as the obesity crisis is compromising greater numbers of women throughout the world compared to men. Demographers, in looking at obesity rates, fear both the epidemic of type-2 diabetes and the catastrophic problem of demographic winters sweeping industrialized nations. They now must factor in the serious and alarming implications that obese women are less fertile, and that chronically ill pregnant women give birth to children who are also wired for obesity, type-2 diabetes and cardiovascular disease. The physiologically-based fetal-maternal relationship in utero, favors epigenetic changes that can predispose infants to chronic disease.[6b, 9]

But also, the mother's eating habits are likely to get passed on to the children. The consequence is devastating, at a population level, as families become compromised because of the debilitating effects of chronic diseases.

TABLE-9.1 Countries with an Obesity Prevalence ≥30% of the adult population

COUNTRY	% OBESE WOMEN	OVERALL % OBESITY
1. TONGA	70.3%	58.45%
2. NAURU	60.5%	58.1%
3. SAMOA	63.0%	47.95%
4. KUWAIT	47.9%	42.15%
5. FRENCH POLYNESIA	44.3%	40.3%
6. QATAR	45.3%	39.95%
7. USA	35.8%	35.65%
8. SAUDI ARABIA	44.0%	35.2%
9. PALASTINE	42.5%	33.2%
10. PANAMA	36.1%	32.0%

The ranking of obese nations is based on the mean obesity rates between genders.[19]

Indeed, the fear is that young obese women, who have diabetes and heart disease, will not tend to form families. They will likely experience unusually high levels of depression, fatigue, and will tend to have poor endurance, a formula that spells disaster for childrearing. At the very least, children require parents with energy and endurance, if for no other reason than to be able to work and provide for their physical needs. A morass of diseases and disabilities will more often than not, impede proper child care.

If we examine the crisis by region, then it becomes clear that mostly Polynesian Islands, South American and Middle-Eastern countries tend to have worrisome levels of obesity among women. For instance, in most of the countries bordering the western bank of the Persian Gulf, female obesity prevalence rates vary between 31-48% with an overall mean of 40.54%. Oman, Egypt and Palestine also have obesity prevalence rates that are elevated. These are countries tarred by the oil wealth that has left them wide open to westernized foods and food distribution infrastructure.

Countries with the lowest obesity prevalence—posted below in the parentheses—tend to be those that are or have been affected by at least one of 5 key factors that have compromised their built environments.

First, brutal dictatorships or repressive political parties like Cuba (8.65%) and Albania (9.1%); second, poverty among the populace as in Sierra Leone (9.3%) Mali (5.2%), Haiti (6.3%), Bangladesh (1.7%), and Ethiopia (0.7%); third, high food insecurity, such as in countries like Kenya (7.2%); fourth, poor living conditions, pitiable population health, and a badly managed health care system, such as in Nigeria (6%), despite being an emerging market that has reached, according to the World Bank, middle-income status; and finally, fifth, chronic civil unrest, political instability and civil war like Nepal (1.1%), and the Ivory Coast (4.7%) despite having the strongest economy in West Africa.

This 5 point model confirms that when market economies are weak, and there is difficult access to food, because of poor inventories, and impoverished infrastructure, populations do not tend to overeat. Rather, they eat less and perhaps sub-optimally; it is not unexpected, then, to observe leaner populations in these countries.

> **There is, however, a paradox to this 5 point model, and that is the low obesity rates found in Asian countries despite political stability, strong economic growth, low rates of poverty and malnutrition, and solid infrastructure.**

There is, however, a paradox to this 5 point model, and that is the low obesity rates found in Asian countries like Japan (2.85%), South Korea (2.3%), Indonesia (4.5%), and China (2.9%) despite political stability, strong economic growth, low rates of poverty, malnutrition, and solid infrastructure. What is going on? Asian countries have experienced unprecedented growth over the last 20 years and yet, despite having strong migration from the rural to the urban centers, seemingly greater purchasing power and access to food, the obesity rates are apparently kept in check, or are they?

In July 2008, newspaper headlines announcing that obesity rates were on the rise in China shocked the world. Bloomberg news posted the headline: "Obesity in China has doubled over the last 11 years." Christina Alesci, in New York, authored the story; she reported that the Chinese waistline had significantly grown, with obesity rates in men tripling and those in women doubling since 1989. Doctor Barry Popkin[32] estimated the number of overweight and obese Chinese at 325 million, representing 25% of the total population of 1.3 billion. This was a shocking revelation that caused scientists to project the possibility of that number doubling by 2028, based on current obesity and overweight growth rates.

Popkin's work also uncovered a 20% jump in death rates from cancer and cardiovascular disease, secondary to type-2 diabetes. There are serious health problems brewing in the background of China's booming economy and rising prosperity. Will the government be able to implement effective damage control?

The New Technologies—The problem, so it seems, is that while the prevalence of obesity (2.9%) is nothing but a blimp on the radar, the prominence of overweight adult Chinese (18.6%) is growing at a rate, that is alarming enough, to cause epidemiologists to warn of a public health problem. In fact, the pervasiveness of both the obese and overweight adult Chinese has increased 49.3% between 1992 and 2002, going from roughly 14.6% in 1993 to 21.8% in 2002.

The upsurge stems from new Chinese dietary practices, embraced by mostly the young who are now consuming more meats, dairy, and vegetable oils, in addition to following more sedentary lifestyles—a consequence of prolonged access to new gaming technologies—compared to the Chinese who lived under Mao's isolationist era. Mao Zedong supported a strong agrarian economy that required hard physical labor; he also implemented clear protectionist policies that kept the U.S. out of China's economy and culture.

It does appear that China's recent intentions, at forging western economic alliances and importing western culture, have carried also the unfortunate consequence of letting American fast food and dietary habits pervert the rather distinctly healthy Chinese diet.

So here again we see, not only the impact of prosperity on the growth of obesity, but also the insidious ways in which fast food restaurants and western eating styles, seep into a culture needing to adapt quickly to the seismic impact of sudden wealth and prosperity.

The problem right now in Korea and China, for instance, is not so much the magnitude of the prevalence of obesity, but rather the unusually elevated annual growth rates of obesity which are now exceeding those of the United States in some age groups.

At the pediatric level, alarm bells are going off at all levels. The percent increase per year in the prevalence of obese children in urban China, between 1991 and 1997, was actually greater than in the U.S. between 1971 and 1994.[37]

Much like the U.S., both parents in China's growing middle class are working outside the home in employments that use advanced technology. They return home, at the end of the day, exhausted and uninterested, despite good intentions, in preparing home-cooked meals. The default solution is processed or fast food.

The Chinese story is not unique, as there is also a growing prevalence of obese Japanese boys in elementary school, and an alarming trend of preschool obesity occurring as well in that developed country. The main reason is the drop in the physical activity of young children, who have been captured by the mesmerizing images and story lines of video games and movies.

The reference to gaming addiction is very real, as these children experience high levels of dopamine secretion, in response to the surreal fantasy video sequences. The frequent and powerful stimulation of the sensory pleasure centers of the brain, are behind the compulsive attachments to gaming. It has been likened to gambling addiction. The problem is more serious with gaming because of the tendency to be captured for as long as 4-5 hours at time, thus leading to a substantial decline, not only in physical activity, but in socialization skills. The fear is that they can now grow up as children living in men's bodies.

East Germany posted a childhood obesity growth rate of 2.25% per year, the highest in the world; surprisingly, Canada was in third position worldwide for the fastest growing prevalence of obese children, whereas the U.S. was in 15th position. There is some wonder whether epigenetics are influencing the obesity rates in some countries. Dr. W.P.T James, from the London School of Hygiene, member of the International Obesity Task Force, writes in an editorial in the International Journal of Obesity:[21]

It is becoming apparent that in different parts of the world babies are being born with very different developmental trajectories and that these may reflect not only the classic effects of early imprinting, but also the effects of the epigenetic conditioning of the allelic inheritance that the babies have acquired, not just from their parents, but seemingly also from their grandparents.

Sara Bleich,[7] a research scientist with the Harvard Initiative for Global Health, in attempting to understand the complex issues that muddle our understanding as to why developed nations are becoming obese, concludes in a National Bureau of Economic Research Working Paper #12954:

Results indicate that the increase in caloric intake is associated with technological innovations such as reduced food prices, as well as changing sociodemographic factors, such as increased urbanization and increased female labor force participation.[7]

Paradoxically, in developed nations, the prevalence of obesity tends to be the highest among the lower socio-economic class, whereas in developing nations, obesity is more prominent among the upper social class. In addition, epidemiologists tend to measure higher obesity rates in the urban rather than the rural settings. These different scenarios tend to blur our ability at constructing a comprehensive obesity paradigm.

Interestingly, upper class women of westernized nations—more than men—tend to also be much leaner than the women of lower social classes. There is some complexity here, but is there a general understandable rule or epitome that can be established? The WHO, in 2000, concludes from its analysis of the pandemic:[39]

From a large body of evidence, the global epidemic of obesity has resulted mainly from societal factors that promote sedentary lifestyles and the consumption of high-fat, energy-dense diets.

It is especially the low levels of physical activity, driven by the adoption of sedentary-based technology, that are compromising the U.S. and other countries. In particular, the greatest culprit, if we make comparisons to the 1950s, is the significant drop in physical activity, both at work and away from work.

The National Bureau of Economic Research (NBER) reported their findings in 2007, from surveys that explored leisurely activities of adults around the world between the early 1970s and 2002.[7]

In countries where the adult obesity growth rate was kept very low, such as Canada and Japan, the survey found significant increases in leisurely activity. For instance, in Canada the compiled survey data showed that, between 1994 and 2002, the proportion of the adult population that regularly engaged in moderately active physical activity, rose from 38% to 49%; in Japan, the weekly commitment jumped from 5.5 hours in 1976 to 8.7 hours in 2001. Whereas in countries like the U.S., where the growth of obesity still remains strong, the proportion of physically active American adults increased modestly, from 24.3 to 26.2%. Similarly, in England where a very elevated obesity growth rate was reported between 1994 and 2004, there was only a 4 to 5% increase in the proportion of physically active women (21%-25%) and men (32-37%).

The major limitation with monitoring physical activity is that it is rather difficult to standardize the unit of physical activity that is most meaningful. The Canadian Census Bureau is interested in measuring the number of people engaging in moderate to active levels of physical activity, without defining any time commitment, whereas the U.S. and England measure the proportion of people committing to at least 30 minutes of moderate physical activity 5 times per week. Japan on the other hand, reports

> On average, children and adolescents, spend close to 8 hours per day either in front of a TV or a computer, surfing the Internet, or gaming.

the total number of hours dedicated to physical activity without any mention of exercise intensity.

There is another problem: Total physical energy output over the entire day does not tend to get measured. This is an important deficiency, as it becomes impossible to distinguish between activities that are leisurely, home-based and work related. This is meaningful because a physical laborer can burn extensive amounts calories at work, so that at the end of the day, it is no longer necessary for him to play a sport or go to the gym to workout.

A construction worker in the 1950s could expend up to 2400 kcal/day only at work, and perhaps as much as 4400 kcal by the end of the day. This contrasts greatly with the mere 800 to 1200 kcal/day now expended by online customer support specialists.

The documentary, **Obesity in America: A National Crisis**[6] documents how there have been significant changes in energy expenditure at work and away from work between the 1950s and 2000. Can energy expenditure tell the complete story? It is difficult to answer given that most of the epidemiological research fails to identify the total daily energy output.

Another approach, helpful in quantifying the physical activity of a population, is to monitor the time dedicated to sedentary activities, such as TV viewing, computer or electronic entertainment. In scrutinizing physical **inactivity** between the 1990s and the year 2000, the data demonstrates very little change in the percent of the population classified as inactive; it remained relatively stable between 25 to 32% of the population, yet the growth rate of obesity in the U.S. was at its highest during this period. However, when reviewing the Nielsen Media Research data on television viewing, there is a steady increase in the number of household hours dedicated to TV viewing, rising from 4.75 hours per day in 1950 to 7.75 hours per day by 2000, representing a 63% increase.[35]

In addition, a survey funded by the Kaiser Foundation in 2008, attempted to quantify the time spent, by U.S. youth, using electronic media. On average, they report that children and adolescents, spent close to 8 hours per day either in front of a TV or a computer, surfing the internet, or gaming. Steven Reinberg reports on the findings of the survey in the January 20, 2010 publication of *Business Week*. He writes:[33]

Children spend about four and one-half hours daily in front of the TV, about two and one-half hours listening to music, an hour and a half on the computer, about an hour and a quarter playing video games, and just 38 minutes reading.

What we are examining here, is not so much the degree of physical activity—this can vary from strenuous to moderate to mild levels of intensity—but really the degree to which we have embraced interests that are clearly sedentary. Compared to the 1950s, according to the U.S. Bureau of Labor Statistics, low occupational activities have risen sharply between 1950 and 1990, and have begun to decline slowly leading up to 2000 (**Figure 9.2**). Meanwhile, the prevalence of high occupational activity has remained between 15 to 17% for 50 years. Another, parameter of inactivity that is significant, at a population level, is the number of hours dedicated to housework in men and women. While the hours per week for men, between 1965 and 1995, increased from 5 to 10 hours, there was a 44.4% decline in housework hours for women. However, overall the hours, dedicated to housework in the average household, has dropped from 27hrs/week in 1965 to just 16hrs in 1995. Also, since 1985, the time spent eating also fell, in both men and women, from 9 to 10 hours\week to about 7 hours. There is little doubt, since the microwave found its way into the

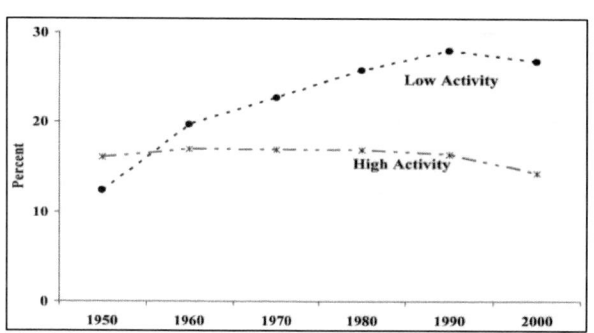

Figure 9.2: Levels of Occupational Activities between 1950 and 2000. Source: US Bureau of Labor Statistics and Census Bureau.[35]

American kitchen, that we now eat faster and in relative isolation from one another to accommodate our busy schedules. But still other problems are affecting us.

Transportation and commuting have also changed in a significant way since the 1960s, as Americans began to own more cars, and travel greater distances per week.

In the 1960s, according to the U.S. Census, 60% of American households owned only one car, and as many as 20% relied on no car; surprisingly, a mere 20% owned two cars. In a 40 year span, the number of Americans who owned only one car dropped to 35%, whereas two and three car ownership rose to 57%. The number of miles that Americans drove weekly and daily has gone up, as more Americans moved to the suburbs; now moms and dads needed to drive longer distances to work. The U.S. Federal Highway Administration reported that the daily miles traveled per person rose from 8 miles/day to 27 miles in 2000.[35] There is ample evidence, at the present time, to support the idea that important declines in physical activity are playing a most significant role in the obesity crisis.

9.1.1 History of Obesity

To comprehend this epidemic, it may be worth stepping back through time to see just when body weights began to expand enough to cause concern. In truth, obesity was historically discussed as far back as Hippocrates, who recommended dietary restrictions, greater exercise and less sleep as remedies to counter the problem.

It was a condition believed to arise from a moral weakness—a contention that was defended for many centuries. There were even documented accounts of morbid obesity by the famous Roman physician, Galen (131-201 CE) who referred to this massive morbid state of corpulence as polysarkia, and saw it as an imbalance in the bad humors; more specifically he perceived it as a problem arising from the surplus of blood.[11]

Although the humor theory of disease has since been proven to be false, many of the remedies recommended by Galen are still used today in the treatment of obesity, notably diet restrictions, exercise and medications that cut appetite. Many of these therapies, according to Doctor Niki Papavramidou[31] from the Department of Anatomy, History of Medicine Division, School of Medicine, Aristotle University of Thessaloniki, in Greece, are still in use today, and are a tragic testament to the stagnation of medical obesity treatments. At a most fundamental level, is the failure of medicine to squelch this crisis, the consequence of no longer recognizing obesity as the main outcome of gluttonous overeating? Are we neglecting to investigate how individuals put those pounds on? Is there a tendency to think of obesity as a metabolic or endocrinological disorder? Are people now becoming obese through no fault of their own?

Obesity has always been seen, from the very beginning, going back to the Ancient Greeks, as an imbalance between excessive calories consumed versus too little exercise. The cause was understood to be from eating more than what the body needed, and it was even clear for the Greeks that death rates were more elevated among obese individuals.

It was the scientific revolution (1473-1772) that opened the door to more methodical approaches to investigating obesity. Although some scholarly works were apparent in the 16th century, it was mostly during the 17th century that significant early breakthroughs in obesity research had commenced. Indeed, Nicholas Bonetus (1679) identified fat cells from the dissections of obese cadavers, and by the 18th century, Morgagni and Haller continued the anatomical descriptions of the obese.[12]

> It wasn't until the 18th century that the first important treatise on obesity was published in 1727 by Thomas Short under the title: *Discourse Concerning the Causes and Effects of Corpulency*. This book promoted the notion that the diet needed to be moderate, sparse and favorable to evacuation.

By the 18th century, the first important treatise on obesity was published in 1727 by Thomas Short under the title: *Discourse Concerning the Causes and Effects of Corpulency*. This book promoted the notion that the diet needed to be moderate, sparse and favorable to evacuation. There was a sense that obesity or corpulence was beginning to be noticeably more prevalent in 18th century Europe, a fact supported by Dr Short's comment:[5]

I believe no age did ever afford more instances of corpulency than our own.

Flemyng (1760) identified four causes of obesity: the first, he attributed to eating excessive food especially of the oily types; the second, he described as being caused by a fragile texture of the cellular membrane of fat tissue; the third, he linked to the blood's predisposition to store fat more efficiently in the vesicles; and finally, the fourth he associated with constipation. He believed that all fluid excreted from the body, whether it be feces, sweat or urine, were comprised of oil and impurities that needed to be eliminated, thus justifying the use of laxatives, diaphoretics and diuretics as part of the treatment.[11]

Early in the 19th century, around 1821, the Belgian statistician, Adolphe Quételet developed a mathematical equation to quantify obesity, by using the patient's weight in kilograms divided by his height in meters squared (Kg/m^2); this became a reliable measure of fatness relative to the height. In this way, he could categorize the severity of obesity in individuals. The premise was that individual measurements could be used to compare to those of an average man, a concept that has carried forward to our present day; indeed clinicians in the U.S. renamed the measurement: the Body Mass Index (BMI). The BMI has been used to categorize fatness in terms of risk levels of chronic disease.[12b] It has been validated as an accurate predictor of morbidity when values exceed 25 (overweight), 30(obesity) or fall under 18 (underweight). Remarkably, this measurement is still called the Quételet equations in several European countries.

The sophistication of our understanding of obesity continued to expand as technology allowed a closer look at human physiology. In reality, Robert Hooke's discovery of the cell as the basic building block of

The sophistication of our understanding of obesity continued to expand as technology allowed a closer look at human physiology. In reality, Robert Hooke's discovery of the cell, using the microscope, as the basic building block of animals and plant tissues, opened the door to the 19th century theory that an excessive number of fat cells was behind the problem of obesity.

By 1850, the adipocyte had been identified as a specific kind of cell in textbooks of microscopic anatomy, thus setting the scene for Hassall (1849) to describe the actual growth and expansion of fat cells. This helped him devise the theory that some obesities could be derived from increased fat cell numbers, an idea which twentieth century scientists like Hirsch and Björntorp would further describe as **hyperplastic** obesity.

However, critical to the medical advancement of the cause of obesity, was the development of this idea of metabolic and energy homeostasis. This was a crucial concept built on the foundation that the body prefers balance. It was Robert Boyle (1627-1691), a 17th century chemist responsible for devising the concept of chemical elements, who introduced the notion that oxygen was critical in metabolic processes. This was a finding he derived from his classic mouse experiment. In it, he housed a mouse within a closed chamber, and noted that it died, shortly after a lit candle extinguish itself. The conclusions he drew from this simple experiment, set the stage for Antoine Lavoisier (1743-1794) to formulate the *oxygen theory,* which recognized the role of oxygen in both combustion and oxidation. He conducted an experiment that involved measuring the heat released from melting ice, and from which the basic principle of calorimetry was derived.

About 100 years later, the German scientist, Max Rubner (1854-1932), devised an adapted version of the *bomb calorimeter,* which had already been created by Pettenkofer and Voit, with the capability to specifically measure carbon dioxide. Rubner deduced that the energy metabolized in the body, from the ingestion of fat and carbohydrates, was identical to the combustion of these macronutrients in the bomb calorimeter. He suspected that both the body and the bomb produced the same amount of CO_2 and H_2O. The more difficult concept, he wrestled with, was the metabolism of protein. It was different from fat and carbohydrate because the energy value, he measured in the form of heat, using the bomb's combustion chamber, was much greater than the energy derived from CO_2 and H_2O produced by the body when protein was digested.[12b]

It was a real problem that could only be explained by the nitrogen component that was unique to protein. Much of the nitrogen, contributed from the ingested protein, rather than getting combusted, as with the bomb calorimeter, was excreted in the urine, feces and as sloughed-off skin. In order to accurately derive the energy in protein, he had to subtract the calories found in the urea nitrogen, the nitrogenous compounds in the feces and in the skin, which in reality were not structurally used by the body. So then by making this adjustment for the lost nitrogen, his bomb-measured energy of 5.35 kcal/g got realigned downward to 4.1 kcal/g once nitrogenous losses from the body were factored in.

> **In Wesleyan College, Middletown, Connecticut, Wilbur Olin Atwater and Edward Bennett Rosa constructed, in 1896, the first human calorimeter, which consisted of a sealed chamber that could measure heat production generated from the human volunteer that resided in it.**

> **The basic rule for weight management is:**
> **Energy in = energy out**

Finding that the energy of the macronutrients could be calculated in food was essential in being able to establish experiments that could measure in humans, whether the first law of thermodynamics could be determined. In 1896, at Wesleyan College, Middletown, Connecticut, Wilbur Olin Atwater and Edward Bennett Rosa constructed the first human calorimeter. It consisted of a sealed chamber that could measure heat production generated from the human volunteer that resided in it. The chamber could measure the energy expenditure of an individual in a steady state, and determine if it equaled the energy consumed. Atwater measured the utilized oxygen in the sealed chamber and the heat output. His book: *The Respiration Calorimeter with Appliances for the Direct Determination of Oxygen* was co-authored by Francis G. Benedict, and published in 1902 by the Carnegie Foundation.

The book's detailed description of the sophisticated apparatus became the foundation for the development of more modern day calorimeters that were able to measure both the oxygen inspired and the carbon dioxide expired.[12b]

Atwater's work confirmed the principle that for the weight of an individual to remain stable, the amount of energy consumed had to equal the energy expended. He derived the modern concept of *energy in* and *energy out* as the basic tenet for weight management.

Conceptually, the more advanced and sensitive calorimeters in addition to the modern technique of using deuterium-labeled water to measure the body's elimination of labeled hydrogen and oxygen (doubly-labeled water) facilitated the most accurate estimation of energy expenditure of humans, in a free-living state. This latter method, confirmed around the second half of the 20th century, that obese people do expend substantially more energy than lean people, and therefore require more ingested calories to maintain the body weight stable. In other words, obese people, in general, eat more than lean people, and are not subject to tremendous slow-downs in metabolic rates. This technique also confirmed that obese people, more than those without a weight problem, underestimate their actual caloric intakes.[12] In the end, the evidence points clearly towards overeating as the main cause of obesity, or consuming calories in excess of what the body requires.

Metabolic abnormalities or chromosomal defects originating from genetic errors can either alter the basal energy levels of the body, change the propensity to store fat or even affect the satiety signals that control appetite. The prevalence of all of these conditions together represents, however, less than 1 percent of the population, and therefore cannot be considered as influential in the current U.S. obesity epidemic. Nevertheless, it is pertinent to briefly review the most important and memorable neuroendocrine and genetic disorders that lead to obesity, as they will help the student to better understand the body's rather complex mechanism for ensuring energy balance.

There are specific **neuroendocrine types of obesities** that can predispose individuals to gain unusually large amounts of weight. The first is referred to as **hypothalamic obesity**, and it occurs when trauma, malignancy, inflammatory disease, or intracranial pressure from a tumor, damage the ventromedial center of the hypothalamus which leads to uninhibited overeating (hyperphagia). The second is called **Cushing's syndrome**. This is an endocrine disease where the patient has an enlarged adrenal glands—the consequence of excessive ACTH (Adreno-corticotrophic hormone) secreted from the pituitary gland.[12c] Weight gain characteristically takes place with the unusual accumulation of fat in the trunk area, the dorsal posterior cervical region and in the supraclavicular fossa (between the collar bone and the chin and jaw bone). The treatment of Cushing's syndrome—this involves the removal of the adrenals—causes cortisol levels to decline and fat to redistribute more uniformly. A third neuroendocrine obesity is **hypothyroidism**; this is a condition that causes, through decreased thyroxin secretions from the thyroid, a decline in the basal metabolic rate, thus increasing the probability of gaining significant weight over the short term.

Another obesity classification is the **genetic causes of obesity**. There are genetic abnormalities responsible for unusual weight gain and fat deposits, but for the sake of keeping the text relevant to an introductory course in nutrition, I will only mention four. The first is called **Prader-Willi syndrome (PWS)**. This is a rare congenital condition that originates from a defect in the father's chromosome, causing mental retardation, hypogonadism, hypotonic muscles, short stature and an insatiable appetite leading to obesity, early in life. Patients with PWS have an average height varies between 4 feet 11 inches and 5 feet 1 inch. These children, if left unsupervised, can eat constantly and gain frightful amounts of weight. This form of chromosomal abnormality, which occurs at a frequency of 1 in every 15,000 to 30,000 births, causes these children to eat and store fat most readily because of a disturbance in the signals sent to the satiety center of the brain. Average female weights have been noted at 176lbs, whereas boys will easily pack on 216lbs. In cases when the chromosomal anomaly occurs on a specific maternal chromosome, the disorder is renamed: **Angleman's syndrome**, which characteristically has a more severe mental retardation without any obesity. The second genetically-based obesity condition is referred to as the **Bardet-Biedl syndrome**. It is recognizable by the symptoms of retinal degeneration, mental retardation, obesity, polydactyly (additional fingers) and hypogenitalism. The third genetic abnormality that leads to obesity is called **Alstrom-Hallgren syndrome**. This third condition bares many similarities with the Bardet-Biedl syndrome, in that it is also characteristically identified by obesity and blindness. To help distinguish the two, additional symptoms have been tagged to Alstrom-Hallgren syndrome: deafness, diabetes mellitus, and the absence of mental retardation.[12c]

Finally, the fourth genetic condition, which was identified by Friedman in 1994 in the obese ob/ob mouse, and subsequently observed in obese cousins of Pakistani descent in 1997, has been identified as **leptin deficiency**.[15] Mutations to the gene responsible for encoding leptin, leads to hyperphagia (overeating), a severe form of obesity (morbid obesity), hypogonadism, and a compromised immune system. Obese individuals who lack the adipose tissue-derived protein, leptin, are unable to utilize the body's normal homeostatic mechanism that recognizes increasing adipose tissue as feedback to shut off the hunger signal. By contrast, leptin-deficient patients, have a persistent uncontrollable appetite, that causes patients with this disorder to eat insatiably without experiencing the soothing effects of being full. Interestingly, when these obese patients were treated with leptin, their appetites normalized, causing significant weight loss to occur.[15]

In all four of these genetic disorders, obesity is often characterized by a disproportionate amount of fat accumulating on the body relative to lean mass. This condition results from a significant loss of protein or muscle and is referred to as **sarcopenia**. There is some evidence, that chronic dieting followed by weight regain—which happens in the majority of dieters—translates into the loss of body protein, followed by the abundant re-synthesis of fat during the weight regain period. If this takes place too often, as in the cases of frequent diet cycling, there is some concern that over a 20 year span, a large proportion of lean body mass (protein) may be lost, only to be replaced by body fat. This shift would invariably cause a significant decline in resting energy expenditure, which is typically seen in sarcopenia, leading to much easier weight gain, and more difficult weight loss.[6]

9.2 The Most Influential Causes of Obesity

Already by the 1960s, America's weight problem was noticeable; roughly 13 percent were obese and 31 percent were overweight. Overall, 44% of adult Americans, 20 years and older, had some kind of weight management problem. There was, without a doubt, a growing concern among public health officials and doctors about the added girth.

The reality is that we sickened ourselves with our lifestyles of physical complaisance, and overindulged in highly pleasurable foods. As early as the mid-1970s, adult Americans began to gain body weight at rates that initially fell under the radar of most epidemiologists and health officials, but which became more apparent by the mid-1980s. In fact the yearly jump in body weight translated into more worrisome population weight increases, between the 1980s and the year 2000. One of those epidemiologists, astute enough to detect the upward weight shift early on, was Dr. Katherine Flegal, a senior researcher at the Centers for Disease Control (CDC). She picked up on the trend when studying the 1988 to 1991 U.S. survey data, which she cautiously published with Kuczmarski in the

> **The risk of becoming obese increases 2 to 3-fold if there is obesity in the family; risk increases further based on the severity of the obesity.**

Journal of the American Medical Association (JAMA) in 1994.[26] Up to that point nobody was really warning or even talking about obesity as a problem at the national level. She was cautious because she had trouble believing the statistical interpretations. It just did not make sense to her that we were getting fat so quickly and in such great numbers.

After the publication of the Kuczmarski paper, medical awareness did rise, but it wasn't until the widespread circulation of the CDC's obesity prevalence charts, around the turn of the new millennium, that medical and public health officials suddenly embarked on a war path.[26] The color-coded prevalence charts described the yearly jumps in obesity prevalence state by state; they documented a changing American landscape in such a visually dramatic way, that it was clear that there was a growing problem, and that something had to be done.

This concern soon changed to alarm after the prevalence of obesity jumped to 35% in 2004. Indeed, the CDC mapped important increases in the prevalence of obese American adults between 1976 to the present (**Figure 9.1**). Interestingly, this increase did not specifically correlate with the prominence of lower occupational activity levels, which really began to be more evident much earlier, around the 1960s (**Figure 9.2**), and attained an apex in 1990. Interestingly, the proportion of Americans engaging in high activity occupations remained relatively stable between the 1950s and 1990s; afterwards a notable decline was observed (Figure 10.2) between 1990 and 2000, as more sedentary positions flooded a market that had become more customer service orientated. Health officials were concerned about the many secondary diseases that were beginning to arise from obesity, notably type-2 diabetes. The documentary, *A Diabetic Nation*, explores the prevalence of type-2 diabetes, and the many secondary diseases.[6b]

9.2.1 Familial Causes of Obesity: Interplay of Environment and Genetics

It was during the 18th and 19th centuries that a familial cause of obesity was being discussed by scientists as it was already evident that obesity was strongly associated with family ancestry. As genetics evolved during the twentieth century, with the important discoveries of Francis H. C. Crick (1916-2004) and James D. Watson (1928-) the notion of a single obesity gene—known as a Mendelian transmission—came into the discussion. Dr. Claude Bouchard, while he was professor at Laval University, in Quebec, Canada, did phenomenal work in the 1988 Quebec Family Study. His team tracked family ties to obesity, and was successful in differentiating between the impact of the environment and genetics.[9, 10]

In reviewing the 1991 Norway and 1998 Quebec studies, he was able to quantify the heritability of obesity to between 25-40% of inter-individual differences in BMI and body fat. Bouchard concludes:

Thus the genetic heritability of the obesity phenotypes accounts for 25–40% of the age- and gender-adjusted phenotypic variances

In other words, family ties appear to increase the risk of a young child becoming obese, but is this because of an obesity gene?

No studies, so far, have been able to confirm a Mendelian transmission that could explain familial obesity. Other studies have established that among obese children, 30% had two obese parents. But just in case the reader rushes with too much haste to conclude that to be obese there needs to be a family history of obesity, Bouchard clarifies that between 25 and 35% of obese cases came from families with normal weight parents.

Nevertheless, research from the early to the mid-1990s calculate that the risk of becoming obese increases 2 to 3-fold if there is obesity in the family, and that the risk increases further with the severity of the obesity. The question that has historically been difficult to answer has to do with the impact of family eating habits on obesity rates in children.

The Bouchard studies were able to quantify that 60-75% of obesity variances, between individuals, were not genetically-based, but rather were tied to the environment in a broad sense. This means everything from accessibility to fast foods, grocery stores, and fresh and affordable produce, to single parent families with low incomes and poor eating habits, right down to individual and family food preferences, in addition to low physical activities, are linked to obesity. In other words, it appears that the genes load the gun, but that it is the environment that pulls the trigger.[9, 10]

As mechanization became part of the industrial revolution that was to make America the industrial mammoth of a new age, so the energy expenditure of individuals began to decline by the late 19th and early 20th century.

It wasn't until around 1920 that the farming tractor—possibly one of the most technological innovations that had incredible economic clout—transformed rural America and liberated a high proportion of the farm manpower, allowing it to migrate to the cities for factory jobs.[34]

> **While the genes may load the obesity gun, the environment pulls the trigger.**

Hence, as greater numbers of the labor force did factory work by 1880, overweight Americans began to make up a noticeable proportion of the population. By the early 1930s, in the aftermaths of the 1929 crash, economic strife hit hard in America, and so the weight gain that took place during the roaring twenties, receded during the 1930s. And not long after, obesity sprang up to be just a nuisance in the early part of the twentieth century, representing at best 2% of the population. It appears that from the outset, the decrease in daily energy expenditure became pivotal in launching the U.S.'s weight management problem.[11, 12b]

Now the intense energy output associated with planting and harvesting greatly declined, and opened the door to some overeating; not all would succumb as energy expended by farmers by the 1950s was estimated still at 2400 kcal/day, which is substantive enough. That amount did not include the tractor driver who was the likely one to gain weight. The NIH data clearly maps a prevalence of overweight adult Americans that barely changed from the 1920s to 2005 (figure 10.1). At best, there was a 2.5% increase in overweight adults over that 85 year period.

This is certainly not substantive enough to create a crisis let alone an epidemic. A 5% obesity prevalence documented between the 1930s to the 1950s, did not constitute any kind of public health problem. In addition, there was barely any kind of noticeable obesity among children and adolescents; at best they were fractional statistics. We have to move forward to the late 1970s and early 1980s to see a sudden jump in the NIH obesity data.

The increasing prevalence of obesity in the U.S. and all the secondary diseases that derive from it, such as heart disease and type-2 diabetes, have set off alarms nationwide; health professionals are warning that obesity and type-2 diabetes have reached epidemic proportions, thus affecting both the adults and the youth, and forcibly changing the quality of life and the health of our nation.

Between 1980 and 2008, obesity prevalence doubled in adults, and most surprisingly, it tripled in children during that time. Pediatric obesity was barely on the radar of most pediatricians in 1960s; the 1963 National Health and Nutrition Examination Survey (NHANES) only detected rates of between 4.2-4.6% in the two age categories 6-11 and 12-19 respectively.[30] However, what unfolded, between 1963 and 2008, reveals troublesome changes in the eating habits and specifically in the lifestyles of American children and adolescents; the prevalence of obesity rose 366% in the 6 to 11 year olds and 293% in the 12 to 19 year old children and adolescents over the following 45 years. This significant jump in pediatric obesity is responsible for putting American youth on an early path of chronic disease.

9.3 The Most Effective Weight Loss Diets

The obesity epidemic has been fueling a very profitable diet industry ever since the 1970s. The solution for Americans becoming obese appeared simple enough to resolve, as the overweight/obesity paradigms were certainly perceived as the consequence of individuals eating excessively. In fact, by the mid-19th century, there was published proof, in the popular media, of weight loss successes achieved through dietary restrictions that were practiced by the general public, in England. A publication in the September 16th, 1933 issue of the high profile UK medical journal, the Lancet, demonstrates that the medical and scientific communities had already been aware of many cases of obesity showing up in English medical practices; it had to be, at some level, acute enough as a problem, that scientists were beginning to recognize types of obesity.[12]

Today, caloric restrictions are still envisioned as viable solutions, and certainly the diet industry has, since the 1970s, marketed all sorts of diets that ranged from very low calorie diets supplying 300-500 kcals per day, to meal replacement liquid meals. In between there were droves of combinations: low fat and high carbohydrate diets, high fat, high protein and low carbohydrate diets, and finally, high protein, low fat and low carbohydrate diets. George Bray argues that the idea that diet books could be seen as effective therapies for weight loss, likely originated from a 19th Century English trend.[12] The English fad was possibly behind the flood of diet books into U.S. book stores by the 1960s and 70s, promising quick weight loss. However, a strange paradox presents itself: If dieting had become such a national pastime, why were Americans still getting more obese?

There is no simple answer, as Americans, in great numbers, have been following diets for weight loss since the 1970s. It became clear, early on, that the weight loss associated with these quick fix diets was short lived; the lost weight was often regained within a year.

Diet books and articles saturated book stores, newsstands, grocery store checkout lines, and TV ads; there was no getting away from the reality that Americans needed to lean down. The U.S. diet industry was born out of a portentous fear of becoming overweight or obese, and success depended, so it seemed, on everyone having a common perception of the perfect body—one that female Americans willingly wanted to embrace, and that American men certainly desired.

> **Rapid weight loss is often followed by subsequent weight regain and is referred to as yo-yo dieting.**

The U.S. diet industry became fueled by this culture with an insatiable thirst to be attractive, a standard set by Hollywood divas, and that was responsible for the sale of many diet books. And yet none of these books caused any significant decline in the prevalence of obesity nation-wide.

Testimonials spoke of rapid weight loss, but failed to report the subsequent weight regain that often followed dieting; as early as the 1960s and 1970s the practice of yo-yo dieting became mainstream and so, medical practitioners and dietitians were warning the public to avoid the practice. Yet, despite the warning calls, millions rode that rollercoaster for years. The idea was that yo-yoing was harmful. The American Dietetic Association advocated slower, but more permanent weight loss. Despite this professional wisdom of slower weight loss, millions loved the idea of quickly losing the fat in order to wear the more fashionable and sexy attire of summer. Marketing the lean silhouette turned out to be more profitable, so it seemed, for both the consumer and the diet industry. The price paid by the consumer, however, over the long term, may have been more than anyone had imagined.

Of the series of diet books that hit the bookstores, the most renowned were: The Scarsdale Diet, Dr Atkins Diet Revolution and the Pritikin diet which were published in the 1970s, followed by the Dean Ornish diet in the 1980s, and more recently, Dr Atkins New Diet Revolution, published in 1992. The Zone Diet hit bookstores in 1995, and finally the South Beach Diet rose to popularity in 2003.

These were certainly the diets that gained notoriety in the public eye and in the medical community, by the controversies they arose, the reported successes, and by the amount of money earned by the authors.

The Zone Diet—The Zone diet consisted of 40% carbohydrate, 30% protein, 30% fat, and a protein to carbohydrate ratio of 0.75, whereas the Atkins diet was based on 10% carbohydrates, 60% fat and 30% protein.

These were two similar diets in that both advocated low carbohydrate for rapid weight loss. The convention of the day, at least in the dieting world, was that carbohydrates caused easy and excessive weight gain, and thus the goal was to maintain carbohydrates in check in order to achieve rapid weight loss.

The premise behind the Zone diet is that it metabolically manipulates the insulin-to-glucagon ratio downwards, thus allowing a more abundant breakdown of fat in the body. The lower insulin levels in the blood are what favor lipolysis (fat burning). The diet also promises a maximal efficiency in the body's metabolism for optimal health, physical and mental performance. Dr. Cheuvront who reviewed the diet writes:[13]

The specific health benefits of the Zone Diet purportedly include, but are not limited to, permanent weight loss, prevention of chronic diseases, enhanced immunity, maximum physical and mental performance and even greater longevity.

While maintaining low insulin levels does favor the stimulation of the hormone-sensitive lipase and subsequent fat loss, the problem is that the author, Barry Sears, fails to point out that carbohydrates, synergistically with protein, cause insulin levels to rise higher than by carbohydrates alone. So then, Cheuvront concludes, the diet does not really help patients achieve this proposed ideal insulin: glucagon ratio.

Using the Alternate Healthy Eating Index (AHEI) to evaluate the nutritional quality of the diet, the Zone diet scored 49.8 out of a possible 70 points or 71% of this nutritional index. In the end, the metabolic changes, that are purported to occur on the diet, have never been substantiated by any research studies.

The Atkins New Diet Revolution—Similarly, the Atkins Diet vilified all carbohydrates whether they were complex starches, starch-like vegetables such as potatoes, yams, or corn, and simple sugars such as sucrose, honey, and corn syrups.[4]

Atkins restricts carbohydrates so severely that in the first two weeks, patients must not exceed 20g of carbohydrates; this represents a mere 4% of a 2000 kcal/day diet. Afterwards, most people are encouraged to maintain total carbohydrates at levels no greater than 40g per day, representing only 8% of a 2000 kcal diet.

The idea proposed by Atkins was that all types of carbohydrate stimulate insulin release from the beta cells of the pancreas, thus favoring fat synthesis. This created a carbophobia of an impressive magnitude. Patients, on this diet, could eat all the meat and fat they desired, but they were not allowed to consume the breads, pasta, cereals, dairy, fruits and vegetables, except for a few.

Dieters began to lose weight more rapidly on the Atkins diet than on the American Heart Association diet, which advocated high carbohydrates and low fat. The success of this diet was based on a few principles of appetite control.

First, low carbohydrates of the magnitude proposed by Atkins, cause ketone bodies to be abundantly generated; this effectively cuts appetite, as ketones have an anorexic effect. The loss of appetite makes it easier for dieters to lose weight; they no longer have to battle with an unrelenting hunger. But it is specifically protein levels of 25-33% of DRI calories that are known to stimulate the body's satiety mechanism.

The second feature of the diet are the elevated protein and fat levels, which cause bile hyper-secretion, especially if fat is consumed as 60% of total daily calories. This would represent, for an average 2000 kcal diet, about 133g of fat, a shocking amount that can overwhelm the biological system, possibly causing nausea and indigestion for many dieters.

Translated into practical terms, this amount of fat would be equivalent to 9 tablespoons of oil. Often eaten over one or two meals, the amount of bile secretions needed to emulsify the fat in the GI tract is considerable, and would certainly contribute towards a certain malaise in some individuals.

To better visualize the fat content of the diet, think about eating 25 strips of bacon soaking in grease every morning, and it becomes evident why the appetite gets turned off. The consequence is rapid weight loss with no purposeful intent at restricting total daily calories. Rather, the high fat and protein provide sufficient satiety and an overall suboptimal calorie intake. Weight loss becomes inevitable, but as many studies have shown, the difference in total amount of weight loss between the low fat diet and the Atkins diet is no longer statistically significant after one year.

> There is simply no evidence to support the use of low fiber, and low fruit and vegetable intakes over the long term, as this kind of diet is inconsistent with long term gastrointestinal health.

More importantly, the fiber content of the Atkins' diet is too low; there is simply no evidence to support the use of low fiber intakes, over the long term, as this kind of diet is inconsistent with long term gastrointestinal health.

Indeed, constipation frequently affects patients that follow this diet; the Alternate Healthy Eating Index (AHEI) gives the Atkins 45g carbohydrate diet, a value of 42.3 out of 70 or a 60% measure of quality.[23]

Dean Ornish's Diet—This diet received a very favorable approval from the American Heart Association (AHA), and an AHEI score of 92% (**Table 9.2**), making it the most healthful diet in the market place, and the most consistent with sound medical advice.[23]

Doctor Ornish vilifies the meats and fats, and identifies them as the main culprits behind the American obesity crisis; he proceeds to not only restrict meat, poultry, and fish, but to also forbid all fats and oils, including healthy seeds and nuts (**Figure 9.3**).

The Ornish diet boils right down to consuming a lacto-ovo-vegetarian diet. This means ingesting all the fruits, vegetables, whole grains, cereals, low fat dairy products and egg whites as desired. The dieters need to know about complementing proteins in order to ensure that protein needs are fully met.

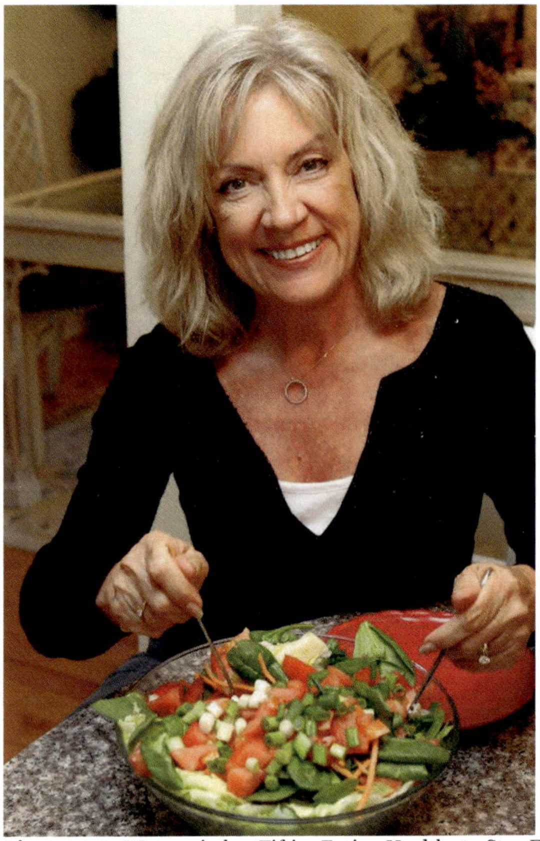

Figure 9.3: Woman in her Fifties Eating Healthy to Stay Fit © Lisa F Young

This diet receives top honors for health because it is consistent with the findings that have emerged from many of the longitudinal cohort studies headed by internationally acclaimed epidemiologist, Walter Willett. He promotes the Mediterranean diet as the most protective against heart disease. In contrast, however, Ornish does erroneously vilify all fats.

So the success of the diet relies on the strong satiety signals that take place from the large volume and weight of food that can be consumed in this diet.

The Pritikin's Diet—This popular diet was published in 1976, and also received AHA approval for its non-vegetarian meal plan. The menu advocates fruits, vegetables and whole grains, in addition to a very low fat content of <10% of DRI calories; protein content is maintained at a normal and healthy 10-15% of DRI calories, but carbohydrates hover around a very elevated 75-80% of DRI calories. Dietary cholesterol should be <25mg on the regression phase, and <100mg/day on the maintenance phase.

In the 1950s, at the age of 42, Nathan Pritikin was diagnosed with heart disease; it seemed like a death sentence at the time since very little was known about the disease. In the 1950s Americans were consuming on average 40% of their calories from fat, and the Harvard studies were identifying total fat and dietary cholesterol as the culprits.

Pritikin created the diet for his own purpose and followed it rigorously. The goal of this diet was not to achieve weight loss, but to diminish the risk of cardiovascular disease. In the end, he reversed his disease, despite very little guidance from the medical community. He proceeded to open Pritikin Longevity Centers by the late 1970s, and his diet received the formal endorsement of the American Heart Association by the mid-1980s.

At the age of 69 he was diagnosed with cancer and committed suicide not long after in 1984. The autopsy report revealed that Nathan Pritikin had no traces of heart disease in his arteries, a finding that was attributed to the rigorous compliance to his strict and stringent diet.

In contrast, **Atkins first Diet Revolution book**, published in the 1970s, was formally condemned by the AHA, but subsequently received support in 2000, when his diet resurfaced as **Atkins New Diet Revolution**. Independent research papers documented important declines in blood lipid risk markers for heart disease, in patients who followed the Atkins regiment. The diet was however, fundamentally flawed in its precepts; it discouraged the use of complex starches, fruits, vegetables and dairy, thus decreasing fiber intake and increasing the risks of suboptimal nutrition and gastrointestinal diseases over the long term.

It recommended increasing the consumption of meats far beyond the limits generally considered healthy; it espoused 25-33% protein and between 45-64% fat. The nutrients, which tended to be suboptimal, were fiber, calcium, vitamin D in northern regions, folate and phytochemicals; the excessive nutrients were the saturated fats, transfats and dietary cholesterol. Total calories, for the induction phase, is estimated at 1750 kcal; for the weight loss phase, 1500 kcal is advised; and the maintenance phase consists of approximately 2170 kcal/day.

The Scarsdale Diet—Written by Doctor Herman Tarnower, who ran a medical clinic in the town of Scarsdale. The book was published in the 1970s, and was based on a diet he devised for overweight patients. This is truly a low calorie diet that contains, in the initial phase, about 1000 kcals. The diet is high in protein (42%), but low in fat (22.5%) and in carbohydrates (35.5%). Patients who followed this diet lost weight because the ketones, generated by the body to compensate for the low carbohydrates, are able to cut the appetite therefore creating a caloric deficit for weight loss[40].

The South Beach Diet—The diet was designed by cardiologist Arthur Agatston and dietitian Marie Almon for patients with heart disease. Published in April 2003, this diet took off when it got popularized as an effective weight loss diet.

Dr. Agatston was trained to recommend the American Heart Association's low fat diet for patients with heart disease. The problem was that his patients experienced a great deal of difficulty remaining on the low fat prescription. They tended to over eat refined carbohydrates and sugars, in order to compensate for the low fat. In the end, patient outcomes were not good as they overindulged in calories and never really lost enough weight to cause a decrease in cardiovascular risk factors. Instead, Dr. Agatston devised a system that identified *good fats* and *bad fats*, and labeled carbohydrates also as *good* and *bad*.

The idea stemmed from the initial findings that obese patients often suffered from insulin resistance—a key symptom characterized by the resistance of the body's cells to the action of insulin—which precipitated physician and University of Toronto nutrition researcher, Dr. David Jenkins, to develop the *glycemic index* (GI) in the 1980s. The index classified a wide variety of carbohydrates based on the degree to which they caused blood sugars to rise in a **postprandial** state.

Bad carbs, to use Agatston's language, are the ones that produce a large output of insulin in response to a surge of glucose in the bloodstream. In turn, the insulin normalizes the blood sugar concentrations. The problem that arises with long term excessive intakes of bad carbohydrates, Agatston writes, is a cycle that causes the patients to form a resistance to insulin, thereby causing elevated blood sugars to persist longer than normal.

The pancreas responds by secreting more insulin, which precipitates a downward drop of blood sugars to below normal levels. These suboptimal levels of glucose, Jenkins discovered, signaled the hunger mechanism to kick-in, leading patients in turn to eat ravenously.

His solution was to eliminate refined carbohydrates and replace them with fruits, vegetables and whole grain products. Likewise, the bad fats were identified as saturated fats and trans-fats, and were replaced by polyunsaturated omega-3 and omega-6 fats. The idea was to eat lean red meats, and poultry, but cut-away the visible fat, and to give preference to nuts, and oily fish.

The authors claim research was done on the diet, conclusively showing its efficacy, but failed to cite any studies. A review of the diet by Drs. Sarah Goff and colleagues, published in the Journal of General Internal Medicine in 2006, concluded that up to 67% of the nutrition facts cited in the book were of questionable accuracy.[17] The South Beach diet appears, nevertheless, as safe and reasonable, plus it scored 72.4% on the Alternate Healthy Eating Index (**Table 9.2**), placing it in third position.[23]

Weight Watchers International—Perhaps the least controversial of the commercial diets is Weight Watchers International. Founded in 1963, by Jean Nidetch, the Weight Watcher diet promotes a low calorie and low fat menu. It provides lip service for exercise, but places emphasis on eating balanced meals that provide between 1200 and 1500 kcal/day using a specific points system. Recently, Weight Watchers retired their old point system in 2010, and initiated a new Point Plus scheme that encourages the consumption of a broad assortment of foods that is consistent with the 2010 Healthy Eating Guidelines.

Foods high in sugar or fat have higher points, and therefore the total daily allotment of points can get used up quickly, if too many bad foods are selected in a day. The major shortfalls in this diet are first, the lack of a clear program that encourages exercise; second, the organization believes that all foods can fit into a healthy diet plan. It is just a matter of being reasonable about portions and frequency of eating. It neglects to recognize that many foods such as soft drinks, highly processed snack foods and meals need to be avoided all together because of their addictive nature and impoverished nutrient content. Nevertheless, the diet's AHEI score puts it in second place (**Table-9.2**) overall.[23]

TABLE 9.2 Alternate Healthy Eating Index (AHEI) for most popular diet books

Weight Loss Diets	AHEI	% of Quality
Dean Ornish	64.6 / 70	92.3%
Weight Watchers High CHO	57.4 / 70	82.0%
South Beach Phase-2	50.7 / 70	72.4%
The Zone Diet	49.8 / 70	71.14%
Atkins 100g carb	46 / 100	65.71%
South Beach Phase-3	45.6 / 70	65.14%
Atkins 45g carb	42.3 / 70	60.4%

Source: Ma, Y, et al.[23]

The long term prospects of remaining on any caloric restrictive diet are, however, not very good. The attrition rate of study subjects, following many of these fad diets, is very high, often in the area of 40%. This means that 4 out of every 10 subjects drop out of the studies because they are too difficult to comply with over the long term.

In the end, these diet books provide hope for weight loss, by recommending restrictive diet plans that often eliminate essential food groups or manipulate macronutrients in ways that tend to be unhealthy over the long term.

In reviewing the weight loss literature, it becomes clear that 95% of dieters regain all of their lost weight at the end of 5 years of follow up. Of the 5% deemed successful, the majority regained significant weight but have managed to remain, nevertheless under their initial weight. A comprehensive review by Mann and colleagues[24] published in American Psychologist in April 2007 conclude that one of the most important conditions for weight gain in later years, and a persistent form of weight problem is previous dieting. This seems almost inconsistent with basic logic. The research essentially concludes that dieting causes weight gain. This does not make too much sense, or does it? In the review, Tracy Mann and her team found that weight loss programs consistently report a loss of 5-10% of body weight over the short term, but significant weight regain in the follow up period. Overall, they report that 33-67% of subjects regained more weight than lost. In one study that had a two year or more follow up period, 83% of patients experienced a weight regain that was greater than the weight lost. More disconcerting was the notion that, even in 4-5 year follow up periods, there was no sense that the rate of weight regain leveled off. Of the 14 studies that met the rigorous standards for the review, most over reported weight loss successes for several reasons: 1- subjects self-reported their weights; 2-diet and exercise were confounded; 3- low follow up rates of 33% favorably biased the results by inflating the degree of sustained weight loss at follow up (the 67% that did not attend follow up meetings were not likely able to keep weight off); and 4- subjects tend to follow other diets, during the follow up period, causing weight loss from the original diet to be overestimated.

The most compelling evidence that dieting alone does not work, is outlined here: First, the observational studies with control groups and long term follow up periods show that those dieters who managed to maintain a weight loss of 29.9lbs after one year, were those who had engaged in regular exercise in the follow up period. The researchers conclude that exercise was the most significant predictor of weight loss maintenance. Second, non-randomized prospective studies have also found that diets were ineffective in managing long term weight loss. In fact, 7 prospective studies concluded that dieting was strongly associated with future weight gain. They report on one study by Korkeila and colleagues, published in the American Journal of Clinical Nutrition in 1999, that showed, in a cohort of 7,729 Finnish adult twins, that a history of dieting was linked to a future mean weight gain of 22lbs, and this after correcting for age, BMI, and several other confounders including energy expenditure at baseline. Another study, important for its sample size of 19,000 healthy older men, for monitoring many aspects of a lifestyle, and for its 4 year follow up period after dieting, concluded that one of the strongest predictors of future weight gain was having lost weight on a diet. This predictor remained significant even after controlling for baseline weight and height, physical activity, TV viewing and eating habits.[24]

A large prospective cohort study followed 14,972 obese or overweight adolescents, over a 4 year period, and found that the group of teenagers who engaged in dieting practices and lost weight ended gaining more weight than the overweight and obese non-dieters. Although most dieters did indeed lose weight, over time they experienced more weight gain than non-dieters. Most important, however, is that fact, that the weight gain could not be correlated to increased caloric or fat intake.

The argument that the practice of following calorie restricted diets is a predictor of weight gain rather than weight loss is further supported by a study by Stice and colleagues. They showed, among adolescent girls, followed over a 4 year period, who engaged in dieting or who had a prior history of weight control efforts, that their risk of obesity was three times greater than the non-dieters.[24]

The conclusions are paradoxical and fly in the face of current therapeutic practices since dieting is indeed the most prominent therapy used to fight obesity. Yet, as early as the 1950s it was clear that the solution to obesity could not be limited to self-regulation of food intake. Mayer (1955) writes:[25]

the hard environment, in which mankind has developed, has made men physically active, resourceful creatures, well prepared to be hunters, fishermen or agriculturalists. Our appetite was never designed as a food-regulating mechanism for persons who spend most of their lives seated on a chair."

The literature is now providing compelling evidence that rigorous and moderately rigorous exercises need to be included on a weekly basis for diet regimens to be effective in weight loss. The Federal Physical Exercise Guidelines for Americans published in 2008, recommend between 150 and 300 minutes per week of exercise of moderate intensity. This represents between 2.5 and 5 hours of week of regular exercise, a commitment that translates into substantive energy expenditure.

DISCUSSION QUESTIONS

1. Why are epidemiologists and demographers becoming increasingly concerned with the growing obesity problem among women specifically?
2. What are some of the costs attached to the rising prevalence of obesity among children?
3. Discuss whether the South Beach Diet is a plan worthy of being recommended for weight loss and overall health, based on the contents of this chapter.
4. Discuss whether the Atkins diet peddles a formula for disaster or improved health. Explain your position
5. Explain why it is that, although obesity prevalence tends to increase in prosperous nations with good social infrastructure and political stability, obesity does not appear to be a problem in China and Japan where obesity prevalence is low despite strong economies and stable governments.
6. What weight loss method would you recommend to a patient in order to sustain long term weight loss? Explain your rationale.
7. Why would you hesitate to prescribe a calorie-restricted diet to an obese person in order to lose significant weight? Explain your position with strong evidence.

References

1. Anderson G, Horvath J (2004)The growing burden of chronic disease in America. Public Health Rep.119: 263-70.
2. Anonymous,(1933) Dietetic Treatment of obesity of the Pituitary type. The Lancet, 222 (5741): 604 - 605
3. Astrup, A., Larsen, TM, and Harper, A. (2004) Atkin's and other low carbohydrate diets: hoax or an effective tool for weight loss. The Lancet 364(9437): 897-899
4. Atkins ,RC. (1998) Dr. Atkins' new diet revolution. New York: Simon & Schuster.
5. Banting. W (1869) Letter of corpulence (4th ed.) London: Harisson,
6. Bissonnette, D.J. (2012) Obesity in America: A National Crisis DVD. Films for the Humanities and Sciences, (run time: 2hrs: 30 min)
6b. Bissonnette, D.J. (2013) A Diabetic Nation: A National Tragedy DVD. Mankato, MN: St-Jude Nutrition Medical Communications, (run time: 2hrs).
7. Bleich, S. et al (2007) National Bureau of Economic Research (NBER) Why is the Developed World Obese? Cambridge MA. NBER Working Paper No. 12954 pp: 43 Working Paper 12954. Retrieved on May 31, 2012 from: http://www.nber.org/papers/w12954 accessed
8. Bloomgarden, Z.T. (2004) Type-2 diabetes in the young: An evolving epidemic. Diabetes Care (4)27:998-1010
9. Bouchard C., Pérusse L., Leblanc C., Tremblay A., Thériault G. (1988) Inheritance of the amount and distribution of human body fat. Int. J. Obes. 12:205–215.
10. Bouchard, C. (1997) Genetics of Human Obesity: Recent Results from Linkage Studies. J. Nutr.127(9): 1887S-1890S
11. Bray, GA. (2009) History of Obesity. *Obesity: Science to Practice* Edited by Gareth Williams and Gema Frühbeck. John Wiley & Sons, Ltd p: 3-18
12. Bray, GA (1990) Historical development of scientific and cultural ideas. Inter. J of Obesity 14(11): 909-926
12b. Bray, GA. (1998) Historical Framework for the Development of Ideas about Obesity. In: Handbook of Obesity. George A Bray, Claude Bouchard, WPT James (eds) New York: Marcel Dekker Inc.: 1-29
12c. Bray, GA. (1998) Classification and Evaluation of the Overweight Patient. In: Handbook of Obesity. George A Bray, Claude Bouchard, WPT James (eds) New York: Marcel Dekker Inc: 831-854
13. Cheuvront, S.N. (2003) The Zone Diet Phenomenon, Journal of the American College of Nutrition, 2003; 22 (1): 9–17
14. Finucane MM, Stevens GA, Cowan MJ, et al. (2011) National, regional, and global trends in body-mass index since 1980: systematic analysis of health examination surveys and epidemiological studies with 960 country-years and 9.1 million participants. Lancet; 377: 557-67.
15. Farooqi, S and O'Rahilly, S.(2009) Leptin: A pivotal regulator of human energy homeostasis. Am.J.Clin.Nutr. 89 (Suppl): 980S-4S
16. Godfrey, JR and Dansinger, ML (2009) Toward Optimal Health: Sorting out the dietary approaches to achieving a healthy weight. Journal of Women's Health. 18(4): 435-438
17. Goff, S.L et al. (2006) BRIEF REPORT: Nutrition and Weight Loss Information in a Popular Diet Book: Is It Fact, Fiction, or Something in Between? J. Gen. Intern. Med. 21:769- 77
18. Harvard School of Public Health. The obesity prevention Source: Globalization. Retrieved June 14, 2012 from: http://www.hsph.harvard.edu/obesity-prevention-source/obesity-causes/globalization-and-obesity/.
19. IASO (January 2012) Global Prevalence of Obesity Sources and references are available from IASO www.iaso.org. © International Association for the Study of Obesity, London
20. International Union for Nutritional Science (I.U.N.S) The Global Challenge of Obesity and the International Obesity Task Force. Accessed on June 4 2012 from: http://www.iuns.org/features/obesity/obesity.htm..

21. James, WPT. (2006). The Challenge of Childhood Obesity. International Journal of Pediatric Obesity. 1: 7-10
22. Kelly T, Yang W, Chen CS, Reynolds K, He J. (2008) Global burden of obesity in 2005 and projections to 2030. Inter J Obesity (Lond). 32:1431–7.
23. Ma, Y et al. (2007) A dietary comparison of popular weight loss plans JADA 107(10): 1786-1791
24. Mann, T. et al. (2007) Medicare's Search for Effective Obesity Treatments. American Psychologists; 62(3): 220-233
25. Mayer, J. (1955). In *Weight Control*. Ames, Iowa: Iowa State College Press
26. Kuczmarski, R J., RD; Katherine M. Flegal, PhD; et al. (1994) Increasing Prevalence of Overweight Among US Adults The National Health and Nutrition Examination Surveys, 1960 to 1991 *JAMA*;272(3):205-211.
27. Maljaars, J. et al. (2009) Effects of fat saturation on satiety, hormone release and food intake. Am J Clin Nutr April 89(4): 1019-1024
28. Mount Sinai Journal of Medicine, Jan/Feb 2011; 78(1):22-48
29. Moyad, M. (2005) Fad Diets and Obesity Part IV: Low Carbohydrates versus Low Fat. Urologic Nursing 25(1): 67-70
30. Ogden C et al (2010) Health E-Stats CDC. Prevalence of Overweight, Obesity, and Extreme Obesity Among Adults: United States, Trends 1960–1962 Through 2007–2008. Retrieved November 6, 2013 http://www.cdc.gov/nchs/data/hestat/obesity_adult_07_08/obesity_adult_07_08.pdf
31. Papavramidou NS, Papavramidis ST, Christopoulou-Aletra H. (2004) Galen on obesity: Etiology, effects and treatment. World J Surg; 28(6):631-5.
32. Popkin BM (2006). Global nutrition dynamics: the world is shifting rapidly toward a diet linked with noncommunicable diseases. *Am J Clin Nutr*; 84:289–98.
33. Reinberg, S. (1/20/2010). US kids using media almost 8 hours per day. Business Week Retrieved June 14, 2012 From: http://www.businessweek.com/lifestyle/content/healthday/635135.html/
34. The Economic History of Tractors in the United States. Retrieved on May 25 2012 from:. http://eh.net/encyclopedia/article/white.tractors.history.us
35. Transportation Research Board Special Report 282. (March-April 2005). Does the Built Environment Influence Physical Activity? Examining the Evidence. Prepared by: Brownson, RC and Boehmer, TK for: The Transportation Research Board and the Institute of Medicine Committee on Physical Activity, Health, Transportation, and Land Use.
36. Van Cleave J, Gortmaker SL, Perrin JM (2010) Dynamics of obesity and chronic health conditions among children and youth. JAMA. 303:623-30.
37. Wang Y, Mi J, Shan XY, Wang QJ, Ge KY. (2007) Is China facing an obesity epidemic and the consequences? The trends in obesity and chronic disease in China. Int J Obes. 31: 177–188.
38. Wang, Y and Lobstein, T. (2006) Worldwide trends in childhood overweight and obesity. International Journal of Pediatric Obesity 1: 11-25
39. World Health Organization (2000) Obesity: preventing and managing the global epidemic. Report of a WHO consultation. World Health Organ Tech Rep Ser. 894;i–xii, 1–253.
40. Wycherley J et al. (2010) Long-term effects of weight loss with a very low carbohydrate and low fat diet on vascular function in overweight and obese patients Intern Med 267: 452–461
41. Yach D, Hawkes C, Gould CL, Hofman KJ (2004) The global burden of chronic diseases: overcoming impediments to prevention and control. JAMA. 291:2616-22.
42. Yoshinaga, M. et al. (2004) Rapid increase in the prevalence of obesity in elementary schools. International Journal of Obesity 28: 494–499.

CHAPTER 10

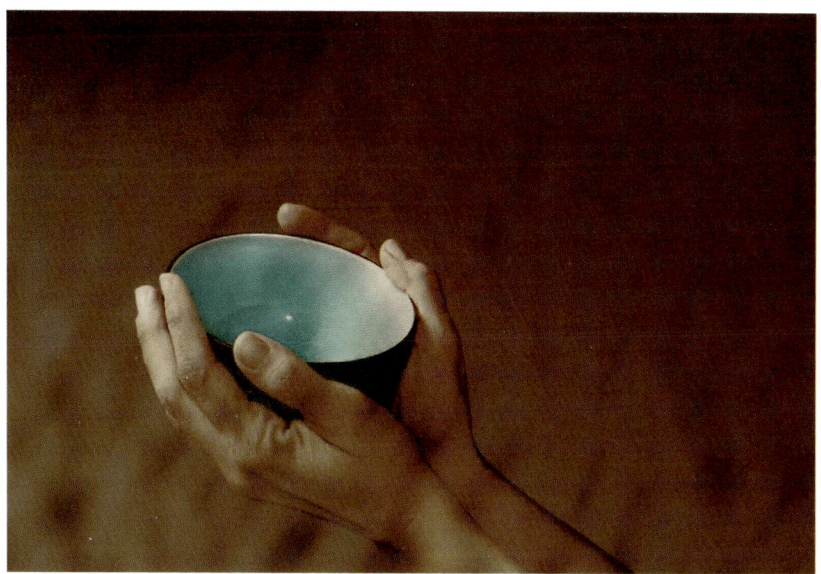

By Suzanne Tucker © Shutterstock__1084137/Shutterstock.com

NUTRITION AND WORLD HUNGER

10.1 Understanding Hunger

Food insecurity is at the source of hunger, and it is defined as the inability to access safe and nutritious foods, in adequate amounts, on a daily basis, to support a healthy life. The Rome Declaration, signed at the 1996 FAO-sponsored World Food Summit, defines **food security** as follows:

Food security exists when all people, at all times, have physical and economic access to sufficient, safe and nutritious food to meet their dietary needs and food preferences for an active and healthy life.[9]

Therefore, food insecurity is not strictly limited to not being able to access sufficient quantities of food, but also quality foods. This is an important subtlety especially within the context of an obesity epidemic that is getting out of hand. Tanumihardjo, a nutrition researcher at the University of Wisconsin, Madison, writes:[13]

Food insecurity is complex, and the paradox is that not only can it lead to undernutrition and recurring hunger, but also to overnutrition, which can lead to overweight and obesity.

The 6th World Survey administered by the WHO in 1996, estimated that there were 841 million individuals worldwide who did not have enough to eat between 1990 and 1992. In 2000, fueled by this shocking world hunger prevalence, many global health agencies came together and wrote the tenets of the *Millennium Development Goals* (MDG) One of the first goals was to decrease, by 2015, the prevalence of hunger and poverty in the world by at least half.[4,9] Progress towards achieving this goal would be measured by the prevalence of underweight individuals and food consumption. However, the number of hungry rose to 854 million between 2001 and 2003 according to FAO data, and then jumped to 1.023 billion by 2009.[11] Despite prevalence values subsequently dropping to 925 million in 2010, it is clear that the UN's strategies, to curb hunger by half, have failed.[9] This failure particularly affects two groups of people the most: First, **pre-school children** are most affected by hunger and malnutrition. Approximately 146 million children under the age of 5 are classified as underweight, representing 18% of all those who are hungry. This can be interpreted either as the consequence of chronic or acute hunger. The WHO reminds us also that there is an estimated 20 million children born every year who are underweight because, throughout pregnancy, their mothers were malnourished. The second most vulnerable group to malnutrition is **women and girls**. In fact, up to 60% of those afflicted with hunger worldwide are female.[11] What is going on that such a colossal increase in hunger prevalence continues to take place?

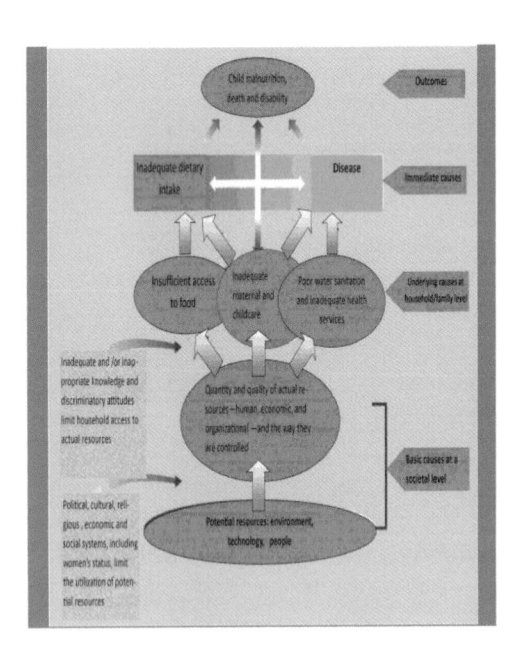

Figure 10.1 Adapted from Fig. 5, Causes of child malnutrition, The State of the World's Children, UNICEF, 1998, page 24.[14]

One of the problems has to do with the illusion created by international humanitarian relief efforts during times of droughts, famines, earthquakes and social conflicts. These disasters tend to be overt and highly publicized. The international relief programs are very successful in creating worldwide alarm and concern, justifiably fuelling relief efforts that garner billions of dollars in foreign aid. The problem is that these crisis situations create **transitory acute hunger** paradigms that only represent 10% of the world's hungry.[9] They live in rural areas and depend on agriculture as their primary source of income. When disasters hit, it is easy to see how the shocks of nature can quickly compromise such a population that has no alternative source of income.[11] They are the ones that are reached by international relief efforts. In truth, 90% of the world's hungry are chronically undernourished, and 75% of them live in the rural areas of developing nations. They are not reached by international aid, and are referred to as the **silent hungry**. They are poor, landless or own small plots of land without the necessary assets needed for regular and plentiful crop production. In many cases the households are headed by low wage-earning women or by adults afflicted by HIV/AIDS. Significant numbers are also orphans without the kind of support needed to be functionally successful in providing for the household's needs.[11]

So then, the problem of hunger can be viewed from two perspectives: first, the Food and Agriculture Organization (FAO) sees the problem of hunger as consequence of the individual not accessing adequate amounts of food, as shown in the small left circle in **Figure-10.1**. Hunger is measured, by the FAO's Millennium Development Goals, as significant weight loss in infants, which is defined as follows:

The percentage of children under-five whose weight-for-age is less than minus two standard deviations from the median for an international reference population aged 0–59 months.[9]

The solution to this problem, as seen through the FAO's lens, is to take steps to increase the food supply through increased agricultural output. The WHO and the United Nations International Children's Emergency Fund (UNICEF), on the other hand, regard hunger as merely the tip of the iceberg, and believe that underneath the surface lies the more compromising problem of malnutrition. Here, malnutrition, not just food availability, is argued as the critical center piece of this whole problem. It requires a far more complex understanding, as it implies that household incomes, health and ability to provide care to the family through nurturing behaviors, are necessary for an overall improved human health.[9] The flow chart, depicted in Figure-68, describes the complex network of causes that lead up to malnutrition, disability and death in children. This, according to the WHO, is the worst outcome, which must be curtailed.

It has been argued that, on a global level, there is ample food available for everyone, and it is precisely the problem of poverty, which limits access to healthy food, and in sufficient quantity, that needs to be resolved.[9, 11] The UNICEF model, depicted in Figure-68, captures, in a few strokes, the causes of this poverty. First the model advances that basic anomalies at a societal level, such as political instability, cultural norms that are discriminatory, economic upheaval or religious intolerances, can seriously limit access, of sectors of the population, to resources such as land, technology and people. As such, the majority of farmers have restricted access to: (a) land for growing crops and earning income; (b) technology assets for plowing the land and applying fertilizers; and finally (c) the manpower to work the fields. They are compromised by the sociopolitical instability that creates fear and unrest, in many cases forcing farmers to flee their lands because of warfare or constant waves of sectarian violence. It is specifically subjugated people, ruled by tyrannical leaders, that makeup an oppressed people, unable to fully utilize resources. Invariably, the household becomes compromised by poverty, from which ensues insufficient access to food, inadequate maternal and childcare, overall poor health services and water sanitation—the consequence of poor quality and quantity of resources at the community level. In the end, the population experiences inadequate dietary intake and disease, which lead to malnutrition, disability and death.[9, 14]
The physiological reality of malnutrition, is not limited to a significant drop in body weight, because of insufficient food intake, but includes nutritional diseases, and debilitating chronic conditions that occur concurrently with visible signs of edema, ascites or physical wasting, depending on the type of malnutrition.

In the case of prolonged protein malnutrition with **edema** and **ascites**, the condition becomes known as "**kwashiorkor**." This is a new medical term introduced by Jamaican pediatrician, Dr. Cicely Williams in 1935. Derived from the African Ga language of coastal Ghana, the term basically means: the sickness that the baby contracts after the birth of the newborn.[17] The infant develops red wiry hair, enlarged fatty liver, dermatitis, no visible erosion of fat or skeletal muscle mass, but a noticeable drop in visceral protein (blood proteins), with a concomitant development of edema[5, 7] (water accumulation in the extremities) and ascites (water accumulation in the peritoneal cavity), causing a protruding belly. It is common to observe higher rates of infections in this condition, as the immune system becomes seriously compromised by a predominantly starch-based diet with suboptimal protein content; the final outcome tends to be death from an infection or diarrhea.

A second condition called **marasmus**, results in

> Both adequate protein and adequate calories are required to combat malnutrition.

advanced emaciation from a total lack of calories, leading to both fat and muscle erosion, but with no edema or noticeable change in blood proteins. In this situation, the person is lacking in both protein and calories, consequently leading to a significant drop in body weight.[7]

These two conditions, at the very least, emphasize the importance of protein and calories in survival. The role of protein cannot be overestimated at the international level. Here in the U.S., we consume too much protein—suboptimal protein intake is almost never seen except as protein-energy malnutrition (PEM) in hospital cancer patients,[5] patients with AIDS, gastrointestinal diseases, alcoholics, and drug abuse.[7]

In contrast, in developing nations, access to protein, especially protein of high biological value, can be a real problem at times. In developing countries, the access to meat is ordinarily restricted, as high prices make it prohibitive. However, in Middle Eastern countries, Mediterranean regions and in Asia, legumes and rice have historically represented excellent food choices for protein complementarity. It is really in countries ravaged by war, dictatorships, and other man-made disasters, that mass migration and poverty force individuals and families to sell properties and their livestock, in exchange for money to purchase staples. It is poverty, rather than a lack of food, that becomes the instigator of undernutrition. Protein foods, in this setting, tend to be more expensive and thus of limited access to a population afflicted by poverty. Internationally, the WHO has however, identified specific micronutrients, such as vitamin A, iron and iodine, as the most prominent deficiencies in the world, but most notably in underdeveloped and developing countries.[15] So prominent are these deficiencies, that they affect up to 33% of the world's population. Consequently, the World Health Resolution WHA45.33 urged Member States, in 1992, to:

establish, as part of the health and nutrition monitoring system, a micronutrient monitoring and evaluation system capable of assessing the magnitude and distribution of iodine, vitamin A and iron deficiency disorders, and monitor the implementation and impact of control programs.[15]

These deficiencies in combination with vitamin D, folate and zinc are responsible for 7.3 % of the world's diseases, and therefore pose a sizable threat to human health, especially in underdeveloped and developing nations.[15]

Iron deficiency anemia—Anemia, characterized by low serum hemoglobin, can be caused by a variety of disorders which originate, worldwide, mostly from either: **a-**blood loss, **b-**poor red blood cell production, or **c-**elevated rates of red blood cell destruction. Iron deficiency, which is responsible for low levels of hemoglobin production, represents about 50% of all cases of anemia worldwide.[15] It is regarded as the most prominent nutrient deficiency in the world, affecting an estimated 2 billion people worldwide, or roughly 40% of the world's population. The bulk of the other forms of anemia result from malaria, which destroys red blood cells (erythrocytes).[15] But most worrisome, is that between 4 to 5 billion people or 66 to 80% of the world population is at risk of suffering from iron deficiency anemia, because of suboptimal iron reserves. Disturbingly, about 90% of those suffering from anemia actually live in underdeveloped and developing countries.[16] The segments of the population where anemia is most prevalent in developing countries are children 0-4 years (39%), children, 5-14 years (48.1 %), all women 15-59 years (42.3%), pregnant women (52%) and finally the elderly, 60 years and up (45.2%).[16] Women are particularly vulnerable to iron deficiency, as they tend to eat less than men, and tend not to be socially favored. There is an estimated 45% of women who suffer from anemia compared to only 25% of men, according to samples taken from various developing countries.[11] In Sub-Saharan Africa, for instance, 90% of pregnant women suffer from anemia, whereas by contrast, 22.7% of women in industrialized nations have anemia.[15] Iron deficiency, prevalent in a population, has been shown to affect the economic output of that nation. This is because it directly hinders the cognitive development of the youth.[16] The most recognizable symptoms are fatigue, tiredness, facial pallor, and lack of zeal. This deficiency disease, in combination with chronic hunger, is responsible for hindering and possibly even halting mental and physical growth and development in children, causing many kids to abandon school. In many instances, when anemia affects infancy and early childhood, iron supplementation tends to not successfully reverse the cognitive impairments.[16]

In addition, anemia affects teenagers and adults, making them more susceptible to infections; their work capacity and productivity tend to noticeably decline; it puts many women at risk during pregnancy, causing 30 to 45% fewer positive pregnancy outcomes. In fact, an estimated 300 women die daily during childbirth because of iron deficiency anemia.[11]
Low thyroid activity is often observed in patients suffering from anemia. Lastly, iron deficiency anemia, predisposes patients to greater absorption of divalent heavy metals such as lead and cadmium.[16]

Retinol deficiency (Vitamin A)—the third most prevalent nutrient deficiency is **vitamin A**. The WHO estimates that about 800 million people, from around the world, are affected by vitamin A or retinol deficiency of which, 254 million are preschool aged children.[15] The risk of vitamin A deficiency is high among those who consume a diet low in dairy products, eggs, fruits and vegetables; individuals with suboptimal nutritional status, high infection rates, notably measles, and diarrheal diseases are prone to vitamin A deficiency.[15] The repercussions of retinol deficiency are particularly concerning as they can involve permanent blindness (keratomalacia) if left unchecked. Moreover, vitamin A status remains the most sensitive predictor of child survival.[15] Overcoming this nutritional problem can be achieved by ensuring animal foods are introduced into the diet--liver, dairy and eggs are preferred. While preformed Vitamin A, in form of beta (β) carotene, is considered a good and acceptable source of vitamin A, the conversion of β-carotene to retinol is only 12:1, whereas other carotenoids have an even weaker conversion of 24:1. Hence, many vegetables and fruits are needed to meet the body's requirement for vitamin A. Synthetic β-carotene, used in processed cereals and foods, actually has a 6:1 conversion rate.[15]

The earliest subclinical sign are growth failure, loss of appetite and night blindness, followed by Bitôt's spots, pale discolored patches, which appear in the conjunctiva of the eye. Not long after, slowly the conjunctiva and the cornea begin to dry out from a lack of lacrimal function (tear production), thus leading to xerophthalmia or non-permanent blindness. There are between 250,000 and 500,000 children that become blind annually.[15] Vitamin A consumed, even at this late stage, can reverse the condition. However, when aid does not arrive in time, a more permanent form of blindness, called keratomalacia, sets in. At this late stage, there is softening of the cornea, a condition more frequently seen in southern and east Asia, in Latin America, in Africa and the Middle East.[5] In international relief efforts, vitamin A supplements--consisting of β-carotene plus oil--have been most efficacious in reducing mortality rates from measles by 50%; this is not surprising given its conversion rate to retinol of 2:1.[15]

The second most important micronutrient deficiency is **iodine**. It could arguably be considered the deficiency with the most significant critical human impact. This is because there 1.989 billion people worldwide, affected by iodine deficiency, and because of its inherent ties with thyroid activity. Epidemiologically, regions that have not implemented salt iodization programs and that have low soil iodine content, exhibit the highest rates of iodine deficiency in its population, in the form of goiter (enlarged thyroid gland) and cretinism (physically stunted with mental retardation).

> The WHO defines iodine deficiency as the most preventable cause of mental retardation in the world.

In fact, the WHO defines iodine deficiency as the most preventable cause of mental retardation in the world. In developed nations, iodized salt programs have been implemented since the 1950s, to ensure a broad protection of the public, whereas in developing countries, there are still many regions who have failed to implement salt iodization to prevent cretinism.[15] There is nevertheless close to 60% of the world's salt supply that is iodized according to UNICEF.[14] The iodization programs around the world have greatly improved the plight of cretinism. In 1990, there were approximately 120,000 children born yearly with cretinism. This number has since dropped, possibly by half as early as 1997.[14] But the magnitude of impact of these programs is felt most impressively in the dramatic decline in the number of children born at risk of some level of mental impairments, resulting from their mother's poor diets. UNICEF and WHO data show prevalence rates of 40 million children born at risk in 1990, dropping to 28 million by 1997.[14] This is an impressive breakthrough in eradicating iodine deficiency disease (IDD). The Ottawa-based Micronutrient Initiative, a Canadian government program aimed at eliminating malnutrition, has significantly contributed technically and financially towards field relief efforts.[14] There are many other nutrients which when deficient produce specific pathologies, but iron, retinol and iodine, according to the WHO, are the three common nutrients responsible for the most devastating nutrition deficiency diseases, currently affecting large populations, and for which public health strategies could be most effective in eradicating.[15]

The solution to eradicating nutrient deficiencies is to: first, eliminate poverty by improving the economy, agriculture and access to a free market; second, to diversify and improve the diet; third, to improve health services and sanitation; fourth, implement a food fortification program; and fifth, widely distribute food supplements.[15]

In the discussion about malnutrition, there are two critical periods, in the life of the individual, during which vulnerability to under-nutrition is quite high. The WHO identifies the period from **conception to age 5** as the critical period for which adequate nutrition contributes greatly to lifelong nutrition security. In this window, they identify the developing fetus as the most vulnerable. It is at that stage that the **fetal-maternal relationship** sets up the epigenetic changes that can forcibly alter the infant's life right through to adulthood.

The lifelong implications become powerfully visible in adults, born premature or as low birth weight babies, as they are most vulnerable to increased rates of obesity, diabetes and cardiovascular disease.[14] It is noteworthy that high rates of fetal alcohol syndrome and fetal alcohol effects in infants are intimately tied to those mothers who consumed alcohol during pregnancy.

The second vulnerable time is the post-natal period between **birth and 3 years**. This is a phase of development that is of utmost importance, as there is continued development of the neuron's myelin sheath; at this time, neurological expansion is exceedingly dependent on the quality of fats ingested in the diet.

The WHO's nutritional focus is placed also on women of reproductive age prior to, during, and after pregnancy while breastfeeding. A nutrition support project in Bangladesh is helping adolescent girls to eat better nutrition, so as to provide a much stronger foundation in anticipation of future pregnancies. Nutrition caregivers, teach teenagers and future mothers about the importance of iodized salt to prevent mental retardation and cretinism in their babies; iron and vitamin A supplements are encouraged to reduce the incidences of anemia and blindness, that can compromise young children. They also instruct them about using oral rehydration therapies on babies with diarrhea.[14] It is during that last vulnerable phase of breastfeeding, that food availability is almost completely irrelevant. Rather, in international nutrition, during the period of breastfeeding, the concern is more about accessing clean water and sanitation, hygiene knowledge and correctly assessing the risks of AIDS /HIV. Indeed, malnutrition can arise from causes, other than not being able to satisfy the appetite. It can be from not providing adequate care or nurturing to children and family members. It's also about the conditions that may physiologically limit access to the micronutrients consumed. So if foods are poorly digested, absorbed or metabolized, there can be clear repercussions on health. So then it becomes important to distinguish between acute and chronic malnutrition, and the impact of infections. UNICEF's World's Children Report describes malnutrition's broad and sweeping impact at a population level:[14]

"It is implicated in more than half of all child deaths worldwide–a proportion unmatched by any infectious disease since the Black Death. It imperils women, families and, ultimately, the viability of whole societies. It undermines the struggle of the United Nations for peace, equity and justice. It is an egregious violation of child rights that undermines virtually every aspect of UNICEF's work for the survival, protection and full development of the world's children.

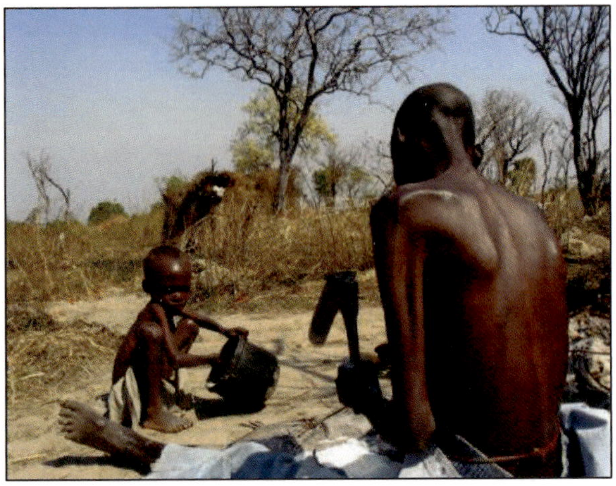

Figure 10.2: A malnourished man and boy working in their Angola village suffering from the effects of civil war. Image by Ton Koene /Visuals Unlimited, Inc. © Getty Images

In **acute malnutrition** there is a dramatic drop in the weight-for-height of the child because of a sudden unavailability of food—a dramatic and acute shortage of food—with perilous consequences as seen in famines (**Figure 10.2**). Weight-for-height percentile charts are very much needed to assess cases of acute malnutrition, as they evaluate the weight relative to the height, so even if the child is short for his age, this method can determine if he is underweight, normal or overweight. If the malnutrition is acute and significant, there will be a downward deviation of two percentile curves below an acceptable median for a specific population;[11] acute and significant malnutrition can also be interpreted if the patient, plotted on the weight-for-height curve, is less than the 5th percentile or fallen below 70% of the 50th percentile weight.[5,7,8] Additionally, a 5% loss of usual weight or greater, by a month, indicates a high risk that the child is malnourished.[8]

In **chronic malnutrition**, the impact is more long term and usually causes stunting in children—a consequence of prolonged poor nutrition from which it is at times almost impossible to completely recover from. The weight-for-age percentile growth charts are popularly used because parameters are fast to measure; but they have a serious limitation: it is impossible to distinguish whether the child's low weight-for-age, for instance, is the consequence of low weight-for-height or of low height-for age. In other words, is the child's suboptimal weight the result of being short for his age or is it more the consequence of being at a normal height, but just low body weight? The correct method to establish the probability of a stunted growth, resulting from chronic malnutrition, is **height-for-age**. If the height-for-age graph indicates that the child is <5th percentile, then he is considered short. If situated between the 5th and 95th percentile, he would be classified as normal height, and if >95th percentile, the child would be tall for his age.[8] Inadequate nutrition, in this situation, results from either insufficient food to meet caloric and nutrient requirements or diarrhea resulting in malabsorption over time; in either case the consequence impacts the rate at which the child grows.[7,8,14]

10.2 Impact of Famines on Populations

Famines are the most advanced form of food insecurity, as they represent an acute, prolonged and widespread food shortage. The United Nation's (UN) Integrated Food Security Phase Classification relies on three criteria in order to accurately identify a famine in a population:[3]
1. at least 20 percent of households must face extreme food shortages (significantly below 2100 kcal/day)
2. acute malnutrition must be diagnosed in over 30 percent of people
3. a minimum of two deaths per 10,000 people every day.

On the one end the spectrum malnutrition caused by famines is observed in developing nations afflicted with droughts (**Figure 10.3**) and floods, while on the opposite end, there is a rising prevalence of obesity in developing nations because of an abundant access to cheap processed foods.

The lack of sufficient food causes large populations to migrate in search of food and safe water. The WHO's World Food Program delivers, on a yearly basis, food relief to an estimated 90 million disaster-stricken individuals. The disasters are, however, often coupled with untenable political instability, which tends to threaten the success of any international food relief effort.

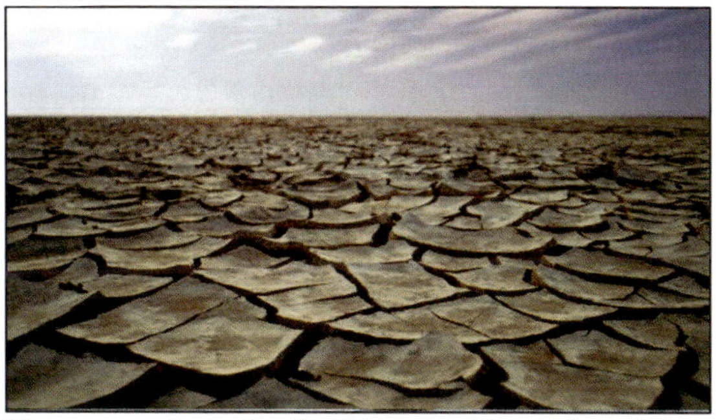

Figure 10.3 Agricultural soil devastated by prolonged drought © Zhuda

Famines in Somalia—In the early 1990s, 300 thousand Somalis died of hunger and malnutrition after fleeing their farms, which were being looted by bandits. Political chaos, general lawlessness and inter-clan fighting created a frightening environment, which led to the mass migration of millions of Somalis to more stable regions. A decade later, again in Somalia, the 2006 drought threatened the lives of an estimated 2.1 million Somalis.

The Guardian's, Xan Rice covered the story from Nairobi.[12] She described a mass migration of 300,000 souls, desperately looking for food and water. Their country was in political chaos, ever since the 1991 coup, during which the dictator, Mohammed Siad Barre was overthrown. Since that time, social and political unrest has kept the country destabilized and on the brink of chaos. After three years of unsuccessful harvests, the country's granaries were depleted and the nation's infrastructure was barely able to distribute any of the international aid. Xan Rice writes:[12]

Today there are few structures in place to deliver aid. The continuing insecurity, including looting, extortion at roadblocks, and kidnappings, has prevented all but the hardiest of humanitarian agencies from operating in many areas. The UN is not immune to the danger: last year Somali pirates hijacked two ships carrying World Food Program rations.

Many died in this tragedy, and like so many other famines, the majority of the population was beyond the reach of international aid. The chaos and the lack of civil authorities, to regulate the distribution of aid, was the main problem.

In 1998, drought and famine hit again, but this time in Sudan and Ethiopia. CNN's Catherine Bond re-

> "Famines do not occur in functioning democracies"
> Amartya Sen, Indian Economist.

ported the story.[2] This time over 1 million, in Ethiopia and Sudan, were paralyzed by famine because nobody could plant the crops; fighting between the Sudanese Liberation Party and the government, created an environment of terror that caused many to be uprooted as they searched for security and food. Bond writes:[2]

They killed our young men, raped the women, burned our homes and schools and stole our cattle,

said Dominic Matiok, the SPLA's administrator in the town of Turalei. He continues:

because of insecurity, we did not farm and now have to depend on wild seeds and roots.

In the south of Sudan, an estimated 250,000 people were at risk of starvation. In Ethiopia, the estimates, according to the World Food Program, were much worse: 800,000 people were afflicted with famine, as they could now only depend on seeds and roots to survive.

Malnutrition swept through the region, but many died because of dehydration, and diarrhea. International food aid, the government contends, was seized by the rebels to feed their armies. The rumor went around the world creating widespread outrage. There is a sense, in the international community, that Indian economist Amartya Sen was accurate when he famously said:

famines do not occur in functioning democracies.

In July 2011, an estimated 12 million people, covering the regions of Sudan, Eritrea, Djibouti, Somalia, Ethiopia, and Kenya, experienced a devastating drought, the worst in more than a half of century, with much of the horn of Africa struggling with hunger. War-torn Somalia, where conflicts have devastated the country's agriculture and economics, and depleted its food supplies, was particularly hard hit by the drought, with 3.7 million people jeopardized by a food crisis. It threatened to cause the greatest famine in decades. At the same time, Western countries were gripped with Wall Street's fluctuating stock prices; the paradox was disturbing, but yet accurately depicted the rift between the Westernized nations' preoccupation with materialism and the depth and breadth of true human suffering. The Somali famine was striking, because Southern Somalia is actually a rich agricultural zone, which has historically produced most of the produce in the horn of Africa. In truth, there was no natural reason for famine in this region of Africa. Tyler Hicks of the New York Times does, however, describe a nightmarish sociopolitical conflict with devastating consequences:[6]

The two parts of southern Somalia, where famine was declared, are controlled by Al Shabab, a brutal Islamist group that is aligned with Al Qaeda. The militants forced out Western aid organizations in 2010. When the scale of the catastrophe became clear, they relented and invited aid groups back. But few rushed in because of the complications and dangers of dealing with them. Many aid organizations are reluctant to venture into Shabab areas because of the obvious dangers—the Shabab have killed dozens of aid workers—and because of American government restrictions. In 2008, the State Department declared the Shabab a terrorist group, making it a crime to provide material assistance to them. Aid officials say the restrictions have had a chilling effect because it is nearly impossible to guarantee that the Shabab will not skim off some of the aid delivered in their areas.

Ever since 1993, there have been dozens of humanitarian aid workers, peacekeepers and American soldiers who have died in, what Tyler Hicks describes as, a cauldron of lawlessness, that has essentially made Somalia a no-go zone. Hence in the midst of the 2011 famine, of all the international aid that was sent, not very much reached the people in need.

The Somalis began to escape to Ethiopia and Kenya, in order to access some assistance but only to be

> In Bengal, the Famine Commission discovered that famine was intimately tied to the extremely low wages of the Bengal worker, coupled with exorbitantly high food prices.

blocked by the Shabab. This escalated the situation to catastrophic proportions with tens of thousands dying of malnutrition.[3]

Famines in Bangladesh—Bangladesh is an East Indian country that was historically hard hit by a series of famines that killed millions. Before its independence from India, it was called the province of Bengal. The first recorded famine in the Christian age was in 1770. It was in fact the worst Bengal famine in the 18th century. The downturn began with a drought in 1769, followed by flooding in 1770, which caused overflowing rivers to devastate all agriculture. It was specifically the rapacious greed of the East Indian Company that heightened human misery after the famine, by commanding greater revenue collection despite Bengal's devastated economy.[1]

In 1866 another famine struck Bengal, causing laborer's wages to sharply drop. For the first time, a government agency with power forms the Famine Commission to investigate the true causes of the famine. In 1896, a mere 30 years later, another famine hits Bengal after a prolonged period without any rainfall.

Although food grain availability was healthy, poor laborer wages did not permit the common folks to access the food, as prices were exorbitantly high. The Famine Commission investigated further and found no government intervention had taken place in an attempt to stabilize prices. The commission uncovered that laborer's wages had not increased in over twenty years, thus keeping the Bengal worker in a state of perpetual poverty.[1]

The Great Bengal famine occurred in 1943, but was really the culmination of a series of crop failures that began as early as 1938, and that worsened with the Second World War. The Japanese takeover of Burma, caused a dislocation of trade—grain imports from Burma were interrupted—and very irregular movements of grains, which were affected in part by regional and district barriers; rationing of grain also took place to help meet the increased demand by the armed forces.

A total of 3.5 million people perished from this famine. The human toll was beyond comprehension, and responsibility rested squarely on the heads of government, due to incompetence and corruption. Out-of-control food prices were fueled by market speculation and hoarding, and threw the local economy into disarray. It was nearly impossible for the common man to afford food. So in this instance, and in many other famines, it was poverty more than food scarcity that was responsible for the many deaths.

The last recorded famine to hit Bangladesh came on the heels of the war of Liberation that took place between March and December 1971. The loss of infrastructure and fixed physical assets from the war, topped $1.2 Billion U.S. dollars. The devastation was so colossal in its impact, that transportation and agriculture were decimated. Add to the fray the cyclones, droughts, floods and other natural disasters, and it becomes clear that the war-torn nation, pummeled by one disaster after another, was afflicted by the soaring unemployment of the industrial workers, small peasants, agricultural laborers, as well as low paid fixed-income earning groups.[1]

Then, in 1974, three important events occurred: A world shortage of food, high inflation, and a monsoon, which caused severe flooding in Bangladesh. These events in combination with a poor food distribution system, created a famine in which over 1 million people perished.

TV cameras from the West, captured the atrocities of people dying of hunger for the first time, and shocked the world into action; funds began to flow generously for relief. There was a mass migration of people from rural to urban centers, desperately searching for food and water; there in the streets, many died of starvation.

The political instability worldwide in addition to the prevalence of extreme weather patterns and natural disasters, have increased the likelihood that famines will continue to strike. Yet, the 2009 World Summit on Food Security has written a clear and measurable objective: to eradicate hunger completely by 2050. This is indeed a daunting challenge with an expected world population of 9 billion.[4]

DISCUSSION QUESTIONS

1. Define food insecurity, and discuss whether this is a problem in American society.
2. Discuss the differences between how hunger is defined by the FAO and the WHO.
3. In the discussion about malnutrition, there are two critical periods in the life of the individual, during which vulnerability to undernutrition is quite high. Identify these two periods, and discuss why they are important.
4. Upon reviewing vitamin A, iron and iodine deficiencies, discuss which nutrient deficiency has the most devastating human impact. Explain your answer.
5. Explain why food availability is not usually the main problem behind populations afflicted by famine and hunger. Discuss some examples

References

1. Banglapedia—The National Encyclopedia for Bangladesh: Retrieved July 3, 2012. http://www.banglapedia.org/httpdocs/HT/F_0015.HTM
2. Bond, C. 1 million people face famine in Sudan, Ethiopia. CNN April 10. 1998. Retrieved November 6, 2013 from: http://www.cnn.com/WORLD/africa/9804/10/africa.drought/
3. Discovery News Undeclared Famine in Southern Somalia July 21, 2011. Retrieved on July 6, 2012 from: http://news.discovery.com/human/somalia-united-nations-famine-conflict-drought-110721.html
4. FAO: The 2009 World Summit on Food Security Retrieved July 22, 2012 from: http://www.fao.org/wsfs/world-summit/wsfs-challenges/en/
5. Gibson, R(1990) S Principles of Nutritional Assessment. New York: Oxford University Press. 691pp
6. Hicks, T. East African Famine 2011 New York Times July 7 2012. Retrieved July 2012 http://topics.nytimes.com/topics/reference/timestopics/subjects/f/famine/index.html
7. Lee, RD and Nieman, DC. (1996) Nutritional Assessment. 2nd edition. New York: Mosby. 689pp
8. Magbool, A. Olsen, IE., Stallings, VA (2008) Clinical Assessment in Nutritional Status In: Duggan, C., Watkins, JB., and Walker, WA. (eds) Nutrition in Pediatrics 4 Basic science, Clinical Applications. Hamilton, ON: BC Decker p5-13
9. McAuslan, I. (2009) Hunger, Discourse and the Policy Process: How do Conceptualizations of the Problem of 'Hunger' Affect its Measurement and Solution? European Journal of Development Research 21, 397–418
10. Mehta, M et al. (2013) Defining Pediatric Malnutrition: A Paradigm Shift Toward Etiology-Related Definitions JPEN 37(4):460-81
11. Pinstrup-Andersen, P and Cheng, F. (2007) Still Hungry: One eighth of the world's people do not have enough to eat. Scientific American 297(3):96-103
12. Rice, X. More than 2 million face famine in Somalia. The Guardian, Wednesday March 22, 2006. Retrieved November 6, 2013 from: http://www.theguardian.com/society/2006/mar/22/internationalaidanddevelopment.famine
13. Tanumihardjo SA et al. (2007) Poverty, obesity, and malnutrition: an international perspective recognizing the paradox J Am Diet Assoc. 107 (11):1966-72.
14. UNICEF (1998). State of the World's Children: Focus on Nutrition. New York: Oxford University Press. 131pp
15. WHO (2006). Guidelines on Food Fortification with Micronutrients. Lindsay Allen, Bruno de Benoist, Omar Dary, Richard Hurrell (Eds). 341pp
16. WHO (2001). Iron Deficiency Anemia: Assessment, Prevention and Control: A Guide for Program Managers. Retrieved January 14, 2014 from: http://www.who.int/nutrition/publications/en/ida_assessment_prevention_control.pdf
17. Williams, CD. (1935). Kwashiorkor: A Nutritional Disease of Children Associated with a Maize Diet. Lancet. 226 (5855): 1151-2. Retrieved January 13, 2014 from: http://www.sciencedirect.com/science/article/pii/S014067360094666X